Discover how to find a woman-centered

Know the four elements every woman's physical exam should include.

Learn how female sex differences can affect your medical care.

Here are some of the crucial topics Dr. Hoffman covers, on which every woman should be her own authority:

- **HEALTHY SEXUALITY**
  A Woman's Way

- **THE HEART DISEASE ALERT**
  It's a Woman's Issue, Too!

- **THE FATIGUED WOMAN**
  Mysteries of the Immune System

- **BE YOUR OWN WOMEN'S HEALTH ADVOCATE**
  It Starts with Choosing Your Doctor

- **PREVENTING OSTEOPOROSIS**
  Don't Become a Little Old Lady

- **TAKING CARE**
  From Mother to Daughter to Mother

- **THE MENOPAUSE YEARS**
  Time to Take Stock

OUR HEALTH, OUR LIVES is a guide to help women negotiate our current medical system. It's a method for reframing relationships with physicians not yet trained to be women's health advocates, and an inspiration for women to start reshaping institutions that don't represent them. With this invaluable resource, you can finally assure the informed, appropriate medical care that is your due.

"A smartly penned, easy-to-follow book that starts with the premise that women's health is a lot more than what goes on below the belt. Dr. Eileen Hoffman's female-centered approach covers everything from women's cancers to eating disorders, from menopause to addiction. . . . [a] great book. . . ."
—*Toronto Sun*

OUR HEALTH OUR LIVES

A REVOLUTIONARY APPROACH TO TOTAL HEALTH CARE FOR WOMEN

Eileen Hoffman, M.D.

POCKET BOOKS

New York London Toronto Sydney Tokyo Singapore

POCKET BOOKS, a division of Simon & Schuster Inc.
1230 Avenue of the Americas, New York, NY 10020

Copyright © 1995 by Eileen Hoffman, M.D.

All rights reserved, including the right to reproduce
this book or portions thereof in any form whatsoever.
For information address Pocket Books, 1230 Avenue
of the Americas, New York, NY 10020

ISBN: 0-671-88086-1

First Pocket Books trade paperback printing March 1996

10 9 8 7 6 5 4 3 2 1

POCKET and colophon are registered trademarks of
Simon & Schuster Inc.

Text design by Stanley S. Drate/Folio Graphics Co., Inc.

Cover design by Christine Van Bree

Printed in the U.S.A.

This book is dedicated to my patients, from whom I learned because I listened. And when their stories were inconsistent with what I had been taught, I listened harder. Validating them, I questioned what I had been taught. This book is the story of my search for a woman-centered medicine.

Acknowledgments

I am grateful to have had the opportunity to write this book and to make a contribution to women's knowledge and empowerment. It is something I have wanted to do for a long time, and I could not have succeeded without the support of many people. My agent, Jane Dystel, gave me the confidence and direction to get the project started. The publishing world is foreign to me, and she has served as an effective guide.

Julie Rubenstein, my editor at Pocket Books, has been an enthusiastic voice. She understood from the beginning the tremendous need for this book and has placed substantial resources and dedication behind getting it published. I am also grateful for the insights and contributions of editor Denise Silvestro, who added much to this project.

Catherine Whitney, my writing collaborator, has been invaluable in helping me to develop a structure and sharpen my ideas. Working with her, I have realized once again how much more women accomplish when they collaborate with each other. I have learned a similar lesson in working with Karen Johnson, a psychiatrist in San Francisco who has been my colleague in the quest for a new women's health agenda. Through our working relationship and friendship, I have been able to pull together all the different strands of my life. Karen has been the "Yes" that has allowed me to emerge from being underground with my ideas.

My family stood behind me every step of the way, even during the long weekends when I was locked in a room working. My husband, Bob Michaelson, and my sons, Daniel and Andrew, have made this project possible by giving me the space, the advice, and the support to see it through.

I am grateful for the professional input from my colleagues: Jim Speyer, oncologist at NYU School of Medicine; Linda Crouse, cardiologist at Mid-

America Heart Institute; Marjorie Luckey, osteoporosis specialist at Mount Sinai Hospital; Brian Levy, endocrinologist at NYU School of Medicine; Suzanne Frye, urologist at New York Hospital; Ann Campbell, a psychiatrist specializing in substance abuse in New York; Jane Lau, gynecologist at Harborview Hospital in Seattle; Leonore Tiefer, sexologist at Montefiore Hospital; Julie Hatterer, psychiatrist at Columbia Presbyterian Hospital; Julie Mitnick, mammography specialist at NYU School of Medicine; Madeline Vazquez, pathologist at NYU School of Medicine; and Jan Werbinski, gynecologist and director of Bronson Women's Health Center, Kalamazoo, MI.

I am also extremely grateful to the staff of the NYU medical library for their enthusiasm about this project and their skill at compiling research information. They served a valuable function to make this book complete and up-to-date.

The climate in which this book is written has been thanks to the efforts of many people, especially those women who are so valiantly leading the new women's health movement within the ranks of medicine: Lila Wallis, past president of American Medical Women's Association and a longtime women's health activist; Janet Henrich, internist at Yale and a consultant to the Office of Research in Women's Health in the development of a women's health curriculum; Florence Haseltine and Anne Colston Wentz, editors of the *Journal of Women's Health;* Jean Hamilton, professor of psychology, social and health sciences, and women's studies at Duke University; Karen Carlson, Women's Health Associates, Massachusetts General Hospital; Ann Moulton, Women's Health Fellowship Director, Rhode Island General Hospital, Brown University; Carol Warshaw, psychiatrist and domestic violence expert, Chicago Cook County Hospital; Charlea Massion, family practitioner and editor of *Women's Health Forum;* and Vivian Pinn and Judith LaRosa of the Office of Research in Women's Health.

A special acknowledgment must be made to the four men in my coverage group—Arthur Lebowitz, Jim Kennedy, Alan Hauptman, and Chuck Slovinski. Without hesitation, they provided the backup I needed in my clinical practice while writing this book.

AUTHOR'S NOTE: This book demonstrates an approach to women's health. I do not claim to represent all women's health issues globally. This edition tries to reflect our American culture with all its diversity. However, since there are limits to the research available on women's health, it is by nature a work in progress.

This book is meant as a guide for women as we navigate our way through a health care system not designed for us. By focusing this way, I do not mean to exclude a discussion of the other determinants of health besides sex and gender. Employment, race, class, citizenship, education, housing, nutrition, and insurance coverage are all critical variables for health and contributors to illness.

Contents

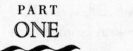

PART
TWO

TOTAL HEALTH IN CONTEXT

PART
THREE

WOMEN'S LIFE CYCLES

PART
FOUR

MIND AND BODY TOGETHER

OUR
HEALTH
OUR
LIVES

INTRODUCTION
A Personal Note

For centuries doctors have been telling women how to lead their lives, in sickness and in health. Who am I to add my voice to this chorus?

I am the perimenopausal woman who is one of the readers of this book. I am the baby boomer with a belief that "I think, therefore I do." I am the woman in my forties come late to motherhood who has lived through the conflict of profession vs. family. I am the working mother who feels the stresses and strains of the economy, the responsibilities of adulthood, and the additional burdens of middle age. I am the caretaker who puts myself at the bottom of the list and asks, "Who cares for me?"

I have been the adolescent who struggled with identity and self-esteem—smoking, drinking, experimenting with sex and drugs. Only when I was doing research for this book did I come to learn that the process I experienced—losing myself between adolescence and adulthood and not putting it all together until my late thirties—is the normal pattern of female development in our culture. I knew that my own lifeline was not linear, as men's seemed to be, but I did not understand why. And I didn't know that I was not alone in my experience.

I have been the young adult, at times called "a piece of ass," at others "a dog," and experiencing both as blows to my self-esteem. I have been the naive young woman losing her virginity when a date pressured me to "go all the way." When I resisted, he exhorted me that it would "be a pity to do a job half-done," as though I would be harming myself by going "halfway." IUDs, OCPs, and PID were abbreviations my generation came to know all too well, while we pursued casual sex as a political statement.

I have been the young woman who struggled with body image, swinging back and forth between overeating and overdieting—always feeling fat unless

1

I was underweight, and too easily sabotaged by the inevitable premenstrual water weight.

I have been the pregnant woman with a ferocious appetite, feeling I had a right to eat ad lib during pregnancy, only to put on eighty pounds and never again be the one-hundred-three-pound woman who bought clothes in petite shops. Not willing to diet any longer, I now pound the pavement instead, running thirty miles a week to avoid adding to those pockets of fat that seem to be parked permanently on my belly and thighs.

I am the middle-aged woman realizing that I have lost my youth—the over-forty person who needs to watch for cancer and high blood pressure and who worries, "Will my next period be my last?" I am the perimenopausal woman asking, "Will I be like my mother when she was menopausal?"—recalling those terrible days of irritability and discomfort. I am the aging woman fearful of her vulnerability, her potential disabilities, and the realities of mortality. I look down the tunnel and consider what my life will look like when my mother has died, my kids are grown, and my husband has passed away—the time when, by default, I will finally put myself at the top of the list and return to a state of "independence."

I prepare myself as I prepare my readers for what lies ahead and how to take control of it.

I am an internist—the product of one of the best training programs that exists. Yet in my thirteen years of practice, I have come to realize how limited I am in the care I can provide to most of my patients, especially the women who are the majority of my practice—as they are for most doctors.

I am a skilled diagnostician, who can order the most specialized tests and who knows how to interpret them. I can pick the most exotic drugs to treat a myriad of illnesses. But in the course of doing all of these highly romanticized things, I have come to see that the drugs I use and the tests I order and the prognostications I make are usually based on research data gathered by studying men. And I worry because I know my women patients need and deserve more.

In my personal experience, I have come to realize how important it is for women to be seen and treated as whole people. I have discovered that, in order to be a good advocate for my female patients, I must know as much as the breast surgeon who interprets biopsy reports, and as much as the mammographer who advises women on the results of their tests. I must know more than the average cardiologist about evaluating the results of tests that are more accurate in men than in women, so I can be sure I am committing my patient to a real diagnosis. I must be alert to the possibility of ovarian cancer in a woman who has nonspecific bowel complaints and include a pelvic examination in addition to an abdominal one. I must be able to advise a woman who has had a total hysterectomy at age thirty-eight due to uterine cancer that we need to assess her risk for osteoporosis and start hormone replacement therapy as soon as we know her tumor is no longer a threat—a consideration many oncologists omit because it is not pertinent to their specialty.

I must make sure that the somatic complaints my female patients bring to me are not their way of indirectly airing psychosocial problems that have no other forum. When I am presented with these problems, I must be sure to elevate them to the level of seriousness it takes to help women integrate their psychic and physical states so they can grow and mature and evolve—instead of giving them the traditional patronizing pat on the back and a sedative to damp down the discomforts.

In my practice I integrate medicine, gynecology, and psychology with nutrition, exercise prescription, counseling, and education. I actively work with surgeons, radiologists, gynecologists, and endocrinologists to pull together the highest quality medical care—to truly be a women's health advocate by blurring the professional turf boundaries and focusing on the woman as a whole person. I have evolved a special practice in women's medicine—a unique application for the female patient, integrating her reproductive functions into the rest of her health care, understanding her in her own right from what we call a "woman-centered" perspective. This perspective takes into account "sex," which refers to women's unique biology, and "gender," which refers to women's unique experience as females in society.

One cannot truly appreciate the health and illness of women without looking at both sex and gender. For example, childhood sexual abuse can lead to gonorrhea and pelvic inflammatory disease, which are sex-specific effects. It can also lead to the gender effects of post-traumatic stress disorder that may manifest itself as depression, dissociation, substance abuse, promiscuity, and more. Another example: On a sex-specific basis, premenopausal women are protected from coronary artery disease, but gender effects are seen in the way their care is managed less aggressively when problems do arise.

I am on the faculty of the Mount Sinai School of Medicine, where I teach medical students, interns, and residents in internal medicine. I am witness to how they adopt an androgynous approach to treating female patients—how breasts and pelvic organs become invisible to them because they are taught that these organs belong to another specialty (obstetrics and gynecology). I interact with students, interns, residents, and attending physicians in gynecology who act as if women are simply "walking reproductive tracts." Doctors in training today are surprised and fascinated to learn that information so long considered universal to both sexes can actually be applied uniquely to treat men and women.

I am part of a political movement dedicated to elevating women's health beyond an *ad hoc* clinical approach; to prevent "women's health" from being co-opted by Madison Avenue marketing; to restructure the way physicians are taught; to advance the art and science of women's medicine. I work within medicine to shift the focus from women's reproductive organs to women as people; to change the professional turf from organs to organisms; to create for women what pediatrics has given to children.

This book reflects my experience as a woman, as a patient, as a physician, and as a female physician. It is dedicated to my patients and the relationships we have, which have inspired my work. Their stories appear throughout, although their names and circumstances have been changed to protect their privacy. It is my hope that this book provides a window through which women can look at themselves, in health and illness, and have a new world view—a view that can help guide them through a medical system not designed for them; a view that can help them reframe their relationships with physicians who have not yet been trained to be women's health advocates; a view that can give them the inspiration to reshape the institutions that do not represent them.

This is just the beginning. As women exert more influence on medicine, by their power as consumers, members of Congress, policy analysts, chairwomen of boards, physicians, and scientists, we will continue to learn and apply new information about women's health. It is the finest legacy we can leave our daughters.

—Eileen Hoffman, M.D.
January 1996
New York City

THE
WOMAN-CENTERED
APPROACH

1

THE MALPRACTICE OF WOMEN'S MEDICINE

Old Systems Die Hard

~~~~~~

Twenty-one-year-old Veronica sat across the desk from Doctor Rose, her shoulders slumping with dismay. She had always been healthy and full of energy, and she couldn't fathom why things had suddenly taken such a turn for the worse. She prayed the doctor would be able to help her so she could get on with her life.

Doctor Rose had been the family physician for many years. A kindly man in his sixties, he listened carefully as Veronica described her baffling symptoms—the feeling of weakness that caused her to drag through the days, the nausea at the mere sight of food, the splitting headaches that arrived without warning, the long sleepless nights. He noted her pale, greenish complexion, suggestive of chlorosis, and the dark misery in her eyes. The young woman sitting in front of him seemed very different from the cheerful girl he had known all of her life.

He completed a thorough physical examination and now he regarded Veronica soberly. "I am concerned about the strain you may be placing on your female parts," he told her. "For now, I suggest complete bed rest."

Veronica grimaced with chagrin. "How can I do that?" she protested. "My studies . . ."

Doctor Rose nodded in understanding. "Yes, you are a student at Smith College. I know this is hard for you, my dear, but I must be frank. Your studies may be at the root of your problems. You are trying to fight nature with a rigorous schedule that stresses your brain. Your efforts may literally be sucking the strength from the other organs of your body. That explains your current symptoms. And if you allow your condition to continue unchecked, things could grow far worse. If you have any hopes of being healthy and living to bear strong children, you must dedicate yourself to regaining your strength. I urge you to quit Smith and save yourself. And we should begin a course of bloodletting as soon as possible."

This conversation was typical of what might have gone on between a woman and her doctor one hundred years ago. At the time, all "scientific" wisdom pointed to the fact that women who pursued educational or career goals beyond the strictures of their traditional domestic roles were in deep danger.

Doctor Rose might have gone on to offer Veronica this stern reprimand: "Being a woman, you are by nature frail and delicate, and your educational endeavors place you at grave risk. Don't you know that your brain is locked in mortal battle with your uterus, struggling each moment so that precious energy may go to one instead of the other? Don't you know that by pursuing these lofty ideas you are in danger of atrophy of the uterus, leading to sterility?

"Studies show," Doctor Rose might add, "that only twenty-eight percent of women who pursue higher education will marry, as compared to eighty percent of women in general. Is it your intention to sacrifice your feminine nature and risk untold ailments, perhaps even mental disease, in the pursuit of your ideas? A new study has shown that forty-two percent of women admitted to insane asylums were educated, like you, compared to only sixteen percent of men. Can't you see that by demanding higher education, you are at risk of being driven crazy? Please take the example of my dear colleague Dr. Margaret Cleaves, who after pursuing a medical education went on to develop a galloping case of neurasthenia. She came to realize only too late that women, and I quote, 'are unfit to bear the continued labor of mind because of the disqualifications existing in their physiologic life.'"

At this point, Veronica would no doubt have felt helpless to argue. After all, "science" had spoken. In spite of her longing to study and make something of herself in the world, the medical dangers seemed real and compelling. She might not have liked it, but it appeared irrefutable that her God-given destiny was elsewhere. If she chose to ignore Dr. Rose's advice, who knew what might lie ahead? A barren life? A worsening of her condition? Insanity? It was a terrible chance to take. Little did she know that doctors had basically created an epidemic out of whole cloth, and their treatments only made things worse. A woman who felt drained and sickly, probably due to a menstrually related iron deficiency, was treated with bloodletting—a "cure" that only added to the deficiency. Such would be Veronica's fate. She had little choice.

This scenario might sound like the stuff of fiction. But it was very real for women of that age. Medical science, as interpreted by physicians, held that a woman's body was literally built around her uterus in a closed-energy system. Any expenditure of energy that was not focused on reproduction (and the accompanying domesticity) compromised a woman's health. As one physician explained in 1870, it was "as if the Almighty, in creating the female sex, had taken the uterus and built up a woman around it."

THE BIG LIE ABOUT WOMEN'S ILLNESS

As I began to study the issues related to women's health in the final years of the twentieth century, I was surprised by how my research kept taking me back in history. It became absolutely clear to me that the way medicine is practiced today is a continuation of the ways women and their health were conceptualized in the last century.

Even though our practice of medicine today is in many ways more advanced, its essential structure is based on nineteenth-century views: Women's health is reproductive health, and all else (heart, lungs, kidneys, etc.) is the same in men and women. We can't transform archaic notions about women, nor the way they are practiced in medicine, unless we return, at least briefly, to the past and come to understand them in their historical context.

The nineteenth-century closed-energy theory supported a social strategy that kept women in line and at home through a campaign of scare tactics. It was a perfect example of the way science and culture intersect.

One hundred years ago, it was considered dangerous to be a woman. This danger came, not from outside forces, but from the body itself—a fragile organism threatened by its own natural processes. Hippocrates' famous aphorism, "What is woman? Disease!" was adopted by doctors during this period, and the "disease" centered in the womb. The Victorian preoccupation with women's reproductive organs enabled men to view women as creatures apart, whose sexuality restricted their activities and dictated the purpose and pattern of their lives.

Being a woman was equated with being sick, a walking set of maladies that began at the point of puberty and continued on until death. Menstruation was viewed as a morbid state, so women by their very natures were invalids. Girls were urged to take to their beds when they began menstruating so that their menstrual cycles would be successfully established. And menopause was the final insult, the "death of the woman in the woman." Virtually every complaint—from nervous disorders to pain—was traced to a dysfunction of the uterus or the ovaries. Sickness was the curse of the woman, especially she who would not be obedient to her domestic role.

But not all women accepted the "logic" of nineteenth-century science. In ever-growing numbers, they went on to college and graduate school, led autonomous lives (some even without husbands), and remained independent within the working world. They were active in social movements as suffragists, abolitionists, and activists on behalf of the poor and workers. They fought for the rights of voluntary motherhood, supporting contraception and abortion.

These women denied that they were either physiologically "unnatural" or socially deviant. They rejected the closed-energy theory, arguing that education, exercise, and careers would strengthen women's bodies and minds. Indeed, they pointed out, it was confined married women, weakened by frequent pregnancies and burdened with large families, who were more prone to hysteria, depression, and gynecological diseases—not their more independent, educated sisters.

They frequently rejected established medicine and looked for alternatives among the so-called "irregulars"—female practitioners who were excluded from "regular" medical training, midwives, homeopaths, and others. Regular medical treatments could be frightening and many women shunned the "cures" that were often more violent than the diseases themselves—leeching, blistering, purging, and the random removal of uteri and ovaries to treat a wide variety of symptoms.

As growing numbers of women refused to subject themselves to the callous methods of traditional medicine, regular doctors became worried that they were losing their patient base to outsiders. Something would have to be done to bring women back into the fold.

Enter the gynecologist. These early "women's doctors" were generally dismissed by their colleagues and were held morally suspect because of their intimate contact with female private parts. With the advent of anesthesia, gynecologists took advantage of an opportunity to elevate the prestige of their specialty and make themselves indispensable. Now Victorian women could be spared both the pain of labor and the embarrassment of being attended by male physicians. With the further advances of antisepsis and aseptic surgery, women could be safely relieved of uteri that were traumatized by multiple birthings and pelvic organs infected by venereal disease. Gynecology established itself as the specialty of women at a time when childbirth and its complications accounted for most of the illness, disability, and death women experienced.

For the first half of the twentieth century, this narrow reproductive focus grew and further consolidated the power of gynecologists in the lives of women. Unable to fight the demand for contraception, gynecologists eventually joined in and by doing so broadened their influence. Gynecologists wielded their power over the lives of women, and women in turn trusted these doctors to know what was best. They allowed their deliveries to occur under anesthesia. They accepted hysterectomies as the solution for all types of irregular bleeding. Gynecologists became the *de facto* women's doctors, and their power cemented the reproductive focus of women's health for most of this century. It also let the rest of medicine off the hook. Since gynecologists were taking care of women and their special needs, the rest of medicine was free to pursue research and therapeutic practices that were based solely on the male.

Even the women's rebellion of the 1960s and 1970s, which led to the establishment of alternative clinics and self-determination on issues like birth control and abortion, was focused on reproductive health as the defining center of women's health. Meanwhile, women continued to be excluded from the mainstream of medical activities.

Contemporary women and their physicians have inherited an outdated system of medical care. But there are signs of change. During the last several years, we have seen the issue of women's health emerge from the limiting definition of reproductive issues to address more comprehensive medical concerns. And women, no longer content to solve their disputes with the medical establishment by seeking alternatives, are demanding that they be heard within the system.

A New Premise for Women's Health

Today, women have the means and the will to reject the dusty old biases that have compromised our health care for generations. In the next hundred years, starting now, we can revolutionize the way our health concerns are handled.

We can begin by recognizing that our focus on "sameness" has led to less effective medical care:

▶ Less research on diseases of singular importance to women, like breast cancer and osteoporosis;
▶ Less basic science that explores sex-specific issues like the influence of estrogen on functions other than the reproductive;
▶ Less application of sex-specific therapies, like medication to treat heart disease in women that is based on their actual physiology;
▶ Less understanding of how the experiences of women's lives can actually produce what doctors label as medical and psychiatric disorders.

We can now demand that women be given their due from a system in which they are the major users.

Women represent about 52 percent of the population, and we account for two-thirds of all medical visits. Nevertheless, we suffer the effects of our historical exclusion from mainstream medicine every time we visit a doctor.

In 1990, the General Accounting Office issued a shocking report bringing the National Institutes of Health to task for failing to include women in clinical trials conducted to study major diseases. The publication of that report started a ground swell of activity and interest in woman-centered health. To date, this activity has been superficial at best—calling for more funding to research breast cancer, osteoporosis, and heart disease. But women are no more hearts, breasts, and bones than they are walking uteri. If we don't improve the way health services are delivered to women, the system will remain fragmented, and the focus will stay locked on the reproductive organs.

Medical doctors are not trained in routine gynecological care and are less likely to perform routine screening tests such as Pap smears and pelvic or breast examinations. But women who limit their medical visits to gynecologists do not receive evaluation or treatment for nonreproductive conditions, such as coronary artery disease, certain cancers, bladder problems, and so on. Women's total health needs are not being met by the specialty of obstetrics-gynecology.

So, while women are the major users of the health system, even for non-obstetrical care, the fragmentation in the system makes them vulnerable to missed diagnoses and inadequate treatment. At best, women's health care is, as one editorial in the *Journal of the American Medical Association* put it, "a patchwork quilt with gaps." At worst, it is life threatening.

Recently I saw a new patient, Rene, a woman in her early thirties. Rene came in for a checkup and I learned that she had suffered from lymphoma when she was in her teens. She was treated with lymph node irradiation that secondarily caused her ovaries to stop working at age sixteen. No one explained that this treatment would have a hormonal effect, and Rene couldn't understand why she was getting hot flashes and feeling so irritable. She didn't pursue it because it was happening at a time when she was rebelling against her abusive parents. She handled her fears, confusion, and discomfort by drinking alcohol, using drugs, smoking, and being quite casual about sex.

Rene was never advised that this kind of radiation might lead to premature ovarian failure and consequently increase her risk of coronary artery disease. Nor was she told that radiation increased her chances of second malignancies like thyroid and breast cancers. She had no advocate to warn her that alcohol abuse would increase her already high risk of breast cancer, or that smoking heightened her potential for heart disease and osteoporosis.

Over the years, Rene avoided regular checkups, and when I met her she had not been to a doctor in over two years. She came to see me about a genital irritation that she feared was a venereal infection. She told me that she came to me after learning of a comment I'd made to a friend of hers. In the context of a visit for a sore throat, Rene's friend described her current stresses—a difficult relationship and the demands of work and graduate school. I empathized, saying, "Just being a woman is hard enough!" That comment, a sign of my understanding, made a big difference to her. She left my office feeling understood, her experiences in life validated.

When Rene heard about her friend's experience, she said, "I know this is the doctor for me." Rene sensed that she would be seen as a woman, not as a disease.

It turned out that Rene did not have a venereal infection. But when I elicited her entire medical history, I was taken aback. Here was a woman who had no idea about her risks, had never been told about the implications of premature ovarian failure, didn't appreciate the added dangers of her behaviors, and avoided regular screening. She told me she was "pretty healthy," that her cancer was a thing of the past. I began the task of gently educating her about her body, and helping her map out a plan for comprehensive preventive care and screening.

Rene's story illustrates the inadequacy of the current health care system in treating the whole woman and in addressing patterns and symptoms in a woman-centered way. Rene's doctors focused only on her lymphoma, and never even raised the issues that were important to her health once she survived the lymphoma—notably, the effects of early estrogen depletion and radiation toxicity. Before she came to see me, Rene said that no other doctor had ever challenged her risky behaviors, and I was also the first to uncover her abusive childhood. Her lymphoma was treated, but Rene as a whole person was uncared for. Fragmented knowledge resulted in fragmented care. She was ill-served by the system she hoped would heal her.

What's the solution? I believe we need an interdisciplinary primary care specialty in women's health that would focus on the woman patient as a whole person, the way pediatrics focuses on children. In addition to including biologically-based sex effects, this specialty would also incorporate gender effects into the understanding of health and illness, the way social context impacts on children's issues in pediatrics. Pediatrics always includes an assessment of children in the context of their social groups—be they family, school, or peers—as a way of determining health. Pediatricians regularly advocate for children socially and even legally when they find dysfunctions in their homes, schools, or other environments. This is because pediatrics focuses on the child, not on the child's organs. Don't women deserve the same?

Medicine as we know it today remains a body of knowledge and practice defined by the male. Even though it is now a widely held belief that women and men are equal, that doesn't mean they're the same, either physiologically or psychologically. Our understanding of disease cannot be studied in the male and applied to the female. And we cannot practice competent medical care without appreciating the effects of gender on women's health. As a doctor, I'm certain that if I did not elicit the history of a patient in the context of her life, I would end up misdiagnosing most of the time. How could it be otherwise? If a doctor doesn't understand the total picture, how could a valid prescription be given? How could a doctor-patient collaboration in pursuit of health or a cure be guaranteed?

I have often wondered why, after so much insult and harm, women keep coming to doctors. I don't know the answer. But my guess is that in a culture where women are the primary caregivers to others, where they are expected to place their interests and concerns behind those of their husbands, children, and parents, health care remains the one arena in which they are allowed to seek care and are given permission to care for themselves.

Furthermore, medicine has insinuated itself so thoroughly into the lives of women that it is hard to separate culture from medicine. Menstruation, contraception, conception, birthing, and menopause—all natural events in the lives of women—have become medicalized. Medical diagnoses have replaced common terms, events are described as pathologic and requiring intervention and treatment, and women's bodies have become marketplaces for profitable technologies.

WOMEN AS PEOPLE, NOT BODY PARTS

Our views about women and how they do and should behave in our society, how they are and should be treated, how they are and are not seen, are gender effects that should be taught in medical schools, included in research literature, and evaluated in health policy decisions. Women use health services differently, communicate differently, and make decisions differently. These differences need to be understood so that all doctors can offer better care to their female patients.

Another recent patient of mine was Penny, a forty-eight-year-old woman who was being treated for high blood pressure. An overweight woman who continued to smoke in spite of her hypertension, Penny exuded a deep misery that made her seem very unattractive—just the kind of woman that many doctors feel impatient with. She was clearly an active participant in her own health problems, and she seemed too defeated to make the necessary changes. Now, she sat in front of me with tears rolling from her eyes and cried, "My hair is falling out!" She reached into her purse and pulled out a plastic baggy filled with hair, which she pushed across the desk. "My previous doctor sent me to a dermatologist," she said, "and she thinks I have alopecia." She reached in her purse again and pulled out a note. "She wants you to check for these blood abnormalities." I took the note and the baggy filled with hair as Penny fought to control the flood tides of emotion that were threatening to overwhelm her.

Instinctively, I knew that this woman had been living on the cusp of a depression—feeling lonely, fat, and ugly. Her hair loss was the latest setback, the final straw that would cement her sense of hopelessness.

I leaned across the desk and looked her in the eye. "Don't let this undermine you," I told her earnestly. "We won't let this happen. If there is no underlying medical cause for your hair loss, we'll make a change in your blood pressure medication. That might be causing it. The important thing to know is, there are things we can do."

Immediately, Penny's facial expression was transformed with relief and hope. It was the response of a woman who had been heard, understood, cared for—and who had found an ally not a judge in her doctor. Her hair loss was a medical problem, but she also needed me to understand what that hair loss meant to her in the context of her life, and to take it seriously.

Women like Penny are used to being parceled out among doctors—from internist to gynecologist to dermatologist to endocrinologist to psychiatrist—with no single caretaker to put all the pieces together and see how they are interrelated.

Indeed, doctors look at a woman like Penny, who needs to become fit and stop smoking, as a problem patient who can't seem to get her act together. They are loathe to stop and consider how defeated she feels, how much she hates the way she looks, how desperately she longs to gain control. Her health problems seem like her own fault, but she is drowning, and she feels that no one really understands. As I saw so dramatically, what Penny needed was to have someone throw her a lifeline by validating her total experience (which was not just her loss of hair), not by retraumatizing her in a callous encounter that might be, "So, you're losing a little hair. At least your blood pressure is under control."

When the medical profession is educated about the special way women use the health care system, how they verbalize their concerns, and how they reach decisions about medical treatment, we can move beyond the old stereotypes of women as complainers and hypochrondriacs (negative value judgments), to a more refined diagnostic ability.

It has been my experience that when a woman complains about pain, anxiety, depression, or exhaustion, her symptoms are real. Yet little attention is given within the profession to the major psychosocial issues that traditionally exist outside the framework of the primary care disciplines: depression, anxiety, the effects of sexual abuse and domestic violence, eating disorders, chemical dependency, and life cycle transitions like menopause. Failure to recognize the impact of these issues on how women commonly use health services leads to inappropriate diagnosis and treatment. Fragmentation of services can make it impossible to treat a problem like domestic violence. Each player in the process attends to a piece of the problem—the blackened eye, the broken bone, the social work referral, the police complaint, the court system—yet it is impossible to get all these pieces working together in a way that helps the woman address this problem in the context of her own life.

This is because the paradigm for medical care is the male gender. Women's health problems are described and understood as being deviations from the male-defined norm. When there is no male model from which to deviate—say, in the case of rape or domestic violence—the system does not know how to respond.

If medicine had evolved with women rather than men as the standard, violence would long ago have been identified as a crisis of epidemic proportions. And it wouldn't be viewed as a woman's problem but as a man's problem.

Just imagine how the epidemic of violence against women might be handled in a woman-centered system. It would be acknowledged as the primary cause of a whole range of disturbances that we now categorize as unrelated disorders, such as borderline personality, eating disorders, substance abuse, chronic pain syndrome, multiple personality disorder, and frequent utilization of health services. Male aggression would become a clinical diagnosis, and millions of dollars would be spent researching and treating this life-threatening disorder.

Our profession is beginning to take note of the sex differences between men and women. Great fanfare has accompanied recent research about hormonal links to disease. There is a new public outcry about the realization that women are excluded from clinical trials and drug testing because their hormonal cycles "screw up the data," while those same treatments and drugs are prescribed to them. But these so-called medical landmarks are merely window dressing that mask the real malaise.

It starts in medical school when archaic images of women's care are reinforced every day—among them the ideas that only OB/GYN doctors ever touch breasts and ovaries, or that depression in a menopausal woman is probably hormonal. As long as women's medical care is focused in the limited domain of OB/GYN practice, and the other specialties fail to customize their art and science to women, there is little hope that we'll ever get comprehensive woman-centered care.

A task of the new women's health movement is to reassemble women as whole individuals within the lens of medicine; to fully appreciate their physiology and psychology in the context of the world they live in; to reframe women's health from female organs to woman as person.

2

GETTING ORIENTED TO WOMAN-CENTERED CARE
A Brand-New Way of Thinking

~~~~

I still remember the way I felt the first time I read *Our Bodies, Ourselves* almost twenty-five years ago. This bulky, oversized softcover, published by the Boston Women's Health Collective, didn't look like most health books. And its prose was unlike anything I had ever read. It was passionate, conversational, easy to comprehend, very personal, and very political. The women authors addressed the reader as a real woman—one with a brain! As I read it, I felt that I as a woman was being treated with the utmost respect, and so was my body.

Our Bodies, Ourselves was a breath of fresh air in an area that had always been paternalistic and preachy. Although its focus centered around reproductive health, it presented a liberating view of the standard topics, riding the new wave of women's awareness and mobilization. For many years after its introduction, *Our Bodies, Ourselves* (and its subsequent editions, *The New Our Bodies, Ourselves* and *Ourselves, Growing Older*) signaled that times had changed for women.

Now, times have changed once again. The language of women's health that served us in the years following the publication of *Our Bodies, Ourselves* needs to be complemented by the language and knowledge of the present era. Our health consciousness must be inclusive of the entire woman. It's time to take *Our Bodies, Ourselves* one step further.

This book introduces an entirely new way of thinking about your body, your health, and your health care. We call this new perspective "woman-centered health." It's more than just a superficial shift toward including a larger menu of women's organs. Indeed, when you look at health this way, it's like transforming a black-and-white picture into a technicolor hologram.

As you read the book, you'll be experiencing your body and the health issues that concern you from a woman-centered perspective. Right away, you'll see that this makes a difference in the design and contents of the book. Most women's health books are topically organized around female issues, and these are dealt with in separate segments: menstruation, birth control, pregnancy, childbirth, baby care, breast-feeding, menopause, and so on. They are, in effect, descriptions of the reproductive mechanics, with women's life cycles being defined according to what is occurring reproductively.

In this book, you will find a more integrated approach. Many topics will show up in unexpected places because of the interconnectedness between reproductive and nonreproductive issues. For example, pregnancy will not just be described as a discrete event, lasting nine months, centered in your uterus and focused on the outcome—your baby. Rather, it will be discussed in the context of its effect on your entire body, both during the pregnancy and for the rest of your life.

Because medicine has always treated pregnancy as a transient physiological event, activated by fertilization and terminated by the production of a child, it has been slow to develop a science of medicine that looks at the underlying hormonal actions. So, unlike most women's health books, this one describes ovarian function not only as it relates to fertility, but also as it relates to healthy hearts and strong bones.

The chapter on pregnancy doesn't talk about it in the usual way—trimesters, symptoms, landmarks, and birthing. That's for a book on obstetrics. This book, with its focus on your total health, will discuss pregnancy from the standpoint of its effect on all the organs of your body, both transiently and permanently. You'll learn how pregnancy predisposes you to other medical conditions, and how it alters the probability of getting certain diseases.

In the same way, you'll find the subject of menopause appearing in our discussion of heart disease and other medical topics, because the depletion of female hormones that occurs at menopause affects your total health, not just your ability to have children.

Issues you might normally find in psychology books, like depression, self-esteem, incest, addiction, and eating disorders, are included in this book because they represent important conditions in the lives of women—conditions that have a different impact on women than on men. They produce symptoms that bring women into every doctor's office, yet often get lost in the male-modeled discipline of medicine.

I frequently see how a so-called psychological or behavioral issue can have serious health implications. Here's a prime example. Nancy was a seventeen-year-old diabetic who had been successfully managing her disease with insulin for many years. But one side effect of insulin is weight gain, and as Nancy grew older and became more sensitive about her weight, she learned to manipulate her doses whenever she wanted to lose a few pounds. She also developed an eating disorder. When I saw her, Nancy's sugar levels were dangerously high. Had I not been sensitive to the psychosocial issue (Nancy's unhappiness about her weight) I would not have been able to treat her diabetic crisis. I might have changed her insulin regimen to poor effect.

In the woman-centered context of this book:

▶ Your body will be examined as a complete and complex entity of its own, rather than as a deviation from the "standard" male model.

▶ You'll learn what tests and procedures are less effective in diagnosing medical conditions in women than in men.

▶ You'll learn how health issues manifest themselves in different ways for women—how unique hormonal actions give you separate pathways to illness and health.

▶ You'll have an opportunity to examine the remarkable ways these hormonal actions impact the cycles of your life.

▶ You'll discover how male-centered models of behavior and psychological development fail to explain female patterns—which is why women so often get labeled as dysfunctional when they fail to behave according to expectations.

▶ You'll learn why good health depends on an integration of mind and body—how your physical self is not separate from your psychological issues or social environment.

▶ You'll begin to see how medicine would function if it served as an advocate for women, and you'll find out how to make that happen in your own life.

THE RISK/PREVENTION/SCREENING TRIO

In each medical chapter, we will follow a basic formula: Defining your risks, reducing your risks through preventive measures, and screening to pick up the early presence of disease.

There are many misconceptions about risk, prevention, and screening, and throughout the book these will be clearly stated. If you're like most people, you probably hear the word "risk" and a red flag shoots up. If you're told you have a risk for a disease, that information may translate in your mind to, "I'm going to get the disease." It's a very helpless feeling!

Actually, the concept of risk is less tangible. When scientists define risks they are simply saying that certain conditions or behaviors seem to contribute to a disease, or have been found in people who have the disease. While knowing about these risks may be a useful reference point, it does not guarantee that you will get the disease. For example, most women who are diagnosed with breast cancer have no known risk factors, despite all the talk about family history contributing to risk.

When reading about risk, you need to be able to translate a piece of information into, "What does this mean to **me**? What is **my** risk?" Simply defined, risk refers to the probability that an event will occur. In terms of the relationship between exposure and disease, it refers to the likelihood that an exposed person will get diseased over time. You might have heard the terminology of risk but not known what it meant.

The term "relative risk" is used to compare disease among exposed persons versus unexposed persons. And the term "attributable risk" is a measure or how much extra risk an exposed person has given the incidence of the disease in unexposed persons. This measure gives you a real number.

The nature of risk is usually presented inaccurately in the public media. It's used as a scare tactic. In this book, I want to help you understand what your specific risk factors are—and how important these risks become over time to the likelihood of disease. But through it all, I ask you to bear in mind that there are many mysteries to disease. Sometimes people with high-risk profiles never get sick, while those with no known risk factors do.

I stress this point to dispel some of the hysteria that often surrounds the word "risk," and also to remind you that there are no absolutes in our knowledge of medical science. Your informed decisions about personal health care need to be made in the context of many factors.

There is also frequent misunderstanding about the distinction between screening and prevention. Many women think that screening is the same as prevention. For example, they view a Pap smear or a mammogram (which are screening procedures) as preventive measures. Just recently, a woman said to me, "I protect myself from breast cancer by getting mammograms." But mammograms do not prevent breast cancer, and Pap smears do not prevent cervical cancer. They pick up disease when it is already present.

On the other hand, eating a low-fat diet may help prevent breast cancer, and practicing safe sex may prevent cervical cancer. Your health plan must include both preventive measures and appropriate screening. The benefit of regular screening practices is that detection improves early treatment outcomes.

Since this book is designed to help you take charge of your health, there will be a heavy focus on risk assessment, practical preventive measures, and screening recommendations. In contrast to some medical books that stress therapies, surgeries, and drug treatments for diseases that already exist, my goal is to give you all the ammunition you need to stay healthy long into life.

USE THIS BOOK IN GOOD HEALTH

In the past, you may have purchased medical or health books as references to put on the shelf in case you needed them. This book contains all the latest and most comprehensive information to make it a thorough and reliable reference book. But before you put it on a shelf, I fervently hope you will sit down and read it straight through. It's the best way to understand and internalize the concept of woman-centered health. It will change the way you approach your own health care and enable you to help change the system to better reflect your needs.

When I first began to think about writing this book, I wanted very much to contribute something important and lasting to the betterment of women's health care. It is a movement in which I have become increasingly active, and I view this book as an extension of my larger commitment.

I have often felt overwhelmed by the sheer size of the dual task of shifting deeply ingrained cultural attitudes and revising systems to be woman-centered. But I have come to see that the best way to contribute to change is to offer individual women the tools to reshape their own health care—to educate and empower them to use the system and take charge of their lifetime health plans. Unlike the women's health movement of the 1960s and 1970s, which encouraged women to seek alternatives to the system that had for so long ignored and betrayed them, I believe that true progress can only be made by laying claim to the system.

As I contemplate the impact of a woman-centered health book, I imagine a scene where women in every city and town across the country start showing up in doctors' offices, clinics, and hospitals, asking educated questions, initiating screening procedures, making demands, and requesting information. It will be like a jolt of electricity to a system that has grown complacent and rigid.

Change takes time. Institutions and attitudes that have been in place for centuries will not collapse overnight. But this book is your invitation to begin that process of change in a personal way.

3

BE YOUR OWN WOMEN'S HEALTH ADVOCATE

It Starts with Choosing Your Doctor

~~~

A forty-year-old woman walks into my office feeling a little shy and more than a little apprehensive. Like many women her age, she has never been to a doctor other than her gynecologist/obstetrician. The sign on my door announcing "Internist" is unnerving; she equates what I do with disease, not wellness.

She happens to be healthy. This medical checkup is a birthday gift she is giving herself. But still, it's a sobering moment because she understands that she has crossed a threshold from youth to middle age. For the first time in her life she feels vulnerable inside her body. When I tell her, "From now on, I recommend a yearly physical beyond routine gynecological care," we exchange a knowing glance—doctor to patient, woman to woman. That glance reflects a host of fears and worries that come with facing the natural but intimidating process of changing and aging.

As she sits in my office, her mind percolates with new and scary considerations. "I remember my mother at forty!" she will say, shocked that she now identifies more with women who are sixty than she does with women who are twenty. Looking down the road, she might speculate about what's in the cards for her, mentally checking off the possibilities: Will she have brittle bones? High blood pressure? Heart problems? Breast cancer? When will menopause arrive, and will it be difficult? Will she need to consider estrogen replacement therapy? Mortality is suddenly very real. How will she know how to take care of herself? Whom should she trust?

If she is like most healthy women, she is totally unprepared for this moment. In her youth, which wasn't so very long ago, she felt physically invincible and the concerns of aging seemed a long time away. Most of her health issues involved "well" concerns—menstrual irregularities, contraception, conception, and vaginal infections. Her body, which served her so nicely in her youth, has suddenly grown unfamiliar and unpredictable. Who is she, now that reproductive health is not her primary medical identity? Are the carefree days of her youth gone? These fears cloud my patient's mind as she undergoes her first full physical.

I use this forty-year-old woman as an example because she is at the age when most women become aware of the broader issues of health. It is also when they usually confront the bitter truth about how inadequate the medical system is to meet their needs.

You may be that forty-year-old woman looking ahead with a dire sense of vulnerability and unease. Or you may be healthy, and feel secure that you are doing all the "right" things to stay that way. You may be an older woman beset with a series of health problems that place you constantly in the hands of the medical system. Or you may be a younger woman determined to avoid the downward spiral that beset your mother—eager to learn how you can stay fit and healthy for life. Whatever your age, you share a commonality with other women by virtue of your gender. Whatever your circumstances, you face an uphill battle in a system not designed to meet your needs.

I am not telling you this to discourage you. To the contrary, when you know where the limitations and inadequacies exist, when you are educated about the system, you can use this information to empower yourself to use it more effectively. It is my goal that this book will offer practical suggestions, medical options, and background information that will arm you with tools and support you in getting the best care possible. It is what you deserve, and it can be done—even in a system that tries to make you invisible.

How to Choose Your Doctor

I have learned as a doctor that I have a lot of power. Sometimes a word I say or a decision I make literally changes a person's life. It can be one of the most rewarding aspects of my profession. But since I know that the best way to treat women patients is to make them partners in their own care, this perception of power can sometimes get in the way.

My profession has traditionally been quite reluctant to exchange power for collaboration. And people, especially women, have allowed doctors to be in charge of their care. Women trust and depend on their doctors for many things. When the doctor is supportive, this relationship can be one of the most important in a woman's life. However, when a doctor doesn't listen or teach or enlist the woman as a partner, the experience can be frustrating, harmful, and humiliating

A woman once told me frankly that visiting her gynecologist was "like having sex without emotional intimacy." She said, "I go in, strip down, he checks my blood pressure, examines my breasts, puts me in those awful stirrups to do a Pap test, and that's it. The whole time, he doesn't say a word and I don't say a word. I know he's a competent doctor and I guess I'm getting what I pay for, but . . ." her voice trailed off wistfully. She didn't know how to articulate what she thought was missing, but I knew what she was talking about. For women, medical care is more than a disembodied service; it's a personal relationship.

Unlike men, who tend to visit a doctor only for specific services when they're sick, women use the doctor-patient relationship in a broader way. Women see doctors for normal life events, including menstrual irregularities, birth control, pregnancy, and menopause. They want more than a technically competent physical checkup. They want to be heard and understood. They want their concerns to be taken seriously, even when those concerns seem tangential to a specific medical issue. Often, they come to the doctor with a hidden agenda that reflects a fear or need they can't share with anyone else, or may not even be fully aware of themselves. Usually, they are eager to be partners in their care, if only they are allowed the opportunity.

Today, women find themselves in the position of being more educated than ever about their bodies and their unique medical needs. Ironically, they are far ahead of the medical establishment, which is still locked in traditional ways of providing care.

How do you go about finding a doctor who will be your partner in maneuvering through the baffling world of health and medicine? What signs, both overt and subtle, should you look for that will tell you whether a doctor is going to be interested in being your full partner?

The usual advice when choosing a doctor is to look for someone with excellent credentials. But medical school standing and diplomas on the wall only tell you part of what you need to know.

Currently, there is no way to know if a doctor is truly skilled in women's health. There are no certificates or diplomas to signal competency. Doctors only gain up-to-date knowledge about women's health by learning it on their own. It's certainly not taught in medical schools yet . . . although this is beginning to change. So, your best bet is to find a doctor through the informal woman's health network that exists in your community. Also, ask your doctor if he or she has taken continuous medical education in women's health.

Try to find a doctor who is prepared to give you comprehensive care. If that's not possible, make sure there is sharing of information and consultation between your doctors. In my own practice, I make certain to do this. For example, even though a patient's gynecologist may have ordered and received a mammogram report, I always have it sent to me, too. Not all gynecologists are skilled at interpreting mammogram reports.

Learn to ask the underlying questions that will provide important clues about a doctor's sensitivity and knowledge of women's care:

▶ Can my doctor treat me as a whole person, or will I be parceled out to specialists for each organ?
▶ If my doctor is a specialist, such as a gynecologist, is he or she sensitive to and informed about the interrelatedness of health concerns? Does my gynecologist work in a cooperative way with an internist or general practitioner who understands the full range of women's health issues? If my doctor is a family practitioner, is he or she up-to-date on women's health data?
▶ Does my doctor believe in preventive care? Will he or she be looking beyond my current status to ask questions about my behavior and lifestyle?
▶ When I have questions that are not strictly medical, are they treated with respect? Does my doctor look for links between my life experience and my health?
▶ Do my visits feel rushed or am I encouraged to talk and ask questions?
▶ Does my doctor have a system for tracking my care from year to year? Does he or she know about factors in my own or my family's history that might inform my care?

▶ Does my doctor "know" me? Does he or she remember my name when I come to the office?

▶ Does my doctor "see" me—as a human being as well as a seeker of services?

This point is absolutely crucial. When I see a patient, I am always on the lookout for signs that there might be hidden concerns—a worry my patient has but doesn't know how to talk about directly. It's less likely that a woman will say, "I'm anxious" or "I'm depressed" than that she'll say, "I have headaches" or "I have diarrhea." But in my opinion, these concerns are every bit as valid and important to a woman's health as a more specified pain. And just as I will freely make lifestyle recommendations to prevent heart disease or osteoporosis, I am also prepared to look for psychosocial causes of medical complaints, to recommend stress management, make psychotherapy referrals, or otherwise counsel my patients.

It isn't surprising that many women are reluctant to be open with their doctors about what's going on in their lives. Most likely, they are responding to past experiences that warned them against airing broader complaints.

Indeed, a survey of 253 primary care physicians revealed that attitudes toward women's complaints were often unsympathetic. According to the report, 25 percent of the doctors believed that women were likely to make excessive demands on physicians' time, although only 14 percent believed this of men. Symptoms related by women were defined as psychosomatic 21 percent of the time, versus 9 percent of the time in men. The report stated, "Among purported physicians' attitudes about women, the most frequently mentioned are the conceptions that women are more emotionally unstable and volatile than men, apt to somaticize emotional upsets as physical problems, and consequently likely to have a higher prevalence of psychosomatic illness than men do. Physicians are described as thinking that women are more demanding, burdensome patients, and more difficult to care for than men."

The survey revealed that even when a woman gave as brief as a two-sentence description of a personal problem, that reference colored the doctor's reading of the entire medical complaint as psychosomatic. Clearly, the prevalence of such attitudes prevents women from receiving well-rounded care.

Furthermore, 20 percent of all patients who visit primary care physicians suffer from well-defined mental disorders (40 percent if minor disorders are included), but most doctors are unprepared to diagnose and treat these problems. So, women are caught in a double bind: Their medical complaints are labeled psychosomatic, and their real psychological and social issues are ignored completely.

That brings us to the next question: Should your doctor be a woman? This is a tricky issue. Obviously, not all women doctors are necessarily women's health specialists; they are, after all, trained in the same biased medical school environment. But we have already established that women present a unique profile when they seek medical care.

For generations, we women have heard from male doctors, trained in the male-care paradigm, that many of our concerns were irrelevant. For generations, we have engaged in doctor-patient relationships that were authoritarian rather than collaborative. For generations, male physicians, unaware of their cultural biases and sexism, have used medicine to control women's lives. Even in the best of situations male bias can cloud clinical decisions or enter into the doctor-patient relationship without the doctor even being aware of it. It is only right that you question whether or not you can expect woman-centered care from a male caregiver. After all, although you are a doctor and patient, you are still man and woman.

Recently, I met a new patient, a forty-seven-year-old woman who was a successful architect. Her case taught me a meaningful lesson about what it means for a healing encounter to occur between doctor and patient—and why that is sometimes difficult with a male doctor.

Brenda was in the process of a workup for possible Lyme disease when she decided she couldn't continue with her male physician. She was referred to me. As she sat in my office, she began to talk about more than her physical symptoms. The words poured out of her. She told me how much she had been struggling to make her business work in spite of the recession and how relieved she had been when a male colleague suggested they combine offices. Before long, he began to express interest in her sexually, and when their relationship moved from the professional to the personal, Brenda was elated. She had waited so long, and now, finally, at age forty-seven, she had found a relationship with a man that was both professionally and personally fulfilling—a true soul mate.

Brenda's face was pinched with pain as she went on to tell me how her fantasy was shattered when she learned the man was married. Not only that, but the dream house she thought he was building for a client was really for his wife of fifteen years. The revelations grew worse. She learned he was independently pursuing business outside their partnership. She felt betrayed.

Brenda had earlier described these events to her male doctor; she needed someone to listen. His response was dismissive. Not only did he fail to connect her emotional upheaval with her physical symptoms, he could not grasp why she was feeling tormented and betrayed. "Brenda," he said to her, "I don't understand why you're complaining when you have more with that man than most women have in their marriages. Why can't you just relax and enjoy it." Betrayed again.

My response was very different. She was my patient, and my role as her doctor was to be allied with her. I understood the transgression without her having to defend her feelings of betrayal. I knew it was important for me to reinforce the validity of her anger, to understand why she was responding as she was. I realized the response of her male physician—which was to sabotage her instincts and shrug off her pain—was one that women are accustomed to.

I assume that he wasn't a bad doctor. In fact, he probably thought he was being Brenda's friend—helping her by pressing her to accept the relationship. He was also intent on addressing the overt reason for her visit. He was the tough doctor, saying in effect, "Just the facts, ma'am." Most likely, he saw her the same way he saw his male patients—who would never dream of spilling out their psychosocial concerns in the midst of medical treatment, and who would more readily accept a diagnosis of Lyme disease than a stress-related syndrome. In his eyes, her story of betrayal was irrelevant to her presence in his office. It belonged in the domain of the psychiatrist.

More than that, this doctor was introducing his own personal male bias into the professional encounter. Forming an alliance with the patient is a basic principle of healing. The doctor-patient relationship becomes a context in which healing can occur. Healing cannot occur if the woman experiences yet another encounter where she is victimized by bias and unequal power relations—a setting that mirrors her experience in the larger culture.

While studies on this question indicate no difference in technical skills between male and female physicians, new research indicates that female physicians tend to be more comprehensive in screening practices and ask more questions than male doctors.

A recent study published in the prestigious *New England Journal of Medicine* showed that female doctors more frequently performed breast and pelvic examinations and screened women for cancer. The doctors who did the least amount of female cancer screening were young male doctors. The NEJM speculated that part of the reason may be that young male doctors were uncomfortable touching women's breasts and reproductive organs. That's not so hard to understand when you remember that medical schools don't train doctors to achieve a level of comfort with these examinations.

When I was in medical school, it took me a while to get comfortable doing male genital exams. But I was expected to perform genital and rectal exams on male patients as a standard part of routine medical care. I didn't have the "luxury" of referring that part of the exam to another doctor. But male doctors seldom get this kind of training with women unless they're specializing in OB/GYN. Even then, their training does not include helping male doctors be aware of their biases and discomforts when having intimate access to women.

Other studies have indicated that there's a real difference in styles of communication between men and women physicians. According to a report published in 1987, patients held the widespread perception that women doctors were more caring and more willing to listen. The authors speculated that "like other women in our society, they [women doctors] have been socialized to accept a less directed, interactive style of communication. Women's style of speech is typically characterized by less obtrusiveness . . ." They cited a study of internal medicine residents in New York City in which observers rated women physicians as more egalitarian than males. The study found that male doctors raised 67 percent of all issues discussed, while female doctors raised only 59 percent—allowing patients to speak more freely about their concerns. Female doctors were also found to be more sensitive to psychosocial concerns.

In a fascinating analysis of male/female physicians, Candace West, a sociologist at the University of California, compared typical directive styles. Male doctors, she found, were more inclined to use a command style:

"Just take one of each four times a day."

"Sit for me right there."

Women doctors, on the other hand, tended toward a less directive and more collaborative style:

"Let's talk about your pressure for a minute or two."

"Okay! Let's make that our plan."

While it may not be true across the board (there are surely many women who use the command style), it does appear that female doctors are bringing to the profession a new atmosphere in which women's complaints will get aired.

There is another issue, too. Sometimes women patients find it hard to express their most intimate thoughts to a man, even if he is a medical professional. They worry, "He'll think I'm stupid," or, "He'll think I'm being silly." The basic health issues can get lost in the clouded sense of a pseudosexual encounter, and the female patient's desire to look good to the doctor— either physically or by impressing him with her intelligence and wit. This is something to consider when you are selecting a doctor, because you can't form a close partnership when you feel uncomfortable.

At times, male doctors can be insensitive to the innuendos that signal a sexual rather than a medical encounter. For example, I know of one doctor who, in preparation for performing a breast exam, reached back and unhooked his patient's bra. He wasn't a bad doctor; he just didn't understand that to a woman, having a man unhook your bra has sexual overtones. These overtones came back to haunt him when the patient, angry about something else, lodged a complaint that he had misbehaved.

Although I personally treat both men and women in my practice, it has been my experience that many women come to me seeking an alternative to the authoritarian approach of their male doctors, or because they feel another woman will understand them better. Yet, I would not recommend that good women's health care exists only through women doctors. Rather, it is my hope that the new sensitivity and knowledge many women patients and physicians are bringing to the practice of medicine will influence the very core of our profession, so that both men and women doctors will become more effective advocates of their patients—male and female. As women's health enters the medical curricula, we can hope that all doctors will become educated to the unique ways women come to medical care.

Let me make it clear that I place no special mystique on the sex of the physician. The important thing is the sex of the patient and whether or not a doctor, male or female, can truly address that patient's needs. When we focus on the whole woman as patient, the rest falls into place.

YOUR FIRST VISIT

For starters, your first visit to a doctor should always begin with you sitting fully clothed in the doctor's consulting room. This is a practice that is disliked by many physicians because it takes extra time. But I think it's impossible to establish a relationship of mutual respect and comfort if you're perched on an examination table clad only in a flimsy paper gown. It's a sure sign that your doctor isn't interested in an equal partnership if you're ushered into a room and told to disrobe before you've even been introduced. It also shows that the physician is insensitive to how vulnerable women feel when they are un-clothed.

Women often avoid nongynecological health exams because they are used to seeing a doctor for matters related to "wellness"—Pap smears, contraception, pregnancy, and birth. A general practitioner or internist is viewed as a "sickness" doctor, and the visit is shrouded in fear and mystery. That's a shame, since regular checkups, especially after the age of forty, are an important part of lifetime preventive health care. But the discomfort is understandable.

Although many women have very good relationships with their doctors, regardless of their sex, and feel perfectly at ease, for others the medical exam goes like this: The doctor pokes, prods, takes tests, and makes notes while you sit there with absolutely no idea what is going on. You suddenly become aware of how many hundreds of different things might be wrong with you. You watch the doctor's face for tiny clues and rush to doomsday conclusions if he or she frowns or grimaces. You feel embarrassed about mentioning a marital problem, a work-related stress, or how tired and depressed you've been. You hesitate to say that you don't understand what's going on, and you are unaccustomed to the passivity of being a patient.

It is ironic that your body, which is the one thing that truly belongs to you, is so mysterious. Yet the medical establishment has cultivated this air of mystery and encouraged your dependence.

I want to demystify the process. We'll be talking about not only the current research related to women's health, but also about the ways you can use that information—how you can learn to tell the difference between good and bad advice, and between old views and new information. We'll place you at eye level with your doctor as you both learn about women's health.

TRUST YOUR INSTINCTS

There is a reason why you go to a doctor at a particular point in time. Maybe you're worried about a specific symptom or symptoms. Or maybe you're just getting a checkup. Be aware that even if it's the latter, something or someone has motivated you to do it now, as opposed to a year ago or next year. Give it some thought in advance and be prepared to fully describe your symptoms, preexisting conditions, and health history. A medical evaluation is like a piece of computer software; you need to input the right data to get the most accurate output. One of the best things you can do to assure good care is to be vigilant in taking stock of yourself. Women have a tendency to comply with the fragmented health care system by deleting information they think has no bearing on their specific complaint, or by sorting out information they think belongs to one doctor and not giving it to another.

Karen, forty-eight, is a woman who ignored the most obvious symptom. She went to the ballet one night and when she rose at the end of the performance, she felt dizzy and nauseated. Her heart started pounding, she broke into a sweat and passed out. She was taken to the emergency room. The doctor who examined her couldn't find any abnormalities, but he decided to keep her overnight to monitor her cardiac functions. I went to see her first thing the next morning. As we talked, she told me she'd been having cramps during the day that felt like menstrual cramps. She hadn't mentioned them to the emergency room doctor because they didn't seem relevant to her symptoms, and he had focused almost entirely on her heart rhythm.

I performed a pelvic exam and found a fullness and a tenderness in the area of her right ovary. I ordered a blood count and found it extremely low. A sonogram revealed there was fluid in her pelvis. The diagnosis: She had ruptured an ovarian cyst.

It didn't occur to Karen to tell the ER doctor about her menstrual-like cramps, which were the most vital clue to what was wrong. Nor did it occur to him to ask.

Sometimes symptoms are taken out of context, either by the patient or the physician. This "decontextualization" will usually send the physician off on the wrong diagnostic path and cost the patient a good deal in worry and money.

Decontextualization is a big problem in emergency rooms, where crises need to be assessed rapidly. This is particularly true for the one in five women who frequent emergency rooms because of battering. I recall a particularly poignant case from my residency. A young woman arrived in the emergency room on a "2PC"—a "two physician consent."

In New York, that's a circumstance under which you are admitted against your will because you're considered a danger to yourself. I was told the woman had taken an overdose of medication, although she seemed alert. I watched her grow increasingly agitated as she was strapped onto a gurney, and I went over and quietly began to ask questions. Sobbing, she told me that she had not taken any medication. The real story, she said, was that her husband had beaten her and it was she who had called 911 in desperation and fear. When the police and emergency vehicle arrived, her husband told them she'd taken an overdose. Refusing to listen to her protests or her demand to speak to a woman officer, the police had ordered her to be strapped down and sent to the emergency room against her will.

When the woman realized I was listening to her and treating her story with respect, she calmed down and began to tell me about her history of being battered and how afraid she was. This encounter opened my eyes to how vulnerable a woman can be when her experience is decontextualized. Over time, I have learned that this is the norm, not the exception, and it permeates all care. Doctors tend to focus on a patient's "chief complaint"—as we are taught to do. Taking a medical history is a process of choosing certain bits of information and discarding others. It is a narrow biomedical model that transfers symptoms out of the patient's context and places them in the doctor's context.

Judy, a patient of mine, might have traveled that same route had I not made an effort to place her symptoms in context.

Judy was a thirty-six-year-old woman who came to me because she'd been having severe headaches for several months. She described the headaches as throbbing, and accompanied by nausea and lightheadedness. She also felt lethargic and had trouble concentrating. She tried taking aspirin, but it didn't help. The headaches did not coincide with her menstrual cycle, and she wasn't taking medications, such as oral contraceptives, that could be a trigger. There was no history of migraines in her family, nor had she ever had them before. She was terrified that she had a brain tumor, and it took all her courage to come for a checkup. She was expecting the worst. I performed a medical exam and found no obvious problems. At that point, I might have ordered a brain scan—at a cost of about one thousand dollars.

Instead, I sat down with Judy and asked some questions about her life. She didn't think the headaches were stress-related because she was happy with a new man she was seeing and things were going very well at work. "It's definitely not work," she said. "I never have the headaches there—only on weekends." I began to explore what might be happening on weekends that was different. In the course of our conversation, Judy told me her new boyfriend was an observant Jew. She respected his Sabbath rituals by not preparing food or going to the store before sunset on Saturday, thereby foregoing her usual cups of coffee on Saturday mornings. *Voilà!* No brain tumor. Just caffeine withdrawal. My prescription: "Get an automatic coffee-maker with a timer you can set before sundown on Friday." Judy did so, and later reported her headaches had disappeared.

That was one problem easily solved. But I went on to probe for reasons why Judy would be so worried that her headache indicated a brain tumor. It was quite a leap for her to make! Further discussion with Judy revealed her anxiety about the fact that things were going so well in her romance she was afraid something would sabotage her happiness. She was unconsciously acting out in such a way as to place strain on the relationship. Another problem solved. By calling it what it was, we achieved the perfect resolution to the problem without resorting to high-cost tests and treatment. When I respected Judy's anxiety about her relationship as much as her caffeine withdrawal headache, a truly healing encounter was able to occur.

When you seek medical care, I want you to remember something: There is no such thing as an imaginary symptom. If you feel it, it's real. Sometimes the cause can be easily determined. Other times, it's more complex. Trust your instincts if you think something is wrong, and learn to be a good observer of the way you feel. Take charge of your health care by helping your physician put all of your concerns in context.

THE PHYSICAL EXAM: WHAT SHOULD IT COVER?

I recommend that every woman have yearly complete physical examinations after age forty. This is a comprehensive exam that should include the four elements outlined here.

Go to the exam armed with the knowledge of what you should expect. This is an area where you can be your own advocate, since not all doctors recommend the screening tests we now know are so important for women's health.

A thorough physical should include the following:

1. A COMPLETE HISTORY: This includes a discussion of inherited risk factors, previous health problems, pregnancy and menstrual history, risk-associated behaviors, occupational exposures, and any symptoms you've been experiencing (from pelvic pain to shortness of breath to irregular periods to fatigue).

2. CARDIOVASCULAR EXAM: The full exam includes the following: A blood pressure reading to check for signs of hypertension (several readings if the first one is high); listening with a stethoscope to your heart and lungs; an examination of the blood vessels in your eyes, neck, abdomen, groin, and

feet for irregularities that might signal diabetes or other vascular problems; blood tests to measure cholesterol and sugar levels, as well as assessing menopausal status if it's not obvious; and an EKG to measure heart rhythm and to serve as a baseline against which damage to the heart muscle or enlargement of heart chambers can be checked. (Note: The EKG is not always accurate in women, so any problems suggested by this test must be checked through more sensitive tests before a diagnosis is made.) Sometimes a chest X ray can provide important information about heart size and function.

3. CANCER SCREENING: There are five major cancers that should be screened for in a regular physical: breast, lung, colon, gynecological, and skin cancers.

BREAST: A breast exam should be done by a physician yearly. Keep in mind that a thorough breast exam takes time. Sometimes my patients get nervous because they think if I'm spending so long examining their breasts there must be something wrong. On the contrary. Be concerned if a breast exam is brief! You should also examine your own breasts each month after your period. (See Chapter 6 to learn how to do it correctly.) Mammograms should be done yearly after fifty, and yearly after forty for women with a family history of breast cancer. Controversy currently exists about the value of screening mammograms under age fifty. This will also be discussed in Chapter 6.

LUNG: The doctor should carefully listen to your lungs and look for other physical signs of compromised lungs, like expansion of the chest, use of extra muscles for breathing, and deformities of your fingernails. If you smoke, live with a smoker, work in a hazardous environment, or have ever had respiratory problems, a chest X ray may be prescribed.

COLON: After age forty, all women should have a rectal exam and be given stool cards to take home (these show whether there is hidden blood in the stool); after age fifty, you should receive a screening sigmoidoscopy every three years—a simple office procedure that looks for polyps, which can grow to become malignant. If you're at high risk for colon cancer because of family history or a personal history of ulcerative colitis or polyps, you should have a full colonoscopy every three to five years.

GYNECOLOGICAL: Your exam should include a full pelvic exam to check for irregularities in the uterus, ovaries, and vagina, and a Pap smear to screen for cervical cancer.

SKIN: Your entire body should be checked for skin cancers or precancerous lesions. This should include an inspection of your vulva for carcinomas that can appear on the vulvar skin.

4. PREVENTIVE COUNSELING: The final part of the exam should be educational: What steps must you take to stay healthy? Are there additional tests that need to be done? What are the consequences of risky behaviors? How can the doctor assist you in changing them? Has your risk for abuse, either physical or sexual, been assessed? Have your risks for illnesses in later years been identified and has a plan for prevention been formed? Are lifestyle issues, like exercise and diet or taking supplements addressed in the prevention plan? Have you been given information about menopause well in advance so that you can begin to consider hormone replacement?

BE YOUR OWN ADVOCATE

I encourage you to be an investigator of your symptoms. This will help your doctor give you better care. Consider the onset, duration, quantity, quality, and associated symptoms. Also consider what you do that makes you feel better or worse.

Whether you're visiting the doctor for a checkup or because of specific symptoms, take some time to make notes about your medical history. The journal in the appendix will help you do this on an ongoing basis. It's an important tool. You'd be surprised how often women forget things or don't consider them relevant to a general health exam. I once asked a woman if she had ever had surgery and she said no. Only during the examination did I discover she'd had a Caesarian delivery some years earlier. That's major surgery, but she had forgotten it. She told me, "I've never thought about it as an operation. I wasn't sick."

Menstrual histories and pregnancies are important to the doctor, too; don't just save that information for your gynecologist. The traditional bifurcated medical system, which reserves certain body parts and functions for certain doctors, will not advance your total good health. Your pregnancies are very relevant to your overall health, since there are many common nongynecological implications. Being pregnant changes your body, not just for nine months, but forever. For example, it is very relevant to evaluating cancer risks later in life. Likewise, the history of your menstrual cycles trace a pattern that may be a hint that you have polycystic ovary syndrome, which is a risk factor for coronary artery disease.

It's also important that you be honest about admitting to social habits that might be putting you at risk, such as smoking, drinking, drug use, and unsafe sex. Many physicians avoid eliciting this information because they are untrained in doing so or feel inadequate in responding to the information. Prevention, nutrition, addiction, and violence are inadequately covered in medical schools, and physicians don't do what they're not trained to do. Yet, most alcoholic women are hiding in doctors offices; battering and incest cause medical problems seen in every doctor's office, but are rarely included in medical history taking; the fear of weight gain is the primary reason women do not stop smoking, yet facts about good nutrition and avoiding weight gain are not given.

Even when your doctor is a good women's health specialist, you must be a full partner in the process. It is empowering to be an advocate for yourself and to know that you are doing everything you can to assure good health for the future.

TOTAL
HEALTH
IN CONTEXT

4

THE FEMALE BODY
Knowing How It Works

~~~

When I started medical school, I assumed that what I learned there would be accurate and true of the human condition—be it male or female. But almost from the start, I saw a blatant disregard for the study of the female body. One of the first courses in medical school is gross anatomy. I can still remember the shock I felt when the instructor told us that female breasts were a hinderance to dissection: "Cut them off and throw them in the trash, and then we can move on with our study of the thorax," he called out breezily. The breasts seemed quite relevant to me, but apparently they were not viewed that way when it came to studying the normal (male) body.

Recently, I was telling this story to a group of students from one of the nation's leading medical schools. They groaned with recognition and assured me that the practice was alive and well to this day. Imagine that! In the mid-nineties, medical school anatomy classes are discarding the study of women's breasts as though breasts just get in the way of exploring more important areas.

Later, I learned that a study examining anatomy textbooks being used in the United States revealed that texts usually depict the male anatomy as the norm against which female structures are compared. This discovery only strengthened my resolve to teach women about their bodies. If established medicine was not going to set the pace, women themselves should.

Why is it so important? You'll see more clearly as you read the following chapters and explore the medical issues that are especially relevant to women. I believe it is impossible to fully understand the issues surrounding women's heart disease, cancer, diabetes, osteoporosis, bladder disorders, or immune system failures if we use the male, not the female, body as a reference point. To do so is just as ludicrous as treating a child like a small version of an adult. Thanks to pediatrics, we have come to see that children are prone to different medical conditions—infections, heart problems, cancers—than adults. They respond differently to medications. And although children may get some of the same illnesses that adults do, these illnesses often manifest themselves differently, and they certainly must be treated in a child-centered context.

I can understand why it's so hard for us to reframe our references and develop a female model. For most of history, the basic human prototype was a male. He was the biological reference point, the perfect anatomy from which all others digressed. Women were considered lesser versions of men whose smaller anatomical structures and brain size made them both physically and mentally inferior.

Scientists and scholars preached that everything about women's physiology, including their reproductive system, was a case of arrested male development, and female sex organs were stunted versions of male organs. Aristotle, considered one of the great scientific minds of human civilization, was secure in the premise that a female was nothing more than "a mutilated male." It was Aristotle's contention that a woman's weaker, colder, and less vibrant physiology generated insufficient heat to transform menstrual blood into the heartier, more viable semen.

If these theories sound ridiculous to modern ears, keep in mind that anatomical differences were historically used as a means of promoting particular ideologies. When scientists looked at the female body, their aim was to reinforce popular notions of dominance.

Most people view medicine as a strictly scientific (and therefore "objective") pursuit. But when we take a look at the history of women's medicine, we see that virtually all dogma has had distinctly social and cultural roots. The entire notion of women's health has a political and social past that vividly demonstrates how lacking in objectivity science can be.

Indeed, science has always been guided by ideology. Throughout history, doctors and their medical practices have often been the vehicles through which cultural myths about women were reinforced. They have always played a pivotal role in our culture as the translators of science into flesh and blood. They have been strategically placed to take the prevailing science, pass it through a cultural filter, and apply it to people in the clinical practice of medicine. For example, when early anatomists noted that women's skeletal structures were different—wider pelvises, smaller rib cages, smaller skulls— they used this information to conclude that women had less brain capacity than men. This conclusion neatly supported the position that women were devolved—that is, frozen in evolutionary time—because their biological function of reproduction limited their ability to diversify and develop. The hierarchical model of biology placed white males at the top and women on an inferior plane. It's a model that, unfortunately, remains in place.

Today, when I see medical schools ignoring the study and dissection of female breasts in gross anatomy classes, I can't help wondering to what extent our efforts to understand the subtleties of breast cancer and its predisposing conditions are hampered by the fact that doctors don't learn the basic anatomy of the ductule system of the breast. I wonder how we can hope to improve our knowledge of the natural progression of the disease when there are so few autopsy series conducted.

Such casual disregard is unthinkable for diseases that afflict men alone. Take prostate cancer. Thanks to autopsy studies (the very kind not done on women's breasts), we know that increasing numbers of men develop small areas of cancer in their prostates as a normal age-related process—an under-standing that has motivated a massive education, screening, and treatment effort related to the prostate. These anatomical studies have taught doctors the need to distinguish between aggressive, life-threatening cancers and those that are more indolent. We should have this same knowledge about breast cancer. It seems clear to me that when we treat the male anatomy as the norm and pay scant attention to critical aspects of the female anatomy, we are left with aggressive treatment for men and lackluster treatment for women.

Cardiovascular disease is an example of how research and clinical experi-ence with men cannot be automatically transferred to women. Medicine has virtually ignored the presence of coronary artery disease in women. All the major clinical trials have been done with men, as have studies tracking the natural history of the disease. Yet heart disease is the number one cause of death in women.

Coronary artery disease is often misdiagnosed in women because the commonly used noninvasive tests are more accurate in men and may not be applicable for women. Likewise, cardiovascular pharmaceuticals have all been developed based on male physiology, without concern for women's higher proportion of fat and its effect on fat-soluble drugs, how effects might vary throughout the menstrual cycle, or whether they are influenced by hormone therapy.

Millions of dollars are being spent to study the effect of estrogen on heart disease by using the male model of the disease. These studies analyze estrogen's role in altering blood fat levels instead of looking at the direct effect of estrogen on blood vessels or estrogen's ability to block incorporation of cholesterol into vessel walls. If we instead pursued a sex-specific understanding of the disease process, we might learn better how heart disease progresses differently in women than in men.

More recently, the AIDS epidemic has highlighted the dangerous consequences of assuming that diseases in women manifest exactly the same signs and symptoms as they do in men. Until 1993, the Centers for Disease Control (CDC) criteria for AIDS were based on men. HIV-positive women who presented with cervical cancer, pelvic inflammatory disease, and vaginal thrush were diagnosed much later in the disease process because they did not present with Kaposi's sarcoma or Pneumocystis carinii as men did. Not only did these uniquely female presentations of the disease delay treatment and thus shorten life expectancy, they often caused undue economic hardship for women, since a prerequisite to receiving public assistance was that patients meet the CDC criteria for the disease.

There's a misconception that what it means to see women as whole people is to study their hearts, lungs, livers, and colons in addition to their reproductive organs. Recently, a woman told me cheerfully, "My doctor knows about women's health. He always checks my heart when I go to see him." But the whole purpose of woman-centered health is to discard the focus on organs and view a woman's total physiology in the context of her environment. Before we can understand how to stay well—through prevention of heart disease, cancer, diabetes, hypertension, osteoporosis, depression, or by addressing other health issues—we have to understand female physiology and psychology.

WHOSE RIB IS IT, ANYWAY?

Forget everything you ever learned about males and females and who's dominant. Modern science has revealed a shocking twist to the old story that the male physiology is superior to the female. Not only are females not derived from males (as in Adam's rib), but technically the reverse is true. Males are derived from females!

Every human being begins its life journey as a female. It isn't until between the twelfth and twentieth week of gestation that masculinization occurs in fetuses that have the Y chromosome. Biologically, the female is the norm and the male is the derivative. Although the male fetus goes on to develop a specific anatomy and brain function, influenced by testosterone, both male and female brains contain receptors for estrogens (female hormones) and androgens (male hormones). The activity of these receptors is influenced by the predominance of male or female hormones circulating in the system.

The presence of male androgens eliminates the brain's ability to drive a monthly reproductive cycle. Hormones affect behavior—such as sexual behavior—which differs in each sex. Increased levels of androgens are associated with more aggressive behavior.

Historically, research into behavior, hormones, and brain function was conducted with an assumption that women were inferior. Today, we know this premise is wrong. We also know that there is more difference within the sexes than there is between the sexes in matter of brain power and intelligence. It is hard to separate the effects of social and environmental factors from biology. However, many behavioral differences between men and women seem to be linked to hormones. Estrogens may create a tendency toward verbal and organizational skills in women, while androgens may enhance mathematical, constructional, spatial, and motor skills. Testosterone is responsible for libido, and although female hormones have often been considered to be the culprit in irrational behavior, androgens might be the real "raging hormones." In the form of anabolic steroids, androgens can cause excessive aggressiveness, anger, hostility, and psychotic behavior.

Of course, knowing about hormonal influences on behavior doesn't give us the entire picture. For example, although males have a tendency toward better math skills, a woman-sensitive learning environment can produce the same results in females. New research shows that women learn better math skills and perform better when they are in all-female classes. In girls' schools, 80 percent of the girls study four years of science and math, compared with the national average of two years in coeducational environments. In fact, graduates of women's colleges perform better than female graduates of coeducational colleges in test scores, graduate school admissions, numbers of earned doctorates, and salaries.

WHAT A DIFFERENCE YOUR HORMONES MAKE!

Female and male hormones exert different influences on the body. How can we protect our health if we don't know what's normal? These are some of the main ways hormones affect the picture.

▶ In the cardiovascular system, female hormones increase dilation of the arteries, affect vascular spasms (as in migraines), and generally improve cardiac function. Male hormones increase heart size, but have no other recognized effects.

▶ In the liver, female hormones inhibit the production of triglycerides and LDL ("bad") cholesterol, as well as free glucose, while male hormones do the opposite. Female hormones decrease the metabolism of drugs, prolonging the action of sedatives, caffeine, and alcohol, while male hormones increase the metabolism of drugs and shorten their active life.

▶ In the fat tissue, female hormones encourage fat deposits in the breasts, hips, and thighs and suppress the movement of fat from these areas. Male hormones contribute to less body fat, especially in the lower body, and favor deposition of fat in the abdomen.

▶ In the gastrointestinal system, female hormones slow down motility—a factor in gallstone formation.

▶ In the respiratory system, female hormones increase the respiratory rate and basal body temperature.

▶ In the musculoskeletal system, female hormones enhance bone density, which is why postmenopausal women are at risk for osteoporosis. Male hormones also insure bone density and strength.

▶ In the immune system, female hormones enhance antibody production and suppress T-cell mediated processes, which are involved in graft rejection. This ability also prevents the rejection of "foreign" matter, such as sperm and a developing fetus.

▶ In the blood, female hormones suppress red blood cell development, lower hemoglobin levels, and increase blood coagulation. Male hormones increase red blood cell development and hemoglobin levels.

▶ Dermatologically, female hormones increase skin vitality, collagen, and water content, while male hormones promote body hair.

THE BENEFITS OF BEING FEMALE

Rather than view the female as derivative of or inferior to the male model, we should marvel at the remarkable adaptability of female physiology. What makes the female body unique is the way it can change to accommodate the pregnant state. This adaptation and the potential for adaptation make a lasting impact on a woman's body, and I believe they give women a unique pathway to health and illness. This is true both during pregnancy and in the nonpregnant state. Unfortunately, until now this pathway has remained largely unexplored in research. Similarly, doctors do not use knowledge of the way reproductive hormones interact with every other system in their understanding of illness or in the general treatment of women. Our data base and health care delivery are fragmented, separating out the reproductive and seeing it only as something that affects childbearing.

Last year, Janice a thirty-three-year-old Catholic nun, came to see me for a second opinion about getting a hysterectomy. Her gynecologist had recommended it because of an ongoing problem Janice had with uterine fibroids. After giving Janice a thorough exam and reading the medical background her gynecologist had supplied, I sat down with her and told her I was very concerned about her getting a hysterectomy. "Your fibroids aren't dangerous," I told her, "and there are other ways they can be controlled, if not eliminated altogether. I'm worried about a woman your age getting a hysterectomy."

Janice looked surprised. "Why? I'm a member of a religious order and I'm not planning to have children. My gynecologist and I discussed this and we both felt that the greater problem was the fibroids."

I realized that Janice was a woman who really needed an advocate! As far as she was concerned, her uterus and ovaries were only relevant if she chose to have children. No one had told her that the hormone depletion caused by a hysterectomy (and the removal of ovaries usually done at the same time) would have a severe effect on her health for the rest of her life. Her gynecologist was urging her to forsake the protected estrogen-rich environment of her natural female state and put herself at risk for, among other things, early heart disease and osteoporosis. Janice was a very bright woman. Once I explained my concerns, she decided that a hysterectomy was premature. "I had no idea," she told me in wonder. "We certainly never learned this in school."

"Don't feel too bad," I said. "Your doctor didn't fully understand the implications, either. But now that you know, you can make informed choices. That's the important thing."

Pregnant or not, the female body's ability to become pregnant gives women special hormonal benefits. It didn't matter that Janice wasn't planning to have children. It was her potential to have children that mattered—a point often missed by doctors who recommend hysterectomies and removal of the ovaries (oophorectomies).

The vast physiologic changes that accompany pregnancy tell us something about the female organism. Only women's bodies are so constructed that they can adapt to a radically different state—a state that involves a tremendous increase in blood volume, enlargement of the heart chambers, greater cardiac output, immune system suppression, and so on. (The full range of changes that occur during pregnancy is explored in Chapter 12.) The hormonal effects that bring about such remarkable changes during pregnancy have an ongoing effect on every organ. Even in the nonpregnant state, female sex steroid hormones affect the severity of many conditions and the way women respond to them. That's one reason women have traditionally been excluded from clinical trials, and also why tests and treatments that work for men often need to be different for women.

For example, basic differences in anatomy have long been appreciated, but they've never been fully incorporated clinically. In addition to the visible differences in height, pelvic structure, and bone and muscle mass, the size of our internal organs differs from men's, as does the thickness of our hair and skin. Most of medicine is geared toward the larger male. Likewise, surgical instruments, designed for men, may be less effective for women. Perhaps that is one reason why surgical outcomes in procedures like coronary bypass have poorer results for women.

The artificial division of medical turf—OB/GYN for reproductive issues, internists and family practicioners for everything else—can be a recipe for disaster when a woman presents with a complicated medical problem. Take the evaluation of abdominal pain. Although there is a clear division of academic, political, and economic turf between the internist and the gynecologist, no clear anatomical distinction exists between the abdomen and the pelvis. It is one continuous cavity where intestines pass through the pelvis and may stick to the ovary; or endometrial tissue may migrate outside the uterus to bleed at distant sites. Yet the woman with abdominal pain must visit at least two physicians, each of whom examines her only partially before sending her to the other, without continuity of thought or continuity of care. That's if she's lucky. She might not be sent to the other physician at all and be left with a misdiagnosis and mistreatment. Or she may be sent to still a third physician—the psychiatrist who says the pain is psychosomatic. While a family practitioner might be able to integrate all three, giving the appearance of more cohesive care, lack of specific training in women's health may still lead to a misdiagnosis.

We gain a powerful tool for better understanding women's health when we fully appreciate the sex differences in biology. Here we have a choice: We can use what we know about differences to reinforce cultural biases, or we can use our knowledge to maximize the quality of life for everyone.

Consider some of the important improvements in women's health care that would come from a better knowledge and understanding of female sex difference:

▶ It would influence the way we treat asthma in women during the low hormonal weeks of menses when their bronchial tubes spasm more.

▶ It would affect the way we counsel diabetics about their insulin requirements premenstrually when carbohydrate craving is triggered by progesterone.

▶ It would alter the time frame for scheduling mastectomies, assuring that they are performed at a time in the monthly cycle when there is less risk of cancer spreading.

▶ It would change the way we design work environments to accommodate the 55-kilogram (121 pound) woman instead of just the 70-kilogram (154 pound) male.

▶ It would make a difference in the way we prescribe medicine, given women's greater proportion of body fat and the influence of oral contraceptives or hormone replacement therapy on drug metabolism.

▶ It would change the way we design research questions that might produce different information in women.

In recent decades, women have spent a great deal of energy moving toward a gender-neutral position and stressing the absence of differences between men and women. We thought being gender neutral was the only way we could gain equal footing. Now we see that when it comes to health and medical care, gender neutrality has resulted in making women invisible.

Sex differences do exist. Let's acknowledge them, understand them, and use the differences for our benefit.

I have often thought that the experience of a woman who enters the health care system is similar to a woman looking into a full-length mirror. But instead of seeing her own reflection, she sees the features and contours of a male. We must change this picture so that the vision a woman sees when she looks in the mirror of medical treatment is her own.

5

THE HEART DISEASE ALERT

It's a Woman's Issue, Too!

~~~~

Teresa was a bright, vigorous sixty-year-old woman who had always been in good health. But for several months, she had been experiencing chest pains almost every day. They didn't seem to be related to exertion, so Teresa didn't even consider a heart problem. She believed she had heartburn, and when she called her family doctor, he agreed. He suggested that Teresa moderate her diet to avoid spicy foods, caffeine, and other possible irritants, and said he'd schedule an appointment if that didn't help.

Teresa made some drastic changes in her diet, but they didn't seem to have any effect. She still had chest pains. By now, her husband was growing alarmed. He was afraid his wife had an ulcer or a gallbaldder problem that was going untreated. Teresa agreed to see the doctor if things didn't get better soon.

But one night, Teresa woke up with pain that seemed worse than usual. She stumbled to the kitchen and took a couple of antacid tablets, but they didn't give her any relief. Frightened, Teresa woke her husband who quickly bundled her into the car and took her to the hospital where it was determined that she was having a heart attack.

I'm certain that if Teresa had been a man, she would not have casually discounted her chest pains. And her doctor's reaction would more likely have been, "I'll meet you in the emergency room," rather than, "Stop eating spicy foods." But Teresa's experience was typical of the frustrating lack of attention that is given to women and heart disease.

Although coronary artery disease (CAD) is the number-one killer of women, and 250 thousand of us die from it every year, the overriding attitude has been that it is a man's disease, with little sense of urgency when it comes to women. Underdiagnosis, overdiagnosis, and misdiagnosis are par for the course. Until recently, there were virtually no studies or clinical trials that isolated sex-specific issues related to CAD and women. We now know that estrogen appears to protect most premenopausal women against CAD, but we haven't fully explored the implications of that knowledge. Nor have we developed an appreciation of the unique ways CAD manifests itself in women. Since doctors don't know to do otherwise, they continue to address CAD in women just as they do in men. It's a striking example of the profession's androgynous approach to medicine—the assumption that men and women have similar profiles when nongynecological problems emerge.

You might think that the risk of CAD among women is a new phenomenon, since it's only been recently that the issue has made an appearance in the public press. But only our awareness is new, not the threat itself. Since 1910, more American women have died of heart disease than of any other cause. Yet, when the American Heart Association held its first public conference for women in 1964, it focused on how they could help protect their husbands' hearts.

The main reason CAD has been considered a men-only disease is that it typically appears in them when they are in their forties or fifties, much earlier than it shows up for women. During the 1960s and 1970s, there was an amazing mobilization of technology and services to address the crisis of so many young men dropping dead of CAD. The Framingham, Massachusetts, Heart Study, the largest and most widespread of its kind, which has tracked a group of 2,282 men and 2,845 women since 1948, initially fed the bias that CAD was a male problem because the men in the study were dying so much younger than the women. Women usually didn't develop heart problems until a decade or more after menopause, and because the profession was insensitive to the problems of the elderly, there was no mobilization to address the crisis of older women. In fact, it wasn't unusual for doctors to ignore the possibility of heart disease altogether. A woman might arrive at a hospital emergency room manifesting all the symptoms of a heart attack, only to be told she was suffering from anxiety. Cardiovascular screening was (and often still is) rarely part of a woman's normal checkup. When a man goes to the doctor, it's foremost in his mind and the doctor's.

The diagnosis of CAD in women is complicated by a number of biological sex-specific effects. The Framingham Study demonstrated distinct female differences in certain risk factors such as cholesterol levels, obesity, and cigarette smoking. Furthermore, when women seek help, they frequently present with different symptoms from men's, and sometimes these symptoms are more difficult to evaluate with standard tests. Once heart disease is diagnosed in a woman, her treatment is far less aggressive. One reason is that women present with CAD at a more advanced stage, so the common treatments used for younger men are less effective. Balloon angioplasty and bypass surgery work wonders for many men with CAD, but are less successful for women, in part because of their smaller hearts and arteries. The profession has yet to develop surgical or medical methods and instruments that are woman-specific. Furthermore, when older women show up with heart problems, it is often too late for them to receive certain treatments. One example is an aggressive intervention called thrombolytic therapy, which dissolves a heart blockage while it is in an early stage. This therapy must be given within six hours of the onset of pain. But women tend to delay going to emergency rooms because they don't know they're having a heart attack, and by the time they get there, it's too late for thrombolytic therapy. Established cutoffs have normally excluded women over seventy, the group most likely to get heart attacks.

Gender bias invades every part of the process. When women do seek help for heart problems, their symptoms (such as chest pain or palpitations) are more likely to be interpreted as psychosomatic. In one study, a research team investigated the ways doctors responded to five medical complaints common in both men and women: chest pain, back pain, headache, dizziness, and fatigue. Researchers found that across the board "men received a more extensive workup than women for all complaints studied." Doctors' decisions to perform more thorough workups on men were not based on the medical facts, which were the same in both men and women, but on the doctors' interpretation of the seriousness of the complaints. The judgment of the researchers was that when men complained of a medical problem, the attitude was, "It must be serious if he's complaining." Women's complaints were not given the same credence.

One doctor told of a sixty-two-year-old woman who came to the emergency room describing chest pains radiating down her left arm and into her jaw. She was diagnosed with anxiety and sent home. A similar presentation in a man would have put him in the coronary care unit.

Even I, who am always on the alert for the special signs of heart disease in women, have been caught off guard on this issue. Not long ago, I was delayed at the hospital one day, and returned to my office to find three urgent messages from a forty-three-year-old woman I had seen once as a patient. I barely remembered Marian. Her messages were verging on hysterical. She was complaining of severe, crushing chest pain. A fourth message, from a friend, told me Marian had been taken to the emergency room.

I called the hospital and talked to the ER nurse, while I quickly perused Marian's chart. When she had consulted me two years earlier, she had been overweight and somewhat hypertensive. Still, I didn't consider a heart problem. It was almost unthinkable for a woman Marian's age who was still menstruating. I told the nurse that Marian was probably having a panic attack.

A half an hour later, I received a call from an emergency room doctor who told me Marian had had a heart attack. I was shocked, until he added the information that her blood sugars were sky high. Then it made sense. In the years since I had last seen her, Marian had become diabetic. I had never known her as a diabetic, so I'd missed the connection. Diabetes is a condition that can lead to heart attacks in premenopausal women.

I was relieved that Marian was receiving immediate care, but the incident served as a sobering reminder for me. Even a doctor sensitive to gender bias had suggested that Marian's problem might be a panic attack.

For these reasons, when women develop CAD, they do much worse than men. Women are more likely than men to die from heart attacks after a few weeks, and they have a 39 percent chance of dying during the first year after a heart attack, versus a 31 percent chance for men. The rate for African-American women is twice that of white women. Women also have a higher death rate following coronary bypass graft surgery and angioplasty than men. In a study from Cedars Sinai Medical Center in Los Angeles, of 2,297 coronary bypass surgeries performed, only 28 percent were women, and they were usually referred for surgery at later stages of the disease than men—only after they had experienced congestive heart failure, unstable angina, or heart attacks. They were older and much sicker than the men referred for surgery, and that might have contributed to their poorer outcomes.

Although, overall, women use the health care system far more than men, this usage drops dramatically among the elderly and poor. Economic considerations, such as a lack of health insurance, and accessibility factors, such as having no transportation or child care, mean less preventive and diagnostic care for the very women who need it the most.

The best way to protect yourself is to learn how to recognize the risks and symptoms, and to be an advocate in your own health care. That means understanding preventive measures, your risk profile, and proper screening procedures according to your age. It also means demanding that you be treated seriously if you are a woman with a risk of coronary artery disease—and knowing how to recognize the options and potential pitfalls in diagnosis and treatment.

CORONARY ARTERY DISEASE, SIMPLY DEFINED

Your heart is like a central dispatcher, pumping the blood needed to sustain life to the rest of your body. It is an exquisitely designed system that assures the regular delivery of oxygen and nutrients. When your heart or the arteries through which blood flows are not functioning, your entire body suffers the effects.

Coronary artery disease occurs through the process of atherosclerosis, or clogging of the arteries that feed the heart. This is caused by an accumulation of substances called plaque (mostly composed of cholesterol and fibrous tissues) along the inner lining of medium and large arteries. It is now believed that eating a diet high in saturated fat and cholesterol is the principle cause of plaque formation.

Over time, plaque hardens and grows larger, protruding into the artery and narrowing the vessel. When plaque forms in the coronary arteries, which deliver oxygen and nutrients to the heart muscle, the eventual result of oxygen deprivation may be a heart attack.

Blockage of an artery can also be caused by a spasm in the vessels around the plaque or a plaque dislodgment that creates an obstruction. Whatever the cause, the part of the heart muscle that is fed by the damaged artery can become oxygen starved and die.

In themselves, blood vessel spasms are not uncommon to women. They occur monthly to produce menstrual flow, and they're also the cause of migraines, which are more frequently suffered by women. But when there is plaque, a normal spasm can further narrow an already narrow artery and create a total blockage. Sometimes a spasm can occur without plaque, accompanied by similar symptoms. Women also have a threefold greater chance than men of rupturing their heart muscles after a heart attack.

For men, the most common manifestation of CAD is a heart attack. It is not the same for women. Women most often present with angina or atypical chest pain syndromes. These often have different characteristics from men's "typical" angina, which usually occurs with exertion.

Women who were included in the Framingham Study developed angina at least twice as often as heart attacks, and the rate for African-American women was even higher. Over the years, women have suffered tremendously as a result of their different symptoms and because noncardiac conditions causing chest pain are more common, especially in younger women. Perhaps if they were having heart attacks at the same age as men, some of the diagnostic bias would not exist.

We really should be comparing the forty-year-old man with the sixty-year-old woman, not with the forty-year-old woman. When we use the forty-year-old woman as a comparison, the conclusion is drawn that angina in women is usually a benign condition, but this is certainly not the case for an older woman. New studies have demonstrated conclusively that while angina in younger women is not necessarily a sign of CAD, up to 90 percent of older women with chest pain have CAD. Untreated, they go on to have heart attacks that are more likely than those in men to be fatal. So, chest pain in women should always be treated as a potential coronary crisis, especially in older women. Private physicians and emergency room doctors need to view a sixty-five-year-old woman who has chest pains with the same urgency they would give a forty-five-year-old man.

STAY AHEAD OF YOUR RISKS

Although plaque buildup is a primary cause of CAD, many other factors affect your level of risk. It is my firm belief that if women understand their risk factors and take preventive action, their incidence of CAD can be drastically reduced. This is self-empowerment. By taking control where we can, women can overcome many of the limitations of the medical system. Our goal is primary prevention, which means avoiding getting CAD in the first place; and secondary prevention, which means reducing the impact of the disease once it's present, or eliminating a factor often seen in people with the disease. In the following section, I will describe the known risk factors and tell you how they relate to your screening and prevention program.

YOUR CAD RISK FACTOR CHECKLIST

1. **A family history of heart disease.**
2. **Low HDL/high LDL cholesterol, plus high triglycerides.**
3. **High blood pressure.**
4. **Smoking.**
5. **Diabetes.**
6. **Obesity, especially high ratio of abdominal to thigh fat.**
7. **Sedentary living.**
8. **Stress.**
9. **Postmenopausal estrogen depletion, or premenopausal ovarian failure.**
10. **Social isolation.**
11. **Race.**

---

1. Is There Heart Disease in Your Family?

If your father had a heart attack before his early fifties and your mother had one before age sixty, you have a familial risk factor. As a rule, the younger your parents or grandparents were when they had heart attacks, the greater your risk. Even if your mother never had heart disease, you can inherit the risk from your father. Race is also a factor; African-Americans have a higher incidence of heart disease than Caucasians and a higher mortality rate from CAD.

Obviously, you can't prevent or change your genetic predisposition, but knowing you have a familial risk can alert you to the need for regular screening. It might also influence your determination to avoid other risks—such as those imposed by diet or smoking.

2. Do You Have High "Bad" Cholesterol?

The most significant primary risk factor for CAD is the accumulation of blood fats, mainly cholesterol, in the arteries.

In itself, cholesterol is not bad. It's a necessary part of your body's operation. Cholesterol is present in every cell, and it's important to many of your bodily functions—for example, the formation of sex hormones, digestive juices, and skin oils. Cholesterol travels from cells to the liver and back again through the bloodstream. It only becomes a problem when too much of it is left behind in the arteries. How does this happen? Cholesterol is carried by lipoproteins, which are produced in the liver and are distinguished by their density. High-density lipoproteins (or HDLs) are strong carriers that efficiently remove cholesterol from arteries. Low-density lipoproteins (or LDLs) are weak carriers that don't remove as much cholesterol and tend to leave it behind in the arteries. If you've heard the terms "good cholesterol" and "bad cholesterol" that's a reference to HDLs and LDLs.

Most experts believe that the percentage of HDL cholesterol to LDL cholesterol is a better determinant of heart risk than total cholesterol, and this seems to be particularly true for women. Whereas total cholesterol and LDL cholesterol are valid indicators for men, they are not as strong a marker of disease in women, especially premenopausal women, because estrogen prevents the incorporation of cholesterol into plaque and slows the growth of plaque. Estrogen is anti-atherogenic. So, qualitatively, a higher LDL level will not have the same effect on a woman as it does on a man. However, a low level of HDLs, which remove and transport cholesterol more efficiently, is a big risk factor for women. Various people suggest it should be at least one-fifth of the total. Others evaluating the absolute number say no less than fifty.

The data about dietary restriction and lipid levels are confusing. Although dietary restriction of fat and cholesterol has been found to significantly lower blood cholesterol levels and heart disease in men, the data in women are less clear. Also, lowering fat in the diet may incidentally cause a lowering of HDL cholesterol, a more significant factor in women than in men.

When you have a blood test to measure cholesterol, it should also include a measurement of your triglyceride levels. Triglycerides are a measure of your body's fat stores, and if you have levels above 200 mg/dl, it increases your risk. This is true for women and not for men.

Lipoprotein lipase, called Lp(a), is also a risk factor for CAD in both men and women. This lipid protein complex can increase the tendency toward forming blood clots on top of atherosclerotic plaques. High levels of Lp(a) increase CAD risk. Estrogen given to women in hormone replacement therapy and to men as a treatment for prostate cancer has been found to significantly lower Lp(a) levels.

3. Is Your Blood Pressure High?

High blood pressure, or hypertension, is a secondary risk factor for CAD. That is, it does not cause the disease, but it is often present in women who have it, and it can accelerate the CAD process. Hypertension is a condition, usually without any symptoms, in which too much pressure is placed on the walls of the arteries, either by increased blood volume or constriction of the arteries. Over time, hypertension strains the heart and weakens the artery walls.

About half of all postmenopausal women have elevated blood pressure, which often begins in their forties. African-American women have hypertension a good ten years earlier than Caucasian women, and have significantly higher death rates from stroke and heart disease. Rates among Native American women, Alaskan native women and Puerto Rican women are somewhat less; rates in other Latina women are significantly less. You are also at greater risk if you have a family history of hypertension or have experienced it during a pregnancy. It's very important to get regular screening, especially if you're at risk, because there are usually no symptoms until secondary problems like heart disease, blindness, kidney failure, and strokes occur.

Most people have had their blood pressure taken at one time or another, as part of a regular exam. When I take it in my office, I usually do it two or three times during the course of the exam. That's because blood pressure is acutely affected by anxiety or nervousness and many people are nervous when they see a doctor. There's even a term for it: "white coat hypertension." That's the tendency of a person's blood pressure to rise on the doctor's examining table. If a doctor tells you that you have high blood pressure, you should be sure he or she has made several readings, perhaps over the course of two or three visits. Don't have caffeine or tobacco for at least thirty minutes prior to having your blood pressure taken. Make sure that a large cuff is used if you have a large arm; otherwise, a falsely elevated blood pressure may be noted.

What do the blood pressure readings mean? Although there is no "normal" number at which blood pressure is considered safe, the range used by the American Heart Association to indicate high blood presure is 140 over 90.

The first number is the systolic pressure—the pressure that results when the heart contracts to pump blood into the arteries. The second number is the diastolic pressure—the pressure exerted on the walls of the arteries between beats. Both numbers are significant, but if the second number is high, there is greater risk since it means there is significant pressure on the arteries even when the heart is relaxed.

I consider a high blood pressure reading in a woman a very serious matter that requires a careful investigation. I examine the retina of the eye, which is the window through which the body's small blood vessels are viewed. When there is hypertension, these vessels have a changed appearance, becoming narrower; there is a danger they can hemorrhage or burst. I then examine the large blood vessels in the neck, abdomen, groin, and feet by feeling for the strength of the pulse and looking for the narrowing that is caused by cholesterol plaques. These plaques can lead to strokes if they are in or near the brain; kidney failure if they occur in the abdomen; or loss of a limb if they occur in the leg. Peripheral arterial disease (PAD—blocked arteries in the leg) increases the risk of death from CAD. Women with PAD need to have a thorough evaluation for CAD and possible bypass surgery before considering surgery for a blocked peripheral artery.

There are two kinds of high blood pressure—essential and secondary. Most high blood pressure is essential; that is, no contributing cause can be found. When high blood pressure is unresponsive to treatment or appears in a very young or elderly person for the first time, it might be secondary to a medical condition. I once saw a seventeen-year-old girl with high blood pressure, which is very unusual. The cause was a narrowing in the artery going to the left kidney. The artery was enlarged and her blood pressure returned to normal soon thereafter.

Hypertension can affect virtually every bodily system. And, as we'll see later in the chapter, it may damage the heart in other ways besides coronary artery disease.

4. Do You Smoke?

About 27 percent of American women smoke, and there is substantial evidence that women who smoke are high risk candidates for heart disease, especially prior to menopause. According to a report in the *Journal of the American Medical Association,* cigarette smoking may account for two-thirds of heart attacks among women under age fifty. The Nurses Health Study, which tracked female nurses between the ages of thirty-five and fifty, showed that women who smoke as few as one to four cigarettes a day increase their risk twofold; heavier smokers (more than twenty-five per day) substantially increase their risk. Smoking overrides the protective effects of estrogen, and smokers tend to reach menopause earlier than nonsmokers, heightening the risk. Time and again, women have come to my office and made the remark, "I'm worried that my smoking will cause lung cancer." Rarely do they realize that their risk for heart disease is just as great and usually even greater. Smoking is also the reason that women over age thirty-five who take oral contraceptives have high risk for heart attacks. Tobacco is a potent blood clotter in the presence of oral contraceptives.

The good news is that the risk for CAD dissipates once you stop smoking. According to a report by the Surgeon General, the risk to smokers declines by as much as 50 percent during the first year after quitting. Within five years, the risk factors for heart disease approach those of women who have never smoked. This is a different pattern than for lung cancer where the risk is never completely eliminated.

5. Do You Have Diabetes?

Remember Marian, the forty-three-year-old woman who went to the emergency room with a heart attack? CAD is rare in premenopausal women unless they have diabetes, but then the chances skyrocket. Why is this? Although estrogen protects most women from CAD, for some reason that we don't fully understand, it fails to protect you if you have diabetes. CAD is the leading cause of death in diabetics, especially diabetic women, among whom the mortality rate is 25 percent higher than in nondiabetic women.

High insulin levels are thought to be the link between hypertension, obesity, and abnormal lipids (elevated triglycerides and low HDL). When diabetes is added to the others, they become what is known as "the deadly quartet."

An interesting study showed that in diabetics with other established risk factors like high triglycerides and hypertension, the presence of depression further increased the risk of developing CAD. In Chapter 7, we'll explore the risk, prevention, and management of diabetes in full detail.

6. Are You Overweight?

Obesity increases your risk of high blood pressure, diabetes, high cholesterol, and CAD. Significantly overweight women have a greater incidence of heart attack, stroke, congestive heart failure, and death from all heart related causes. Today, one in five U.S. adults (some thirty-four million people) are obese—defined as being 20 percent over the recommended weight range. According to an eight-year study conducted by Harvard Medical School and the Brigham and Women's Hospital, as much as 70 percent of CAD among obese women was related to their excess weight. The Framingham Study concurs, showing that obese women under age fifty have a two-and-a-half-times greater risk of CAD.

Additional studies suggest that the distribution of fat, not the amount, might be the real killer. People with excess android or belly fat (known as apple-shaped) have a higher risk than those with excess hip and thigh fat (known as pear-shaped). The apple-shaped woman with fat around the abdomen is at greater risk for CAD because android (abdominal) fat is associated with low HDL, high triglycerides, and resistance to insulin, as in diabetics, leading to higher insulin levels. African-American women are more likely than Caucasian women to have this pattern. The pear-shaped woman, whose excess fat is in the lower body, does not share this risk because hip and thigh fat is less easily mobilized; indeed, it serves as stored energy to be used during pregnancy, for breast-feeding, and for enhancing estrogen levels after menopause.

It is interesting to note that abdominal fat tends to be deposited when cortisol, the stress hormone, is high. Studies in women with abdominal fat show an excess secretion of cortisol during periods of stress. Obviously, behavior modification must be considered, in addition to calorie consumption.

Most women have gone on diets at least a few times in their lives. Unfortunately, they often diet to reduce hip and thigh fat, which women naturally have in greater abundance. While overall obesity is a risk factor for CAD, the danger lies in the amount of android fat.

7. Do You Get Enough Exercise?

Growing evidence shows that inactivity might be an independent risk factor for CAD. Unfortunately, few studies have been women-specific; only five in forty-three even included women. But initial reports indicate that low fitness levels are associated with obesity and other CAD risk factors in women, especially African-American women. High fitness levels have been associated with lower blood pressure and better lipid profiles and lower insulin levels.

Heart-healthy exercise is aerobic. Aerobic activities include walking, running, biking, swimming, or cross-country skiing. Aerobic exercise creates the type of heart muscle contractions that improve cardiovascular conditioning.

Since a sedentary lifestyle is a primary risk factor for coronary artery disease, it's important for you to make regular aerobic exercise a routine part of your life. If you are not currently active, don't try to do too much at first. Start slowly and gradually increase the level. You can even incorporate exercise into the normal flow of your life—for example, walking instead of driving, or walking up a flight of stairs instead of taking an elevator.

8. Are You Under Stress?

Stress is a tricky thing to define and diagnose, and unfortunately, it too often has not been taken seriously as a coronary risk factor—especially for women. Again, stress has typically been identified as a man's problem. But the Framingham Study and others have begun to appreciate that women experience stress, too, and it has harmful effects on their blood pressure and hearts. As many women find themselves juggling multiple roles, stress is likely to receive more attention as a risk factor. Be clear that it is not the multiple roles themselves that add stress. Indeed, many women thrive in this environment. Stress can affect women when there is tension or lack of support at home, or when they are in a job with little control or autonomy. The stress response includes high levels of chemicals that make the heart work harder by raising blood pressure, increasing heart rate, and enhancing the force of contractions. Stress hormones, including cortisol, counterbalance the work of insulin and cause higher blood sugar. In order to keep blood sugar normal, the body adjusts by raising insulin levels, and this may be significant in the development of cardiovascular disease and adult diabetes.

Social isolation can be a heart damaging stress factor. In one study conducted at Duke University, 1,368 patients who underwent coronary angiography from 1974 to 1980 were followed through 1989. Patients (male or female) who were unmarried or had no close partner or confidant had only a 50 percent five-year survival rate compared to 82 percent among those who were married or had a close confidant. It was believed that the stress caused by being alone and having no strong support system contributed to their poor results.

In the general population, three out of four men over age sixty-five are married, while three out of five women are living alone. Since most of the research on social isolation has been done with men, we don't know conclusively what unique factors might be present for women, whose social network may add burden to blessing.

A dramatic illustration of the effects of social isolation was presented in a research study of seventy-seven female cynomolgus monkeys (the animal model for CAD). All of the monkeys were fed the same moderate heart-healthy diet. However, thirty of the monkeys had been in an experiment in which they were housed in single cages; the other forty-seven lived in social groups. In spite of a similar diet, the female monkeys housed in single units had significantly more heart disease than those who lived in social groups.

Furthermore, those who had income levels below ten thousand dollars had worse five-year survival rates than those with incomes above forty thousand dollars. Again, the stress of having financial worries seemed to contribute to the results.

The poverty rate for elderly women is 19 percent, the highest of any group in the United States. Over the past three decades, poverty has become feminized. The number of female-headed households has doubled, and these are four times as likely to be poor than other families. Among those poor households, African-American and Latina women are twice as likely as Caucasian women to be heads of households. Women of color have higher rates of diabetes, high blood pressure, and cardiovascular disease. Women without health insurance have higher blood pressure than women with health insurance coverage. Poor women who may be homeless, unemployed, or struggling to make ends meet, usually find it more urgent to put food on the table than to get their blood pressure checked. But their risks are heightened by stress, smoking, alcohol abuse, and high-fat diets.

After they suffer heart attacks, women experience greater anxiety, depression, guilt about being sick, and sexual dysfunction than men. These factors are important when we consider heart disease, and our assumptions must be refined to be relevant to women. For instance, although marriage predicts increased survival in men, it has been associated with higher rates of depression in women—even more so for married African-American women in higher socioeconomic groups.

9. Are You Postmenopausal?

Heart disease is rare in women before menopause, although it can occur if other risk factors are present, or if a woman has suffered premature estrogen depletion. Doctors have to be alert. I've seen menopausal women with mild risk factors have unexpected heart attacks. I've also seen heavy smokers or hypertensive diabetics who developed heart conditions in their forties. We have to remember that when we talk about risk factors, it's not the same as saying, "You will get CAD," or "You won't get CAD."

There is compelling evidence that estrogen replacement therapy (ERT) results in a highly significant decline in the risk for heart disease in postmenopausal women. Studies have shown that estrogen inhibits the incorporation of cholesterol into blood vessel walls. It raises HDL and lowers LDL cholesterol. Estrogen also increases the dilation of the blood vessels and makes them less prone to spasm.

A widely reported study by Dr. Trudy L. Bush and her colleagues at the National Institutes of Health's Heart, Blood and Lung Institute followed 2,269 women, ages forty to sixty-nine for an average of five years to determine the effects of ERT. The death rate of those on ERT was only one-third that of the subjects who were not taking estrogen.

Women who have had premenopausal hysterectomies, with or without removal of the ovaries, also have a high risk of CAD if they are not receiving estrogen replacement. For this group, there is evidence that ERT makes a remarkable difference. In the NIH's study, the death rate among women whose ovaries had been removed before menopause was ten times lower if they were receiving estrogen.

We are just beginning to see prospective research on the therapeutic use of estrogen for women. The Women's Health Initiative will be a major advance in the long-term study of various hormone replacement protocols. Reports are already coming in about the increased survival of women with known heart disease being treated with estrogen, and I hope to see more studies looking at the use of estrogen in the treatment of active heart disease in the future. It is interesting to note that we are also seeing articles about androgens and heart disease in men; for example, the possible link between baldness and CAD may be due to a man's androgen profile. In any case, a sex-specific biologic approach to understanding disease will benefit everyone.

Some researchers believe that "compliance bias" is at work in these observational studies of hormone replacement therapy (HRT) and CAD prevention. That is, it might be true that women who use HRT are generally taking better care of themselves, getting regular checkups, exercising more, and eating healthier diets. It is hoped that the Women's Health Initiative will settle this question by looking at hormone use in a randomized controlled study.

There has been a great deal of controversy surrounding the advisability of ERT. Fear of developing cancer of the breast or uterus has discouraged many women from taking estrogen after menopause. We will explore the relative risk factors in detail in Chapter 13. For now, I will give you a simple answer: Most women on ERT gain far more benefits than they incur risks.

CAD PREVENTION CHECKLIST

1. **Significantly reduce saturated fat and cholesterol in your diet.**
2. **Maintain normal blood pressure.**
3. **Don't smoke.**
4. **Keep blood sugar levels in check.**
5. **Maintain a healthy weight.**
6. **Exercise regularly.**
7. **Reduce stress in your home or workplace.**
8. **Consider HRT after menopause.**
9. **Maintain a rich social network for support and connection.**

WOMEN'S HEART PROBLEMS AREN'T ALWAYS CAD

Grace, a fifty-eight-year-old woman, was convinced she had coronary artery disease, although she didn't have any of the standard risk factors. There was no history of it in her family, and she was a basically healthy woman whose vegetarian diet and exercise regimen kept her cholesterol and blood pressure at excellent levels. Furthermore, she was experiencing no chest pains or other dramatic episodes. Given her profile, heart disease would have seemed unlikely, but Grace was caught in a diagnostic process that almost proved disastrous.

When she was in her late forties, Grace's prior physician discovered she had an abnormal cardiogram—a slowdown in a part of the heart's electrical conduction system, which coordinates contractions. Because of this abnormality, the physician sent Grace to a cardiologist, whom she then saw on a regular basis for several years.

On one of her visits, the cardiologist asked if she had any symptoms. Grace searched her mind and came up with something she thought might be a symptom. She told him that she sometimes grew short of breath walking up the subway steps. Based on that symptom, the cardiologist performed an echocardiogram, which is a sound-wave picture of the heart. It showed that a piece of the heart wall was not moving properly. After that, he ordered a thallium stress test, which showed another abnormality, but in a different region of the heart muscle.

On the basis of these tests, Grace's cardiologist made a diagnosis: "You have a heart condition." And he put her on medication used to treat CAD.

When Grace came to me, she was very frightened, and her normal confidence was shaken by the idea that she was a woman with a life-threatening disease. But I was perplexed by the diagnosis because Grace had no CAD risk factors, and the two tests revealed different abnormalities. It became clear that she did not have angina or blocked arteries—what one typically thinks of as being a heart condition. So, what was going on? I had three different doctors review the echocardiogram and thallium stress test, and I got three different readings on them.

After some investigation, I discovered that the disturbance in Grace's electrical conduction system, which had caused the abnormal electrocardiogram, also caused a false positive (an abnormal reading when no abnormality was present) on the thallium stress test. My question was: Did Grace have a heart abnormality that was not coronary artery disease?

I spoke with Grace's cardiologist and he said, "Well, let's do a tie-breaker," and he ordered a third test. That test showed that Grace's heart muscle wasn't functioning strongly—something we already knew—but it didn't show anything else. We decided to take her off the heart medication and follow her condition over time. In the course of two years, Grace developed other wall-motion abnormalities, but her problem had nothing to do with blocked arteries. It wasn't CAD and, in fact, the medication given to her initially would have worsened her condition. With time, we were able to achieve a proper diagnosis and treat Grace's real heart problem—a weakness in the heart muscle. But think about it. Had the original diagnosis of CAD held, Grace would have been treated with the wrong medication. Worse still, she would have lived as a person who has been told she had CAD, a factor that would compromise her quality of life and rattle her confidence. Grace's original internist and cardiologist hadn't considered the inconsistencies in her presentation or tried to investigate them. They made the diagnosis based on what was often seen in men: Shortness of breath with exertion was a sign of CAD.

Doctors normally refer to chest pains as either "typical" or "atypical." These terms are solely based on research conducted with men and have little relevance for women. So-called "typical" chest pains are those that accompany heavy exertion. That's the usual way men present with angina. But women tend to have more atypical chest pain—that is, pain not associated with exertion. The good news is that the causes are not necessarily very serious and can often be treated without drastic measures. The bad news is that sometimes a diagnosis of CAD is missed because a woman's chest pains will not be associated with exertion.

However, it is useful to familiarize yourself with some common female heart conditions that are not CAD, since a misdiagnosis can work both ways.

A common cause of non-CAD chest pain in women is mitral valve prolapse. This is a genetic condition that can be hard to pinpoint since its symptoms tend to mimic CAD's. Women with mitral valve prolapse suffer nonanginal chest pain, heart palpitations, dizziness, and fainting. But the cause is not a weakness in the heart muscle or blocked arteries; it is a malformation in the heart valve located at the opening of the left ventricle, which is your heart's primary pump. When the valve is malformed, it does not close tightly, and sometimes small amounts of blood leak backward—the way air leaks through a loose doorframe. If the leakage remains insignificant, there may be no problem at all. But if there is too much leakage, it can ultimately lead to a backup of pressure into the lungs and a weakening of the heart. This is a rare course for mitral valve prolapse.

The major complication of mitral valve prolapse is infection of the heart valves (endocarditis). This occurs because bacteria that have found their way into the bloodstream during certain procedures, like dental work or gynecological surgery, can settle out in areas of turbulent blood flow such as the area around a poorly closing valve. That is why doctors recommend antibiotics at the time of these procedures. While women more commonly express the gene for MVP, men are at higher risk for these complications.

Women have typically had a difficult time getting an accurate diagnosis for mitral valve prolapse, in large part because of palpitations and chest pain, which can also be seen in anxiety and panic attacks. MVP and panic disorders are two conditions common to women. These symptoms often lead physicians to suspect a psychiatric reaction, rather than a physiological cause.

A diagnosis of mitral valve prolapse requires that a physician listen to the patient and resist assuming that reports of chest pain, anxiety, and panic are imaginary. Sometimes mitral valve prolapse can be detected by listening to heart sounds with a stethoscope. A snapping sound can often be heard. That, accompanied by a late systolic murmur, is suggestive of mitral valve prolapse. This can be further documented on an echocardiogram.

There is a clear genetic component to MVP, as 30 to 50 percent of first-degree relatives also have it. Furthermore, the genetic tendency is modified by sex—more than twice as many females as males have the condition. Although you are born with MVP, it will usually take years to manifest itself and may even disappear in women after age fifty. First-degree relatives should be screened with echocardiograms.

Severe complications occur in a minority of cases, and these might require surgical repair of the valve. However, most cases of mitral valve prolapse are asymptomatic and require no treatment at all. Sometimes medication can be taken to ease chest pains and irregular heartbeat.

Mitral valve prolapse is sometimes the reason for another common condition, heart arrhythmia. Arrhythmia is an abnormality in the heart rate that causes palpitations, shortness of breath, and dizziness. These symptoms can be very worrisome, but often they aren't serious. For pregnant women, they are usually normal, since pregnancy involves changes in the blood volume and heart capacity. Arrhythmia can also be the result of too much caffeine, stress, or a thyroid condition.

Another chest-pain syndrome in women is called Syndrome X. The name itself gives you a clue about the confusion surrounding this disorder. Its formal description is microvascular angina—chest pain not caused by CAD, which involves the larger blood vessels in the heart. In the past, doctors often assumed that the pain was psychological, since it afflicted women of all ages and was not accompanied by other signs of heart disease. Today, we know it is real, and also that both men and women suffer from it—although it's more common in women. These patients have atypical chest pain and may even have abnormal EKGs and stress tests, but if they get worked up aggressively and have cardiac catheterization, they are found to have normal coronary arteries. An interesting study done at Yale showed that most of these women had been surgically put into menopause, and their chest pains disappeared when they received estrogen replacement therapy. These patients usually respond well to medications that block vessel spasms (called calcium channel blockers).

Despite the frequency of noncoronary chest pain syndromes, women who report chest pain should be treated seriously. CAD should always be considered, with a sex-specific analysis of risk factors and test results made during a diagnostic workup. And physicians should always account for other conditions that can cause symptoms that feel like chest pain—such as ulcers, gastrointestinal disorders, esophageal spasms, gallbladder disease, and blood clots to the lung.

HYPERTENSIVE HEART DISEASE

Pain-related syndromes aren't the only non-CAD causes of heart problems. In addition to being a secondary risk factor for CAD (as we discussed earlier), hypertension can serve as an independent factor for heart failure. When you have hypertension, your heart must work harder to adjust to the increased pressure. This is more so in women than men. Over time, the constant stress leads to thickening of the heart muscle and then heart failure.

Noncoronary factors such as hypertension play a more important role in the development of congestive heart failure in women than in men. Women are more susceptible to the development of a thickened heart muscle (called left ventricular hypertrophy or LVH) than men; they have more LVH at all levels of blood pressure. As we age, our heart muscles thicken. The average increase is 54 percent in women compared to 25 percent in men. Hypertrophic cardiomyopathy of the elderly (thickened heart muscle that loses its elasticity as a pump) is predominantly seen in women, especially African-American women with high blood pressure.

When controlling for all other factors, race is still significant in the risk of developing hypertension. Some studies have shown that African-Americans have less decline in blood pressure during sleep. Perhaps this physiologic difference, giving African-Americans a more consistently elevated blood pressure during a twenty-four hour period, can explain their higher rates of heart failure, liver failure, stroke, and blindness.

There are studies that suggest sex-specific factors that combine with genetic tendencies toward high blood pressure. For example, women with high blood pressure are more sensitive to the fluid retention caused by salt when they have a family history of hypertension than women with high blood pressure with no family history of hypertension. This relationship is only seen in women. Clinically, we have also found that African-American women with high blood pressure are more responsive to diuretics.

High blood pressure is the most common factor leading to renal failure and a need for hemodialysis—an area where gender bias exists in access to care. African-American women are more likely than Caucasians to need this treatment, perhaps because of the earlier onset of hypertension and the increased severity of blood pressure.

Hypertensive heart disease can manifest simply with shortness of breath on exertion. This is not caused by a blocked flow of blood to the heart muscle, as in CAD, but by a stiff heart muscle that is unable to relax as it fills with blood before a contraction. The stiffness causes the pressure inside the heart to rise, which leads to congestion in the lungs, where blood may back up. This is called diastolic dysfunction.

I have often wondered why my well controlled hypertensive patients and some of my nonhypertensive elderly patients have LVH. Not until I did the research for this book did I get confirmation of what I was seeing in my practice: Women are different.

Differences also appear when we look at the benefit of treatment for hypertension. Treatment clearly benefits men and to a lesser extent African-American women. No benefit has yet been seen in treating Caucasian women, and several studies have even shown that Caucasian women are harmed by standard treatment—although this may not apply to very elderly women. Obviously, more sex, age, race, and ethnically sensitive studies need to be conducted.

Hypertension affects other parts of the body. Hypertensive women are particularly at risk for strokes—the number three killer of women after CAD and cancer—a condition that can occur when the arteries feeding the brain are under too much pressure. Strokes are eight times as likely if you have high blood pressure.

A stroke occurs when a blood vessel in the brain closes off or bursts, leaving areas of brain tissue without oxygen; ultimately, these areas will die. The warning signs include dizziness or a loss of balance or coordination, fogginess of speech, difficulty understanding what others are saying, sudden blurred or decreased vision, unexplained numbness or weakness on one side of the body, loss of consciousness or sudden drowsiness, or a sudden, severe headache.

Early signs might resolve within a day, not leaving you with a fixed defect. This is called a transient ischemic attack (TIA), a warning that a stroke could come, the way angina is a warning that a heart attack could come. Immediate treatment is urgent, since 50 percent of the people who experience TIAs go on to have a major stroke within a year. Even when a stroke is not fatal, it can be extremely debilitating, and may leave permanent neurological

KNOW YOUR RISK FOR HYPERTENSION

▶ Family history of high blood pressure, diabetes, high cholesterol, and early CAD.

▶ History of oral contraceptive use. If oral contraceptives were discontinued, was it because of high blood pressure? The real risk for heart attack or stroke increases for the over-thirty-five woman who smokes.

▶ History of toxemia or high blood pressure during pregnancy.

▶ History of diabetes.

▶ Other CAD risk factors: obesity, smoking, or low HDL cholesterol.

▶ High salt intake.

▶ High alcohol intake. Three or more drinks a day can both raise blood pressure and increase resistance to hypertensive therapy.

▶ Psychosocial and environmental factors, such as a stressful family situation or work conditions. (Interestingly, lack of medical insurance has been correlated with high blood pressure.)

▶ Obesity. There is a direct relationship between weight and blood pressure; weight loss can significantly lower elevated blood pressure.

▶ Sedentary living. Sedentary obese women have a 20 to 50 percent increased risk for developing high blood pressure. This can often be treated with moderate physical activity.

▶ Pregnancy. High blood pressure can be transient, mild, or develop into a severe condition. See Chapter 12 for more information.

▶ Smoking. Although nicotine can raise blood pressure acutely, it does not cause sustained high blood pressure. However, it is a significant risk factor for stroke and brain hemorrhage in women.

▶ Use of medications that affect blood pressure—oral contraceptives, steroids, anti-inflammatory drugs, cold remedies, and appetite suppressants.

▶ Low levels of potassium and calcium seem to exacerbate hypertension. These abnormalities can even be caused by diuretics used to treat hypertension.

problems including speech impairment, weakness or paralysis, and difficulties in mental capacity and memory.

Seventy percent of stroke victims survive the event—women more so than men. Since women tend to suffer strokes later in life than men, female stroke survivors often become nursing-home dependent owing to the absence of a suitable caretaker at home.

Other sex-specific risk factors for stroke include toxemia of pregnancy, postpartum cerebral hemorrhage, hypercoagulative blood conditions, some autoimmune diseases, severe mitral valve prolapse, and oral contraceptive use by smokers. Observational studies have shown that estrogen replacement therapy reduces the incidence of strokes by 50 percent. Heart arrhythmia (atrial fibrillation) can also cause strokes in men and women. Unfortunately, most studies looking at the benefit of anticoagulation in preventing stroke have been done with men.

For the elderly, strokes can be even more frightening than a diagnosis of heart disease because they so often mean an end to independent living. So, while avoiding hypertension is important in reducing your CAD risk, it also has implications for your overall health.

SCREENING FOR HEART DISEASE

Even now, little is being done to address the practical ramifications of treating female heart problems as aggressively as those of males. It is urgent that we begin to diagnose CAD earlier in women, a change that will only occur with better physician training, patient information, and diagnostic tools that are woman-sensitive. Unfortunately, when the conventional methods of diagnosing heart disease are used on women, they produce a high degree of false positive (abnormality on the test with no disease present) results and some false negative (test fails to pick up an abnormality that is present) results. It is important to realize that women have different physiologic responses to exercise than men. Women do not increase their ejection fractions (how much blood is actually pumped out of the left ventricle) as men do, and this single factor is often used as a sign of CAD in stress testing. What is normal in women may be considered abnormal since it is so in men.

Let's look at the common tests and discuss their effectiveness for women.

Electrocardiogram (EKG)

DESCRIPTION: The EKG is a graph of the electrical activity in the heart. It is a painless procedure, administered by placing electrodes over the chest, arms, and legs. These are attached to an electrocardiogram machine. The EKG enables a doctor to assess heart rhythm, electrical conduction abnormalities, thickness of the muscle, the possibility of enlargement of the heart chambers, and injury to or death of cardiac muscles.

ACCURACY FOR WOMEN: Women's autonomic nervous systems seem to have a more pronounced effect on the EKG, causing false positives, so this test alone is insufficient. Mitral valve prolapse, thickening of the heart muscle, and gallbladder disease can all cause changes on the EKG. The EKG done at rest can also fail to show ischemia (lack of blood flow), present only during exercise. However, combined with symptoms such as chest pain, an abnormal EKG can indicate the need for further testing. And a normal EKG is no guarantee of the absence of CAD.

Exercise Stress Test

DESCRIPTION: This test combines vigorous exercise on a treadmill while being monitored on an EKG to determine whether the heart is receiving enough oxygen during times of physical stress.

ACCURACY IN WOMEN: The Exercise Stress Test has a 33 percent false positive and a 26 percent false negative rate for women, and should rarely be done in a premenopausal woman since the rate of accuracy is even worse. In my opinion, it is unfortunate that many practitioners continue to rely on this test for women when it is accurate less than 50 percent of the time. A flip of the coin would be just as accurate.

Thallium Exercise Stress Test

DESCRIPTION: The thallium stress test is more accurate than the exercise test alone. First, the patient exercises on a treadmill until maximum heart rate is achieved. Then, a radioactive substance called thallium is injected into a vein, and a special camera monitors the distribution of thallium into the heart cells. If a portion of the heart does not receive thallium, it is likely that the area is blocked from receiving blood. The test is repeated several hours later when the person has not exercised. If the second test is normal, that means the heart is being denied blood only during periods of exercise, which is suggestive of blocked arteries. If both tests are abnormal, that indicates part of the heart may already be permanently damaged.

ACCURACY IN WOMEN: Thallium stress tests show false negative results in about 25 percent of women. Sometimes women's breast tissue interferes with a clear reading and it comes up false positive. Sex-specific analysis for thallium imaging is being developed and may improve the validity of this test in the future.

Stress Echocardiogram

DESCRIPTION: This is a painless test that bounces sound waves off the heart, providing a picture of the heart's structure during rest and exercise. A wand is passed over the chest that produces a two-dimensional picture on a screen. (It's the same technology that is used in a sonogram, a common test for pregnant women that shows a picture of the fetus.) An echocardiogram shows the size of the heart chambers and movement of the heart valves, and reveals any part of the heart muscle that isn't contracting properly.

ACCURACY FOR WOMEN: This is probably the most accurate noninvasive test for women, giving correct readings nearly 90 percent of the time. The cost is reasonable, and the test gives a physiologic picture of the heart's ability to work under stress. Unlike an EKG, an echocardiogram allows a clear view of abnormalities in the heart muscle itself, without exposure to radiation.

Cardiac Catheterization

DESCRIPTION: This is a serious invasive procedure that is only indicated if other tests suggest CAD, or if a person has rapid progression of cardiac episodes. It is performed in a hospital under local anesthesia. A plastic tube is passed through a blood vessel in the arm or thigh into the heart. A dye is injected into the catheter and an X ray traces the flow of the dye through the arteries and into the heart.

ACCURACY IN WOMEN: This procedure is highly accurate. However, it is also invasive and can be dangerous. It's only indicated for people who are very sick or are candidates for heart surgery. There have been many cases reported of women who were subjected to this invasive test based on faulty results from exercise and thallium stress tests, and who were not found to have CAD. On the other hand, gender bias often keeps women from getting this definitive procedure and delays access to bypass grafting and angioplasty.

I consider tests to be tools that, combined with other factors, enable a diagnosis. But single tests must always be viewed with caution since they are so often inaccurate in women. I hope that in the near future we will have gender-specific tests that are more accurate. Until that time, beware the diagnosis based solely on these tests and advocate on your own behalf for the best woman-specific workup you can get. Always be aware that your physician might not know everything there is to know about woman-centered care, especially when it comes to CAD. Be your own advocate by staying alert and informed.

COMMON QUESTIONS ABOUT HEART DISEASE

My doctor says I shouldn't worry about heart palpitations during my pregnancy. Is that right?

Women usually aren't aware (because no one has ever told them) of the scope of changes that occur during pregnancy. Pregnancy isn't limited to the uterus. As your uterus enlarges to accommodate the growing fetus, your other systems adjust to meet the extra demand. Increased blood volume and blood flow might result in symptoms that mimic heart disorders. Coupled with the fatigue and episodic light-headedness that sometimes occur with pregnancy, you might think these symptoms spell heart trouble. Chances are, they're perfectly normal side effects of a very physiologically demanding condition. Always be sure, however, to tell your doctor about any symptoms. Don't just assume they're not important. (See Chapter 12 for more information on the changes and complications associated with pregnancy.)

Can CAD be reversed once I have it?

CAD is usually considered irreversible, especially if there is damage to the heart muscle. Arteries and organs are not capable of rejuvenation. However, if heart disease is diagnosed and treated early, and if you make the lifestyle changes necessary to avoid further progression or damage, you can effectively reverse the disabling consequences of CAD, if not the disease itself.

I take birth control pills. Do I have an increased risk of heart attack?

If you're over age thirty-five and smoke, you do have a risk of heart attack and stroke on the pill. But if you're not a smoker, there's little or no risk, in light of the new low-dose pill formulations.

Some predisposing factors should be reviewed prior to oral contraceptive use and the following women should be observed during their first year on the pill: Women with a family history of stroke, African-American women, women with kidney disease, obese women, women over age forty, and those who have suffered high blood pressure during pregnancy. Most women who become hypertensive on oral contraceptives will normalize their blood pressure within a few months of discontinuing use.

I have slightly elevated blood pressure. Should I stop drinking coffee?

There is no evidence that moderate consumption of caffeine is harmful, even if you have high blood pressure. When you drink a cup of coffee, your blood pressure might experience a small temporary rise. However, the real danger of hypertension isn't the minor ups and downs, which are normal, but rather a long-term, steady condition. The risk factor is not your moment-to-moment blood pressure, but your average blood pressure over time.

I've heard that taking large doses of vitamin E can reduce my risk of heart disease. Is this true?

Two Harvard Medical School studies have shown lower incidents of CAD in people who use vitamin E supplements. In addition, the Nurses Study demonstrated that women with the highest consumption of vitamin E over a period of two years (mostly from supplements) had a one-third reduction in risk, compared with those who took little or no vitamin E. While these studies did not fully consider other risk factors, they are promising enough to demand further study. If you take vitamin E supplements, keep in mind that large doses might be hazardous. Vitamin E is fat soluble; unlike vitamin C or the B vitamins, the excess does not get excreted in your urine. The Recommended Daily Allowance for most people is only 400 IU. Vitamin E can be found in nuts, green leafy vegetables, and wheat germ.

Other antioxidants have been found to protect against heart disease in men. (Studies have yet to be concluded for women.) Flavonoids in black tea, onions, and apples were found to significantly protect men in the Netherlands against death from coronary artery disease. Flavonoids are also found in red wine, and may be the reason for lower CAD rates in France.

If I have high blood pressure, do I need to avoid HRT?

No, quite the contrary. Estrogen has been found either to have no effect on blood pressure or to lower elevated blood pressure. It has also been found to decrease the incidence of stroke.

My mother had breast cancer. Should I avoid estrogen replacement therapy?

Most doctors would not prescribe estrogen replacement for a woman with such a strong familial risk factor. It's likely that your breast cancer risk will increase with long-term estrogen use, especially if your mother had her breast cancer before menopause. However, I ask you to consider your relative risks before making a decision. For many women, including those with family histories of breast cancer, the benefits of hormones in reducing heart disease, stroke, and osteoporosis might outweigh the risk of breast cancer. On the other hand, many women prefer to reduce their CAD risks without incurring others. They feel more comfortable avoiding HRT. See Chapter 6 for more on this.

I have high cholesterol. Should I take cholesterol lowering drugs?

Since there have been virtually no drug trials that include women, it's difficult to give a definitive answer regarding heart-related medications. For severe familial hyperlipemia (a blood abnormality not treatable by diet), these drugs may be helpful, but they carry many potential side effects and are not safe for use during pregnancy or while breast-feeding. Furthermore, drugs don't "cure" the condition; they only control it. The best and safest way to lower "bad" cholesterol is by reducing saturated fat and cholesterol in your diet, exercising, not smoking, reducing stress, and taking estrogen replacement at menopause. The National Cholesterol Education Project states that estrogen is the drug of choice for treating elevated cholesterol in postmenopausal women.

Will an aspirin a day help prevent heart disease?

Low doses of aspirin (one to six tablets per week) have been shown to prevent heart attacks and strokes in men. There have been no studies specifically conducted with women, but the Nurses Study hinted at benefits for women who take small amounts of aspirin. Once again, the best way to protect yourself is by making the lifestyle changes I've recommended in this chapter. Sometimes when we think there's a magic pill that eliminates risk factors, it diminishes our motivation to do the things we know will work. Also, for women with mitral valve prolapse who have TIAs (transient symptoms of stroke), aspirin may prevent tiny clots forming around the valve that are assumed to break off and cause the TIA.

Do anti-hypertension medicines affect sexual function?

Studies on the side effects of these medicines have been done almost exclusively on men. However, a few reports mention instances of menstrual abnormalities, decreased vaginal lubrication, and nipple discharge. Only one study to date has looked at sexual function in both men and women, and that showed improved sexual functioning in both men and women when they changed from other drugs to captopril.

I have high blood pressure. How can I keep track of it on a regular basis?

If you have been diagnosed with high blood pressure, you might consider purchasing a home blood pressure kit. This will help you monitor your blood pressure on a more frequent basis. Blood pressure fluctuates throughout the day, and the average blood pressure reading is a better predictor of risk than the one-time reading in the doctor's office. When my patients have high blood pressure, I usually encourage them to purchase their own machines and keep a diary of readings at home. Then I ask them to bring their machines into the office, and we compare their readings with those that my machine gives. Home monitors are easily available at a moderate price from medical supply stores. There are three widely used models:

Mercury meters: A straight glass tube with a reservoir that contains mercury, which is linked by tubing to a pressure cuff.

Aneroid units: Metal bellows that respond to pressure from the cuff and move a needle across a calibrated dial.

Electronic arm models: A microphone senses sounds from the arteries during deflation of the cuff and measures the beat-by-beat force of the blood flow.

For more information about monitoring your blood pressure at home, call the American Heart Association (800-AHA-8721) and ask for the publication, *Buying and Caring for Home Blood Pressure Equipment.*

I have high HDL cholesterol. Should I drink alcohol to lower my risk of CAD?

A recent study showed that women between the ages of forty-five and seventy-four who drank half an alcoholic beverage or less a day had a 20 percent decreased risk of heart disease; 40 percent if one-and-a-half to two drinks a day were consumed. But you have to weigh this information against the possible connection between alcohol and breast cancer, as well as the other down sides to drinking, which occur at lower doses and within a shorter period of time in women.

RESOURCES

ORGANIZATIONS
American Heart Association
1615 Stemmons Freeway
Dallas, TX 75207
214-748-7212

National Heart, Lung, and Blood Institute
9000 Rockville Pike
Bethesda, MD 20892
301-496-4236

National Stroke Association
8480 East Orchard Road
Suite 1000
Englewood, CO 80111
800-787-6537
303-771-1700

PUBLICATIONS
Harvard Heart Letter
Published by the Harvard Medical School
164 Longwood Avenue
Boston, MA 02115

Silent Epidemic: The Truth About Women and Heart Disease
Published by the American Heart Association
800-AHA-8721

6
WOMEN'S CANCER
Beyond Breasts and Ovaries

~~~~~

Bridget, forty-seven, was well informed about "female" cancers, and she knew the importance of regular screening. She had a Pap smear every year. She religiously performed a breast self-exam each month. At age forty, she scheduled her first mammogram, which she repeated every two years. When she came to me for a physical, she was prepared with a complete family history and a list of relevant questions. But when I asked her if she had ever been screened for colon cancer, she drew a blank.

"Colon cancer?" she blurted out with surprise. "Isn't that something old men get?"

I smiled because I had heard the same reaction so many times before. It is a common misconception, even among women who are as educated as Bridget. While many women are rigorous about screening for "female" cancers—that is, cancers of the breasts and reproductive organs—they are unaware that lung and colon cancer are female cancers, too. Meanwhile, they go along feeling a false security because they get Pap smears and breast checks.

This lack of perception is another example of how women's health has been genitalized. And the bias is reflected in cancer research. Typically, when men and women have a body part in common, such as a lung, researchers tend to study it in the male. Women are studied for what distinguishes them from men—their breasts and genitals. One argument for the male bias in research is that men are easier to study. They have fewer hormonal and reproductive complications than women and thus are thought to make "purer" subjects. But I find the argument that women aren't fit subjects for clinical trials involving other cancers ludicrous. Women, after all, comprise a majority of the health services users. Rather than treating their differences from men as an obstruction to research, we should be examining how being a woman places them at more or less risk, and how these risks affect diagnosis and treatment.

There is strong evidence that this research bias influences the behavior of doctors. As the *New England Journal of Medicine* recently reported, there is an appalling lack of cancer screening being done on women—especially by young male doctors who, the report said, may be uncomfortable touching women's breasts and genitals. When screening is done, it focuses on breast and gynecological cancers, ignoring the fact that lung cancer is the number one cancer threat to women, and more women die from colon cancer than from any gynecological malignancy.

Medicine often fails to look at subgroups of women, thereby limiting our understanding of how we could do better at prevention and screening. For example, Latina women have markedly lower rates of breast cancer; black Latinas have a 40 percent lower rate than Caucasian women. However, in a recent study of this population, none of the cancers diagnosed were in very early cases—only in later stages of the disease where fewer conclusions could be drawn. Also, white Latinas have different cancer rates than black Latinas. Black Latinas have lower rates of lung, cervical, and bladder cancer than black non-Latinas; while white Latinas have higher rates of cancer of the liver, gallbladder, and cervix than white non-Latinas. A similar issue exists in the study of African-American women, who have lower rates of breast cancer but higher mortality rates. What can we learn from race-sensitive research? And how can we incorporate cultural and economic factors into cancer screening recommendations and availability? We have a long way to go in this regard.

Women diagnosed with cancer suffer disproportionately within a system that is not designed for them. Since different medical specialties hold primacy over different body parts, treatment is almost always fragmented. The work of prevention, screening, and treatment cries out for a woman's health specialty, where women are seen as whole beings without undue emphasis on reproductive parts.

The current system defies all logic. Your breast and reproductive screening is usually monitored by your gynecologist. Not only is your gynecologist not a cancer specialist, but he or she is not trained to screen for signs of cancer in other organs. Chances are, your gynecologist hasn't even been screening for lung and colon cancer. Furthermore, if tests conducted by your gynecologist indicate cancer of the breast or genitals, you're sent directly to a surgeon, who is not trained in internal medicine and cannot guide you about long-term issues such as estrogen replacement or screening for second malignancies. And often the surgeon limits treatment to surgery, and doesn't offer the expanded views and up-to-date information that an oncologist would. If you try to do your own research, you'll find little available in the way of practical information. Much of the writing about women and disease focuses on the psychosocial impact, not the medical implications—as if to say, men have bodies and women have feelings.

All in all, this might seem like a discouraging picture. How can you feel empowered in your medical treatment when there are so many unknowns, when your chances of receiving proper screening and diagnosis are hampered by the biases and structure of the system, when you're shuttled from doctor to doctor with no single specialist monitoring your comprehensive care? The tendency among women is to get angry at the system. You feel betrayed by people who you feel should be protecting you. Cancer is so intimidating that it's tempting to go along with everything you're told, to be driven by fear into docility at a time when you most need to become an activist for your care. One of my patients brought that lesson home to me in a striking way.

Chloe was a fifty-three-year-old woman who had been seeing her gynecologist every four months for the past twelve years because of a benign lump that was removed from her breast. In every way, Chloe presented herself as a self-confident, informed woman, assertive about her health care. She took pride in being an involved patient, and she never accepted her gynecologist's recommendations without asking many questions. She later admitted that she didn't particularly like the man, but she went to him because he had "an excellent reputation for being a good technician."

During one of Chloe's routine visits, she discovered that the mammogram she'd had taken four months earlier had noted a change, yet she'd not been informed. Her gynecologist shrugged off her alarm, saying that he didn't think the description of the change warranted further intervention. "Don't worry," he told her. "I'm watching things."

Chloe was not comforted by his paternalism. In fact, she was appalled that he could be so casual. After all, he was the one who had been telling her for twelve years that she needed to be screened every four months! Chloe stood up to her gynecologist and demanded to be referred to a surgeon who performed a breast biopsy. The finding was intraductal carcinoma, a potentially curable stage of breast cancer.

It was at the time of Chloe's biopsy that I became involved with her care. My job was to be her advocate, steering her through the maze of pathology reports, treatment options, and choice of surgeon, and to help her decide whether or not to see an oncologist. Together, we managed the emotional fallout not only of the diagnosis, but of the betrayal Chloe experienced within the health care system.

Chloe's story was a clear example that women must be their own advocates; they can't count on the system to do it for them. Had Chloe accepted her doctor's advice and decided not to worry, the result might have been fatal. Your best weapon is your knowledge of risk factors, preventive measures, screening for early detection, and the options available for treatment. In this case, knowledge is empowering. And finding a woman's health clinician to help you navigate your course through the system is an invaluable aid. Many women are frightened when they learn about the gaps in medical care and start assuming responsibility for themselves. It's better to have a partner in the process.

WHAT IS CANCER?

Fifty years ago, cancer was such a fearful subject that you rarely heard mention of it. A diagnosis of cancer was like receiving a visit from the Grim Reaper. It was an automatic death sentence. Today, although we have yet to discover definitive causes for cancer, much less an all-purpose "cure," our enhanced medical knowledge has made many cancers manageable, and public education has given us new options for avoiding risks.

The reason cancer is so baffling to scientists is that it is not a single disease. Your body contains literally trillions of cells, and the abnormal growth that signals cancer can occur in many distinct ways. You can be genetically predisposed. Or environmental toxins and viruses can stimulate a change in a cell's growth. Or cofactors can enhance a deranged cell's ability to grow or travel.

Our ability to understand cancer is further complicated by the fact that not all abnormal cell growths are malignant. Some are benign and therefore not cancer. Even among malignant cells there are wide variations in appearance; some can be hard to detect.

Malignant cancer cells damage the smooth operation of the group of cells to which they belong. They also begin to divide, and if the process of division continues, the cancerous cells can quickly number in the billions. Unlike normal cells, which keep to their own terrain, cancerous cells can travel throughout the body, interfering with the cell patterns in other regions. When cancer cells spread to other parts of the body, the result is called metastatic cancer. Early screening is designed to catch the abnormal cells before they grow and travel.

THE WARNING SIGNS OF CANCER

The American Cancer Society recommends screening if any of the following signs appear:

1. **A change in bowel or bladder habits.**
2. **A sore that doesn't heal.**
3. **Unusual bleeding or discharge.**
4. **A thickening or lump in your breast or elsewhere.**
5. **Indigestion or difficulty swallowing.**
6. **Obvious changes in a wart or mole.**
7. **A nagging cough or hoarseness.**

KNOWLEDGE IS POWER

To the average layperson reading the papers and watching the news, it can sometimes seem as though everything you do places you at risk for cancer. That's because, as much as cancer has been studied, scientists have been unable to pinpoint exactly what causes it. Certain high risk factors have been identified, including heredity, smoking, diet, environmental exposure, and viruses. However, not all people who have known risk factors get cancer, and many people with no known risk factors do get it. Your educated response to this morass of confusion is to understand what is known about each cancer, take preventive measures within your control, and follow a regular screening regimen.

There are many types of cancer, and each has its own profile. In this section, my focus is on those cancers that most affect women, in order of their lethality: cancers of the lung, breast, colon, reproductive organs, and skin.

Lung Cancer Is Number One with Women

Although it has now surpassed breast cancer as the leading cause of cancer death among women, some official medical organizations still suggest that it's not cost-effective for doctors to regularly screen for lung cancer. Like other "androgynous" diseases (CAD and colon cancer), lung cancer was always thought of as a man's disease. While it's true that it appears about three times more often in men than in women, I believe there are two reasons for this historical bias:

First, women are only now smoking at the same rate as men. Since World War II, more women began taking up smoking—one reason why between 1950 and 1985, lung cancer death in women increased 500 percent. Since smoking is a factor in about 90 percent of lung cancers, it's likely that women will achieve parity with men as long as they continue to smoke—and female smokers are expected to outnumber male smokers by the year 2000. The tag line of a popular cigarette manufacturer, "You've come a long way, baby," is reflected in the grim statistics.

Second, the idea that lung cancer was a man's disease has delayed diagnosis in women. This hit home for me a couple of years ago when a thirty-eight-year-old woman smoker came to me with a cough she couldn't shake. No other doctor had taken her seriously, and she'd never been screened for lung cancer because, although she smoked, she was a young woman and didn't fit the classic profile. I ordered a chest X ray, found cancer, and we lost her within six months.

It is imperative that we begin to take lung cancer seriously as a feminist issue and as a women's health issue. The tobacco industry spends $4 billion a year in advertising, much of it specifically targeted to women. The three most common ploys used are weight reduction, desire for independence, and

and appeals to youthfulness. The focus on thinness is especially insidious among teenage girls. Research shows that adolescent girls who start smoking are more inclined than nonsmoking girls to idealize the elongated, painfully thin models in cigarette advertisements. It is not surprising that smoking rates are higher in girls with eating disorders. And the use of diet pills is greater among female smokers than nonsmokers.

I have often found that the same woman who wouldn't dream of forgoing an annual Pap smear for cervical cancer thinks nothing of smoking a pack of cigarettes a day. It's time to get our priorities straight. Lung cancer is killing women. Worse still, statistics show that the greatest increase in new smokers is among teenage girls and young women.

The risk of lung cancer increases the younger a woman starts smoking. In light of that, it is especially sobering that smoking among teenage girls is on the rise. Notably, the incidence is twice as high among high school dropouts. It is predicted that by the year 2000, smoking among women with only high school educations or less will be around 30 percent, compared with 10 percent among women who are college graduates. Given the strong association between educational level and smoking, women of relatively low educational status are likely to be disproportionately represented in future lung cancer statistics.

It's painful to watch our young women set off on a course that we know is disastrous.

These are the facts. If you smoke, you risk lung cancer. But we are also beginning to see that passive smoking—being around smokers—might pose a real danger, too. Studies show that the risk of lung cancer more than doubles for a woman who lives with a smoker for a forty-year period, even if she doesn't smoke.

Women smokers may be at greater risk for lung cancer than men. They get smoking-related lung diseases earlier in life and their tumors are more aggressive.

Race plays something of a factor in risk. Rates are similar among Caucasians and African-Americans, while they are somewhat lower for Latina and Asian Pacific women. However, lung cancer survival rates are lower for African-American women.

There may even be gender effects in the type of lung cancer that women get. Women tend to get adenocarcinoma, even if they are not smokers. It grows quickly and spreads to distant organs. Men are more apt to get squamous cell carcinoma, a less aggressive cancer. Malignant tumors have been reported to have estrogen receptors, which may be of importance in treatment.

Smokers also have a heightened risk if there is lung cancer in their family. They are five times more likely to develop it themselves. Only 10 percent of lung cancers are not related to smoking. The factors involved in these cancers are well known—asbestos, radioactivity, and industrial chemicals, as well as conditions like asthma, emphysema, and tuberculosis. However, our attention should not be diverted from the real culprit, smoking. Recently in New York City, there was an uproar when asbestos was found in public school buildings. Parents were absolutely hysterical about the threat to their children and demanded that the schools be closed until they could be assured there was no asbestos. Yet, many of those same parents would think nothing of smoking cigarettes in front of their children every day—a far greater threat to their health.

Smoking is also related to other cancers—of the mouth, throat, esophagus, stomach, pancreas, kidney, bladder, and cervix, and to leukemia.

CHECK YOUR LUNG CANCER RISK

▶ **Do you smoke?**
▶ **Do you live with a smoker?**
▶ **Did your parents smoke?**
▶ **Is there lung cancer in your family?**
▶ **Do you or your partner work in a toxic environment?**
▶ **Do you have a history of asthma, pneumonia, emphysema, or tuberculosis?**
▶ **In addition to other factors, are you over forty?**

ATTACK LUNG CANCER AT THE SOURCE

Prevention is the key to avoiding lung cancer because by the time a chest X ray reveals an abnormality, there is less chance of a cure. Lung cancer develops and spreads very quickly, and the five-year survival rate for women diagnosed with lung cancer depends on how early it is detected; when detected early, the rate is 53 percent for Caucasians and 45 percent for African-Americans—as opposed to a discouraging 16 percent and 12.6 percent respectively when it is detected late.

Although there is no good screening test for lung cancer, I always look for its presence as part of my medical exam. But once again, screening is not the same as prevention. I have frequently heard smokers express great relief when their chest X rays came back normal, as though that lets them off the hook. But their relief is hardly justified. A smoker might show a perfectly clear X ray and by the following year have a tumor that has already spread throughout her lungs and to other sites in the body. While various methods of early detection are being tried, I must stress that at this point, early detection has little effect on survival. A chest X ray can pick up a one centimeter tumor, but by that time it has divided more than twenty times. Therefore, it might have metastasized by the time of pickup.

Chest X rays can also be falsely positive; not all shadows on an X ray are cancers. All diagnostic tests have problems with false positives and negatives. Medical technology isn't perfect. We have to understand the limits of our technology and make clinical decisions based on educated guesses informed by many pieces of information. And don't forget about luck or exceptions to the rule.

Andrea was a forty-three-year-old nonsmoking woman who grew up in a nonsmoking household. She had a routine chest X ray prior to outpatient surgery for irregular menstrual bleeding. This type of routine chest X ray is being discouraged because of its low yield in terms of affecting the course of treatment or outcome for hospitalized patients. Yet, Joan was "lucky" enough to have a solitary pulmonary nodule discovered this way. At the same time, she was "unlucky" because she had none of the usual risk factors for lung cancer. Once again, risk factors do not provide a crystal ball. Not all those with risk factors will get sick, and some people who get cancer have no definable risk.

Screening can sometimes allow for earlier detection without delaying the time of death. But overall, it seems that the benefits of early detection outweigh the potential disadvantages to an individual, even if it is more costly to the insurance company.

Although the American Cancer Society does not recommend yearly chest X rays in smokers as a cost-effective way of screening for lung cancer, the value to an individual may be incalculable. A solitary nodule might still be removed before it has spread, so there is some reason to promote screening for smokers over the age of forty.

If you smoke, I urge you to study carefully the information in Chapter 17, and take advantage of the methods for quitting.

BREAST CANCER: WOMEN'S GREATEST FEAR

Perhaps no other disease that afflicts women challenges us psychologically and socially as much as breast cancer. The discovery of a tumor in the breast unleashes an entire series of fears that are every bit as traumatic as the fear of death. Many women report that the insult inflicted on their bodies is multiplied a hundred times by the added insult of maneuvering through the health care system—and the traditional failure of physicians who treat breast cancer to adequately outline options and reduce panic. Add to that the fear that losing a breast or part of a breast will affect her sexuality, and it's easy to understand why women feel a growing sense of panic about breast cancer.

A little bit of fear is good. It propels women to get appropriate screening, improve their lifestyle habits, and perform regular self-exams—the best ways of guarding against breast cancer. But I think it's also important that we put the risk in perspective. There's a lot of publicity about the report that each woman has one in nine chances of contracting breast cancer, but the statistic

---

AGE-ADJUSTED BREAST CANCER RISK

By age 25: one in 19,608
By age 30: one in 2,525
By age 35: one in   622
By age 40: one in   217
By age 45: one in   93
By age 50: one in   50
By age 55: one in   33
By age 60: one in   24
By age 65: one in   17
By age 70: one in   14
By age 75: one in   11
By age 80: one in   10
By age 85: one in   9

woman has one in nine chances of contracting breast cancer, but the statistic is misleading, as you can see from the following chart. The statistical risk changes with age. So, while it's true that the risk is one in nine for an eighty-five-year-old, it's only one in 19,608 for a twenty-five-year-old. The statistic one in nine represents an American woman's lifetime risk for ever getting breast cancer. I see no reason to overplay the risk. Suffice it to say that it's great enough for all women to maintain good screening habits.

The truth is, we still don't know as much as we'd like to about the real risks associated with breast cancer, and 70 percent of women who get breast cancer don't fall into any risk categories. But research points to certain facts that we can consider when evaluating risks:

▶ Two-thirds of women who get breast cancer do so after age fifty.

▶ Family history seems to play a role, especially if there has been breast cancer in your immediate family—a mother or sister—and more so if their cancer occurred before age fifty. The older the family members were when they got cancer, the less the risk. For example, if your mother got breast cancer at age seventy-five, you may have a minimally increased risk. Truly genetic familial risk is rare, accounting for only 5 to 7 percent of cases. We are on the brink of being able to diagnose this risk by gene typing. Most familial risk is polygenic and probably depends on multiple "hits" besides genetic predisposition—such as environmental exposures and dietary patterns. Risk can also be transmitted by an abnormal gene in the father.

▶ If you have had cancer in one breast, you have a 5 to 10 percent chance of getting it in the other breast. Also, if you have cancer in other sites—particularly uterine or colon cancer—your risk for breast cancer increases.

▶ High fat diets have been linked to breast cancer in a number of studies. In one, 750 Italian women were studied; those who ate high-calorie, high-fat diets had a threefold risk of breast cancer, compared to those who ate fewer calories and less fat. Studies of Japanese women who eat traditional diets of only about 20 percent fat show they have far fewer incidences of breast cancer. The difference is believed to be fat related, not genetic. One study showed that first generation Japanese women in San Francisco have twice the incidences of breast cancer as their cousins in Japan. An interesting question is whether it is just the low amount of fat in the Japanese diet or the presence of plant estrogens found in soy products and greens eaten by the Japanese that interfere with estrogen's stimulation of the breast. There is another school of thought that suggests the risk factor might be the high concentration of fat-soluble pesticides found in animal fat.

Scientists are just beginning to discover potential links between nutrition and cancer that might have vast implications for prevention and treatment. For example, animal experiments show a connection between high-fat diets and breast cancer, except when calcium and vitamin D are added to the diet. There are higher breast cancer rates in areas of the United States with less sunlight—thereby providing less of the body's own supply of vitamin D. This effect is also seen in homebound elderly women who have little or no exposure to the sun. It is possible that adolescent girls, whose breasts are still developing, may increase their chances of developing breast cancer later if they eat high-fat diets and don't get adequate calcium and vitamin D.

High fat intake is also associated with higher estrogen levels, a risk factor for breast cancer. A high-fiber diet can reduce estrogen levels; wheat bran fiber added to the diet of premenopausal women can reduce estrogen levels by 20 percent. The low-fat, high-fiber diet is now being evaluated in women who have already had breast cancer by the Women's Intervention Nutrition Study. Dietary fat may also be involved in disease progression. For example, Japanese women not only have lower rates of breast cancer, they also have better survival rates—and the reason might be diet.

Obesity itself has been associated with a risk of breast cancer in postmenopausal women. This is probably because fat tissue has the ability to metabolize adrenal steroids to estrogen products, keeping estrogen levels higher in older women. On the other hand, obesity in young women is associated with lower rates of premenopausal breast cancer, probably because of the tendency toward menstrual irregularities that lower estrogen levels. So, the high-risk profile is a slim premenopausal woman who puts on significant weight in her middle years, then gains more weight after menopause. However, this may not hold true for African-American and Latina women, since obesity is more common but breast cancer rates are lower.

▶ Early onset of menstruation and late menopause are potential risk factors, as well as late pregnancy or no pregnancy. The factor here is the number of ovulatory cycles a woman has. One hundred years ago, women started menses at age seventeen, got married shortly after, immediately had children, breast fed for extended periods, and had more children. They had very few ovulations. Today, some girls start menses at age twelve, may delay childbearing until their thirties or later, and have one to two pregnancies. They may have forty years of ovulatory cycles—480 of them. It is possible that exposure to progesterone, which is made after ovulation, is a risk factor. Or it may be some other factor associated with the ovulating ovary. This is unknown.

▶ Hormones: This is still an uncertain area of investigation, since some breast cancers are estrogen-dependent while others are not. There is some evidence that use of birth control pills in the teens and early twenties may slightly increase the risk of premenopausal breast cancer, and the FDA now requires a warning label on birth control pill packets. Diethylstilbestrol (DES), used from the late 1940s until the early 1960s to prevent miscarriages has been shown in some studies to increase the risk of breast cancer later on in life. The literature on breast cancer and estrogen replacement therapy is less clear. Most studies have shown no added risk. A few studies have shown increased risk with long-term use—ten to fifteen years. And a few studies have even shown decreased risk. I realize how confusing this is for a woman who must make a decision about hormone replacement. However, like any other important decision you make about your health, the best method is to weigh your own very personal history and circumstances.

▶ Alcohol: Alcohol intake has been noted to increase risk in more than three dozen studies. Some show that as little as one drink per day increases the risk.

▶ Environment: Recent reports also find a relationship between DDT and breast cancer, with a four times greater risk in women with higher levels. Women with breast cancer have been found to have metabolites of DDT at far greater amounts than other women. An example of the connection might be found by studying Israeli women. Rates of breast cancer, which have normally been very high in women of Jewish heritage, have substantially declined since Israel discontinued the use of DDT. Given the new trade agreement made by the United States with other countries, we must increase our vigilance to assure that products with DDT levels higher than current U.S. standards will not be allowed on imported peaches, bananas, grapes, strawberries, broccoli, and carrots.

Those who cite environmental links to breast and other cancers are often accused of being alarmist. But consider the extremely high rates of breast cancer observed on Long Island, New York. These cannot be explained away by age and ethnicity. A careful study looking at geographical variations of breast cancer rates, proximity to Brookhaven National Laboratory, and the correlation with radioactive releases from nuclear power plants shows an overwhelming connection between radioactive contamination of the air, drinking water, and diet with the high breast cancer rates of that region.

It is interesting that medicine continues to harp on the hormonal causes of breast cancer—as if to say that women's own hormones are their greatest danger—while ignoring environmental causes.

BREAST CANCER RISK FACTORS

Age over fifty
Family history
Menarche before twelve years
Delayed childbearing—after thirty years
Menopause after fifty-five years
Obesity after fifty years
Hormonal exposure
High-fat diet
Radiation and environmental toxins
Predisposing breast conditions
Alcohol intake
History of cancer in one breast
History of uterine or ovarian cancer

There are many benign conditions that do not lead to cancer—such as cysts and calcifications. These conditions complicate regular screening, but doctors and insurance companies should not make the assumption that they place women at certain risk for cancer. Again, much of the panic about breast cancer centers around a sense of doom for those who have risk factors. Remember, being at risk is a relative thing. It does not predetermine that you will get a disease.

Recently, a young woman whose mother and older sister both had breast cancer asked me if there was any way she could protect herself. She felt doomed by her family history, even though she was very careful with her diet, didn't smoke, and had generally good health habits.

The truth is, if you're a young woman who has a strong history of breast cancer in your family—that is, your mother had it, your sister had it—perhaps the best protective measure you can take is to have a baby before age thirty, breast-feed for a lengthy period, then have several more children whom you breast-feed. This is radical advice in a time when women are beginning to realize many different choices. It's also not necessarily feasible for any number of personal and economic reasons. Nor does it seem a very good motivation to have children—as a preventive factor against breast cancer! I hope that in the coming years research will improve the condition of high-risk women, while society learns to be more supportive of women who choose to have their children at a young age and breast feed them.

We are also close to the time when genetic testing will be available for women with familial factors for breast cancer, and those with true genetic risk will be able to make more fully informed choices about risk reduction. To date, very little research has been done on the epidemiology or causes of breast cancer. Medicine has been satisfied with the ability to treat breast cancer with surgery. I wonder, if men were getting penis cancer in large numbers, would they be satisfied with surgery as a solution?

One other risk factor we need to talk about is the role of stress in the evolution and progression of cancer, especially breast cancer. As we will learn in Chapter 10, chronic stress can inhibit our immune system's ability to fend off cancer cells.

A case in point comes to mind. Sandra was a highly energetic, productive woman. Her mother had breast cancer, and as her mother's disease progressed, Sandra's stress increased. At the same time, she lost her job and her marriage fell apart. Then, she found a lump in her breast. In her usual "this won't get me down" style, Sandra tried not to miss a beat in her everyday life. She scheduled her surgery so that she could go on her usual winter ski trip first. She thought her positive attitude would get her through, but her disease progressed. At that point, Sandra did some searches, found a new job, moved to a less stressful city, surrounded herself with a large social network of friends, and got involved in a healthier intimate relationship. Sandra is still not free of disease, but her disease has remained inactive for years. Such resilience is an important factor in decreasing risk.

THE IMPORTANCE OF SCREENING

Good breast cancer screening includes three things: your monthly self-exam, your annual medical checkup, and, after age forty, your regular mammogram. Younger women do not benefit from screening because their breast tissue is too dense to get a good picture and their breasts are more sensitive to X-ray exposure. As you grow older, your breast is less radiosensitive and less dense, allowing a clearer view. It's also when your risk increases. I recommend having mammography every other year during your forties and every year after fifty. If you have a family history of breast cancer, your annual screening should begin at age forty.

There has been some controversy about the advisability of screening mammographies before age fifty. Most studies do show that after fifty, mammographies substantially lower mortality from the disease—about 40 percent at five to seven years. They have, however, failed to show a survival benefit for women under fifty, which is a crucial factor. There are several explanations for this. First, these older studies were not using the same high-resolution mammograms that we now have. Second, these studies often failed to differentiate between premenopausal and postmenopausal women. The denser breast tissue of younger women can cause tumors to be missed. Younger women are also more likely to have aggressive, fast-growing cancers that may arise and spread quickly between screenings. Some experts recommend more frequent screenings for premenopausal women with risk factors; others are concerned that frequent X rays might induce cancer.

While the policy makers concerned with cost issues for large populations may hedge on their recommendations regarding mammogram coverage, we cannot fail to remember that early detection in particular women can mean a cure. Furthermore, early mammographically detected breast cancers are more amenable to breast-conserving surgery. Perhaps it would make more sense to expend effort on finding better treatments for these earlier detected cancers than to quibble about whether or not to screen for them.

There are still many women in their forties or fifties who have never had a mammogram, even though the population is more educated than ever about their importance. Why aren't women following these recommendations? The biggest reason is that their doctors aren't making the recommendations. Current data from the American Cancer Society show that only 37 percent of doctors follow mammography guidelines.

Another reason women don't get mammographies is the very natural nervousness that accompanies this test. Research has shown that fear of breast cancer can be debilitating. One study tracked women whose mammograms had shown abnormalities but who were later found to not have cancer. Even though breast cancer had been ruled out, three months later 47 percent reported high anxiety related to their mammograms, and 41 percent still had breast cancer worries.

A third deterrent to screening is concern about pain and discomfort. Like most medical procedures, mammograms can be unpleasant. But a survey of 597 women in Great Britain revealed that most women found the discomfort less severe than having a tooth drilled, a Pap smear, or giving blood.

Another significant deterrent is cost and the lack of insurance coverage. Until recently, Medicare didn't cover screening mammographies and many women have no insurance coverage at all. In spite of their documented benefits, screening mammograms are still excluded from some policies.

I hope you can see beyond your fear to the importance of mammograms. And please keep in mind that your mammogram is not a place to cut costs. Accurate mammography is an art. It requires good equipment that will clearly show the slightest abnormalities and a skilled reader to detect them. One of the earliest signs of breast cancer can be tiny deposits of calcium called microcalcifications. The problem with screening large numbers of women is that many women have microcalcifications who don't have cancer. A skilled mammographer can detect the abnormal from the nonproblematic calcifications. But a number of women will be sent for breast biopsies who don't have any cancer. Not all mammograms are equal. It is important to get good quality mammography, interpreted by a skillful mammographer. So, even if you have to go outside your health plan to get one by the best mammographer available, it is a wise expenditure on your part. Take responsibility for your health care, and don't assume that what is covered by insurance is best.

In addition, a mammogram won't necessarily detect cancer. Even in the most skilled hands, some 10 percent of breast cancers are mammographically silent. Not long ago, Mary, a forty-two-year-old woman, came to me for a checkup. She was even a little bit embarrassed about taking up my time because she said she felt perfectly well. While I was examining her breast, I detected a very tiny nodule. I sent her for a mammogram and then a fine needle aspiration without waiting for the mammogram results because I knew that mammograms aren't able to detect cancer 100 percent of the time. My philosophy is that any nodule must be pursued aggressively. Mary's fine needle aspirate showed an invasive intraductal carcinoma, even though her mammogram was normal. At surgery, the total lesion measured nine millimeters. Mary was treated with a lumpectomy and radiation therapy.

Once again, let me remind you that screening is not the same as prevention. Screening is designed to pick up cancer when it's already there. Even when lesions exist that are believed to be markers for high risk, there's no way of knowing whether these lesions will turn into a cancer or whether the body's immune system will eliminate them. The purpose of screening is to detect cancer as early as possible, before it has a chance to spread.

Remember, a screening mammogram is not a diagnostic one. This is the problem with mobile screening vans. Women need to be called back for further tests if anything is detected, and a mammogram should always be coupled with a clinical breast exam. It is always better to have your mammograms done where they can be read by a proficient mammographer at the time of the test, so any further diagnostic studies can be performed. This is the highest quality service that women can get—and that is what they deserve.

You may want to schedule your mammogram just after your period so it will be less uncomfortable, but a mammogram can be read with accuracy at any time during your cycle. (Mammograms are not advisable if you are or might be pregnant.)

COMPELLING REASONS FOR MAMMOGRAPHY SCREENING

1. **Mammography is the only screening tool that has been shown to reduce mortality from breast cancer.**
2. **Mammography is the only method that detects lesions that are not palpable at a time when curability is over 90 percent.**
3. **Mammography is safe and effective, with a highly favorable risk/benefit ratio.**

The monthly self-exam is another thing many women fail to do, either because they forget or because they don't know how. I always ask my patients in a neutral voice, "Do you examine your breasts?" The almost universal reaction is guilt and embarrassment. Women say, "I try to . . ." or "I'm not very good at it." I never chastise them because, the fact is, self-examination is a limited screening tool. And manual exams by physicians aren't much better. In one study, doctors performing standard breast exams on a rubber model detected abnormalities only 40 percent of the time.

Overemphasis on breast self-exam, especially when we have access to state of the art diagnostic equipment, puts us in the position of blaming women for unsuccessful self-detection. Let's keep it in perspective. It's good to know how to do breast self-exams, but it's not the only screening tool available.

The best time to do a self-examination is the week after your period. If you're postmenopausal and not taking combination hormones, schedule a day in the month when you always do it—like the first. If you're taking cyclical hormones, the best time for a breast exam is just before starting the progesterone or on the last day of your week without any hormones.

Here's the most effective method. While you're in the shower, place one hand over your head. Then take the other hand and walk it around the opposite breast, as if you are tracing the spokes of a bicycle wheel. Use the flats of your fingers, not the fingertips. Keep the pressure constant, and be sure to go up into the armpit and directly over the nipple. Repeat with the opposite breast. Then, after your shower, do the exam again, lying down on your bed. Hold the resting arm in a relaxed position over your head, not hooked underneath.

What are you looking for? Most women think they're looking for lumps, but this isn't the most important consideration. For one thing, breasts are naturally lumpy. When you examine your breasts, what you're looking for are areas that feel different from usual. If you perform regular self-exams, you'll become familiar with the unique architecture of your breasts so you can distinguish between what's normal and abnormal for you. Look for asymmetry, thickening or puckering of the skin, retraction of the nipple, spontaneous nipple discharge, or areas that are fixed, harder and don't change with your menstrual cycle.

Your breast is composed of fat, glandular tissue, and fibrous tissue. Each woman's breasts are different in the way these components dominate. Normal glandular tissue is like a bunch of grapes; it's mushy and it moves around. Fibrous tissue separates the glandular tissue and gives shape to the breast. It feels like ridges and is especially prominent underneath the breast.

Get to know your lumps. They will vary during your cycle, getting bigger and more tender just before your period. Remember, an unusual lump must be drained and shown to disappear, or aspirated and looked at under a microscope. A negative mammogram isn't sufficient to rule out cancer.

When suspicious microcalcifications are seen on the mammogram without a lump being felt, you'll need an excisional biopsy, done by a surgeon in an operating room. Sometimes, radiologists can use a computerized mammogram machine to "stereotactically" locate the abnormality when a lump is not felt. A needle is put into it to evaluate the area as a surgeon would when opening the breast tissue. The specimen needs to be x-rayed to be sure it contains the suspicious calcifications, and the breast needs to be mammogrammed again after it heals from the biopsy to show that the calcifications have been removed. Most solid lumps, especially in very young women, are benign.

A pregnant woman who detects a lump should have it tested with an ultrasound and drained if it's cystic. If it's solid, a fine needle aspiration should be done for diagnosis without mammography. Pregnancy does not worsen the course for women with breast cancer.

WHAT TO DO ABOUT LUMPY BREASTS

Lumpy breasts are referred to as fibrocystic, a term overused by doctors, mammographers, and pathologists, with everyone meaning something different. Lumpy breasts are normal, especially in young women. Most breast lumps are benign and pose no extra risk for breast cancer. Only in certain cases are they risk indicators—and even then, cancer can only be detected with a fine needle aspirate or a tissue biopsy.

Here's a simple explanation of the types of risk-associated lumpy breasts:

▶ Mammary dysplasia with atypia. Dysplasia is common, but it is not a problem unless it is associated with "atypical" changes in the cells. When atypia is present in a woman with a family history of breast cancer, this can be a high risk situation.

▶ Intraductal carcinoma or DCIS. DCIS is a condition associated with localized cancer cells. It is found on mammograms as microcalcifications (only 20 percent of which are DCIS). We currently have little knowledge of the natural history of DCIS. How often does it stay benign? How often does it regress and go away? How often does it progress to invasive cancer, and in whom and under what circumstances? We do know that when invasive cancer occurs in one breast, DCIS can be found in the other breast almost half the time. Yet only 12 percent of women get cancer in the second breast. So, not all DCIS progresses to invasive cancer. And not all microcalcifications are DCIS. This is another area of concern in the "under fifty" controversy. Are we picking up too many areas of microcalcifications and generating too many biopsies that are not cancer?

If this is so, how do we decide what to do? Should we remove all breasts with DCIS? No! Mastectomy itself has a 1 to 10 percent recurrence rate. That's because the breast is not a discrete organ with clear anatomic boundaries. Some residual tissue can remain in the chest wall or up in the armpit. Current treatment recommends lumpectomy if the lesion is less than three centimeters, although there is a 12 to 15 percent chance of recurrence. A recent study shows that this recurrence rate can be halved by adding radiation therapy. Large lesions are usually treated with mastectomy.

▶ Lobular carcinoma in situ, or LCIS. Not a premalignant lesion in its own right, this breast pathology is a marker for breast cancer that may pop up anywhere in the breast. It may not appear on a mammogram or be felt as a lump but as an area of thickening. Its presence confers a 20 percent lifetime risk of bilateral breast cancer.

Our lack of certainty about the natural history of breast cancer and its precancerous stages is not just due to the lack of autopsy series that examine women's breasts. Pathologists further the confusion, especially regarding DCIS, by using an artificial map when evaluating biopsy material. They divide the breast into quadrants. Multiple lesions in the same quadrant are called "multifocal"; lesions that appear in different quadrants are called "multicentric." These terms are used to measure disease activity and to guide treatment decisions. Yet normal breast anatomy has no such quadrant structure. The ductule system of the breast is tortuous and it corkscrews. What may appear to be in many places on a pathology slide may actually be coming from the same ductule. This is another example of how women are invalidated, and an arbitrary and erroneous norm is established.

Breast cancer treatment is a clear example of an area that cries out for a women's health specialty. Stephanie is a forty-five-year-old patient who had a lumpectomy and radiation for breast cancer. After her treatment, she saw her surgeon every three months, her oncologist every three months, and her radiation oncologist every three months. Stephanie was spending so much time with doctors that I felt guilty every time I urged her not to forget about the rest of her body and see me.

Before her cancer, Stephanie was not a worrier or a person who paid much attention to her body. Now, she was a wreck. She felt her body was about to betray her at any moment, and it seemed as if she spent her entire life seeing doctors. Her emotions rode a roller coaster, dropping to the depths before a doctor visit and riding high after one. Every cold was threatening. A backache was enough to keep her up all night.

Initially, I encouraged Stephanie to check out every symptom that worried her because it might give her the reassurance she needed. But after two years, I realized that it wasn't her breast cancer that was driving Stephanie crazy. It was the health care system! The specialists who insisted that she see them so frequently were making her feel vulnerable. I knew that they were each in their own way being responsible, but the end result was to trap Stephanie in a sense of her illness. After talking it over, Stephanie and I decided on a follow-up plan that felt less oppressive to her. Together, we would take primary responsibility for monitoring her health. I encouraged Stephanie to contact me before consulting a specialist.

This is another example of the need for a women's health specialist—a doctor trained to give comprehensive care. When I took on that role with Stephanie, the cloud of dread that hung over her lifted. Today, she is living a more normal life. No, I am not an oncologist. But I am equipped to care for Stephanie, the person, and focus beyond her cancer to help her feel whole again. Recent studies confirm no significant difference in outcome when women with breast cancer are followed by oncologists or primary-care physicians.

COLON CANCER: A HIDDEN THREAT

Colon cancer—or colorectal cancer, which is cancer of the large bowel, made up of the colon and rectum—is the second most common cancer in women and the third most common cause of cancer death among women, but again, many doctors skip this screening in standard medical exams. I find it interesting that so much publicity has been devoted to ovarian cancer, which is relatively rare, when four times as many women (158 thousand a year) will die of colon or colorectal cancer.

It is also rarely mentioned that women who get breast, endometrial, or ovarian cancer are at higher risk for colon cancer. A woman with breast cancer may focus on avoiding a second malignancy in her breasts, but not be aware that her risk of colon cancer is also increased.

Unfortunately, it's not always so easy for women to get a diagnosis of colon cancer. They have to be aggressive. In a large study conducted among men and women in the Seattle metropolitan area who had recently been diagnosed with colorectal cancer, it was found that, in spite of the fact that women made more trips to the doctor, their diagnoses took much longer. Both men and women reported the same general symptoms, including rectal bleeding, abdominal pain, and general weakness. The researchers concluded that clinicians responded differently to women than to men in following up the same symptoms.

In another study it was discovered that only 6 percent of OB/GYN doctors, 23 percent of general practitioners, and 33 percent of internists recommended colon cancer screening to their female patients. These figures are alarming, especially since more than one-half of all women never see a doctor other than their gynecologist or obstetrician.

The shameful thing about the failure to screen women for colon cancer is that its cure is based entirely on early detection. The American Cancer Society reports more than a 50 percent cure rate when the disease is diagnosed and treated early. In light of that, it's absolutely crucial that doctors discuss the disease with women and begin screening after age forty.

For a long time, scientists thought that certain ethnic and cultural groups had strong genetic predispositions to colon cancer because it occurred ten times more often in the West than it did in the East. Although familial risk can account for 20 to 25 percent of colon cancers, there is strong evidence that the major difference is accounted for by diet, not genetics. Repeated studies show a link between high animal fat consumption, low fiber consumption, and colon cancer.

The Nurses Health Study bore this out for women, showing that those who ate more fat and less fiber were more likely to get colon cancer. In one especially persuasive note, it was shown that women who ate beef, pork, or lamb as a main dish on a daily basis had two-and-a-half times as great a risk as women who ate these dishes less than once a month.

Part of the correlation might be that women who eat more fat naturally consume less fiber as part of their regular diet. There was strong evidence that fiber-rich foods, especially cereals and fruit, decreased the risk. Our Paleolithic ancestors consumed a diet that was about 20 percent fat. This diet also included 100 to 150 grams per day of fiber. Food was consumed in small amounts throughout the day, rather than at several large meals. Our Western diet typically consists of 25 to 40 percent fat and only 10 to 14 grams of fiber. Breast, ovary, and endometrial cancers are related to high fat intake. Also, dietary fat affects the amount of bile acids found in feces. Bile and metabolites are thought to be the cancer promoters in the colon, and a low-fat, high-fiber diet decreases production of these metabolites.

Familial factors also contribute to colon cancer. If it exists in a first-degree relative, the risk is two to three times as great, especially if that relative was young at the time of the disease. There are also a number of familial polyposis syndromes (tendency toward excessive polyp formation in the colon), again rare, that are associated with high rates of colon cancer.

Recent evidence also shows that removal of the gallbladder increases the risk of colon cancer in women, but not in men.

By and large, the biggest risk for colon cancer is the presence of polyps. Polyps larger than one centimeter are also associated with higher risk. It takes about seven years for a one centimeter polyp to transform into an invasive cancer, so good screening offers an excellent opportunity for detection.

EVALUATE YOUR COLON CANCER RISK

1. Do you consume a high-fat diet (more than 10 percent saturated fat and 25 percent total fat)?
2. Do you consume less than 25 grams of fiber per day?
3. Is there a history of colon cancer, or polyps, in your family?
4. Have you had breast or gynecological cancer?
5. Have you had pelvic radiation therapy?
6. Have you had inflammatory bowel disease?
7. Have you had your gallbladder removed?
8. Are you over fifty?

DON'T IGNORE COLON CANCER SCREENING

Jean is a robust professional woman of seventy who has always tried to live healthily. She came to see me because she was feeling heaviness in her chest and shortness of breath on exertion. Her physical exam and EKG were normal, but her LDL cholesterol was high and her HDL was low. Jean had never taken estrogen and didn't want to start, so I suggested a regimen of aspirin and vitamin E, in addition to medication for suspected CAD. Her symptoms went away immediately. After this scare, Jean became avid about her diet and continued to be physically active. Last summer she went trekking in Alaska and had a great time.

Although Jean was very health conscious, I could never convince her to get a screening sigmoidoscopy for colon cancer as part of her preventive health regimen—that is, until she noticed blood in her stool. She immediately scheduled the procedure, and I was horrified to find a large mushroom shaped lesion that was probably a cancer. Jean then had a full colonoscopy to look for other polyps. The pathology report from her biopsy showed invasive cancer arising from a polyp. Jean was lucky enough to be eligible for a partial colectomy and didn't require a colostomy (necessitating a bag). But she was unfortunate in that she had seven positive lymph nodes at the time of surgery. Her heart held up well through all the stress, but she will most likely die from her cancer. Had she received regular screening, her prognosis might have been much different.

I start colon cancer screening at age forty. It includes a rectal examination, stool cards (which you take home) that look for hidden blood in the stool, and a screening sigmoidoscopy. The sigmoidoscopy begins between ages forty and fifty, depending on your risk factors. Many patients say, "But my gynecologist did a rectal exam. Do I need another one?" My answer is yes because about 10 percent of polyps and cancers are within reach of a finger. Many gynecologists do rectal exams as a way to better examine the uterus. They don't focus on the rectum itself or commonly test the stool for hidden blood.

There are two types of sigmoidoscopes—rigid and flexible. A rigid sigmoidoscope is a metal or plastic tube that allows examination of the rectum and the lower part of the colon. It can pick up 30 percent of polyps and cancers. The more recently developed flexible sigmoidoscope is longer and it bends in such a way that a clinician can view the entire length of the left colon with less discomfort to the patient. A sigmoidoscopy with a flexible instrument can detect polyps at least 55 percent of the time. Screening sigmoidoscopy has been shown to reduce colorectal cancer mortality by 70 percent. It is as effective for colon cancer screening as mammography is for breast cancer screening and a Pap smear is for cervical cancer screening.

For greater detection and also removal of polyps, a colonoscopy must be performed. This is a more complex procedure, but it can usually be performed on an out-patient basis. A scope is passed up the rectum through the entire colon. A colonoscopy can detect polyps, collect tissue for biopsies, and then remove the polyps, without surgery.

Symptoms of colorectal cancer include blood in the stool (which isn't always visible to the eye), a change in bowel habits, unexplained weight loss, unexplained anemia (due to unnoticed blood in the stool), black stool, painful defecation, and persistent abdominal cramps. Of course, any of these symptoms might have a number of other causes, but none of them should go unchecked.

Sometimes patients come to see me because they have noticed blood in their stool. They're terrified they might have colon cancer when they really have hemorrhoids. Hemorrhoids are a much more common cause of blood in the stool than colorectal cancer. Usually, the blood is bright red and visible, and bleeding is accompanied by pain or itching. Hemorrhoids are easy to treat. Although cancer is usually not the cause, I recommend a sigmoidoscopy just to be sure. We can't assume that rectal bleeding comes from hemorrhoids, especially after age forty.

Another common condition is diverticulosis, pockets within the wall of the colon. About 20 percent of people over age sixty have this condition. Sometimes the pockets grow infected and can cause pain and altered bowel habits, but, again, this condition is not precancerous, and can be easily treated with antibiotics. It rarely requires surgery.

It is relevant to note that women in the Nurses Health Study who used estrogen replacement had decreased rates of colon cancer. Both estrogen and progesterone receptors exist in the gastrointestinal tract, and this is an area for further study.

EARLY DETECTION FOR CERVICAL CANCER

Cervical cancer was once fairly common. Its 60 percent decline during the last twenty years is a testament to the aggressive campaign to encourage women to get regular screening Pap smears. It is clear that early detection is the key to avoiding cervical cancer. Even so, in 1993, 13,500 cervical cancer cases were diagnosed and 4,400 women died. Cervical cancer rates are rising in young white women, up 3 percent per year between 1986 and 1990 despite regular screening. By comparison, incidence rates are declining in African-American women of every age and in Caucasian women over fifty. So, we have work left to do, particularly in areas of the country where poverty is high and preventive health and screening services are not readily available. Many insurance plans don't cover preventive screening. And some cervical cancers are becoming more aggressive in spite of screening.

Women of color are more likely to have advanced stages of cervical cancer and to die from it because of poor access to screening and lack of early detection. The mortality rate of Native American women is more than twice that of Caucasians. However, aside from the high rates of cervical cancer, Native American women are less likely to get other cancers, probably because they don't live as long. Lesbians can also get cervical cancer—a fact their doctors don't always consider. All women should receive regular Pap tests.

How do you get cervical cancer? By and large, it's a sexually transmitted disease, and a young woman's disease—the average age is twenty-eight. Prostitutes have four times the incidence of cervical cancer as the general population, and certain strains of the human papillomavirus (HPV) or genital warts are found in 90 percent of women with CIN (Cervical Intraepithelial Neoplasia, a precancerous state). The sexual revolution of the 1960s might be the reason we're seeing more cervical cancer today, twenty to thirty years after exposure to HPV. The presence of the HP virus seems necessary, but alone it is not sufficient to cause cancer. Most women with HPV will not progress to cancer unless they are infected with certain strains of the virus (type 16 and 18).

If you smoke, the risk for cervical cancer is even higher, since cigarette smoking seems to weaken the immune status of the cervix, or act as a cofactor in tumor promotion. In fact, smokers are twice as likely to get cervical cancer as nonsmokers, even when the number of sex partners is the same. The simultaneous presence of the herpes simplex virus may be a cofactor in the non-Latina Caucasian population. Immunosuppression by the HIV virus may allow the progression of a very aggressive form of cervical cancer. Women with organ transplants, also immunosuppressed, have similar problems with HPV cancers of the anogenital tract.

CERVICAL CANCER RISK FACTORS

1. **Do you have multiple sex partners?**
2. **Has your partner had multiple sex partners?**
3. **Do you have unprotected sex?**
4. **Have you had genital warts or other sexually transmitted diseases?**
5. **Do you smoke?**
6. **Are you HIV positive or otherwise immunosuppressed?**

Risk reduction for cervical cancer is achieved by reducing your exposure to sexually transmitted diseases. That means choosing fewer partners, and choosing partners who have had fewer partners. Protection involves using condoms, even if you are also using another method of birth control. Oral contraceptives are not associated with an increased risk of cervical cancer, as was once believed. And the use of a diaphragm with spermicide is associated with decreased risk.

Pap Smear: The Best Screening

Most of the women I see in my practice have had regular gynecological checkups over the years, so they're familiar with the Pap smear as a screening test. What they don't fully understand is what a Pap smear shows. The most common misunderstanding is that a Pap smear will pick up the presence of any gynecological cancer, including ovarian and uterine. While a Pap smear may detect abnormalities in other areas of the reproductive tract, it's not a good screening test for these cancers. The Pap smear is designed to detect the presence of abnormal cells in the cervix, which signal the possibility of cancer, or which may become cancerous later if they are not treated. Other conditions noted on Pap tests include infections, inflammation, and atrophy of the vaginal lining (from estrogen depletion).

The second most common misperception is that when a Pap smear shows abnormalities, it automatically means cancer. This belief is so prevalent that most women with abnormal Pap results feel panic stricken. In reality, the development of cervical cancer is a long, slow process, and most abnormalities are not cancer—although they may be precancerous. Every year, 50 thousand women are found to have CIN, the abnormal cell growth that potentially leads to cancer. (It is also called SIL—squamous intraepithelial lesion). But not all abnormal cells are cancerous. Some lesions stay that way for a long time, while others go on to develop invasive cancer. Sixty to 70 percent of HPV lesions go away or regress on their own. Only 1 percent of the lowest grade cervical lesions will ever develop into cancer.

Diagnosticians use a very thorough method of interpretation, called the Bethesda System, to evaluate the characteristics of a specimen. This system determines everything from the quality of the specimen to the level of abnormality—from benign cellular changes to intermediate grades of abnormal cell change to cancer. While any abnormal Pap smear is reason for retesting, don't assume it means cancer.

The third most common misperception is that a Pap smear is foolproof. On the contrary, of every one hundred women tested, if five are abnormal, one cancer will go undetected. If that woman gets tested every year, it may not be a serious problem. Unfortunately, some medical organizations, including the American Cancer Society, state that if a woman has a normal Pap smear three years in a row, she only needs to repeat the test every three years. The American College of Obstetrics and Gynecology disagrees, urging a yearly Pap, especially for women with HPV or HIV, smokers, and those with multiple or new sex partners. I always do a yearly Pap test, especially for young, sexually active women who are most vulnerable to this disease. Why take a chance? It's easy, inexpensive, and given the variables, better to be safe than sorry. Interval cancers do appear—that is, a more aggressive cancer can come up during the year, especially in women who are HIV positive; they should have Pap tests every six months. If you've ever had anything more than low-grade CIN, you should always have a yearly Pap test. Remember, CIN is asymptomatic. Invasive cancer, however, may present with symptoms like discharge, abnormal bleeding, pain, and bowel and bladder irregularities.

Don't assume that you are protected by age. Many physicians are biased against doing Pap tests for older women because of the false assumption that they are no longer sexually active. But consider this: 25 percent of new cases and 40 percent of deaths due to cervical cancer occur in women over the age of sixty. Some older women avoid Pap smears because it is painful to insert a speculum into an estrogen-depleted vagina. The vagina might also have narrowed, making it unable to accommodate a speculum. Using estrogen vaginal cream before the yearly Pap test might help. Also, if your doctor can't insert a speculum, that doesn't mean screening should be abandoned. Often, a moistened Q-tip that blindly scrapes the cervix can produce an adequate sample.

You can improve your chance of getting an accurate reading on a Pap test if you avoid using tampons, birth control foams and jellies, and douches for a few days before your test. Pap smears are not done during your menstrual period.

Doctors also need to know how to get the best Pap smears. Sixty percent of false negative smears are due to doctors' poor technique. Doctors must sample the cervical canal as well as the outer part of the cervix for a complete result. The other 40 percent of false negatives are due to technician error in the lab.

What do you do if your Pap smear indicates an abnormality and repeat tests concur? Abnormal results fall into one of several categories. Once it is established that the problem does not lie with the test itself, it may be diagnosed as anything from an inflammation or infection to a possible cancer.

A very common Pap test reading is "atypia," meaning the cells don't look quite right but they're not abnormal enough to suggest CIN. Benign conditions often cause atypia: postpartum states, atrophic vaginitis due to estrogen loss, or just poor Pap test techniques. An atypical Pap smear should be repeated in three months. If the second Pap is also atypical, colposcopy should be done.

Pap tests don't always detect CIN, so further tests with atypical Paps are needed. CIN lesions seen initially should be pursued with colposcopy and biopsy.

A colposcopy is an examination of the cervix with a magnifying device; a tissue sample is then taken from any abnormal looking area for a biopsy. If the test reveals the presence of mild precancerous cells, your doctor may choose a course of watchful waiting that includes regular Pap smears and diagnostic retesting. If, however, the biopsy confirms that there is moderate to severe precancer (dysplasia), the abnormal tissue should be removed or

---

WHAT TO DO IF YOU HAVE AN ABNORMAL PAP

1. If the Pap smear is technically incomplete or insufficient, repeat.
2. If the Pap smear shows benign (noncancerous) changes and organisms are found, treat for infection and repeat the test in three months.
3. If the Pap smear shows benign changes but no organisms are seen and a woman is asymptomatic, further treatment is not needed.
4. If the Pap smear shows atypical cells of undetermined origin or low-grade CIN, follow-up is needed. Current recommendations range from repeating the test in a few weeks to treating with antibacterial cream and repeating, to referring for colposcopy and biopsy.
5. If the Pap smear shows low-grade CIN or high-grade CIN, have a colposcopy and biopsy or LEEP.
6. If cancer is found, visit a gynecological oncologist, or discuss options with your gynecologist.

destroyed. This can be done with cryotherapy (freezing), which is the least costly method, although it can be hard to control the area of freezing. Laser therapy is more precise but needs to be done in an operating room. A newer method, called LEEP (loop electrocautery excision procedure), is the most definitive procedure. It is performed in a doctor's office and is not very costly. LEEP includes the biopsy and treatment all in one procedure, so every woman who undergoes it is automatically treated for CIN whether she has it or not.

Be aware that all procedures have potential, though rare, complications such as scarring, narrowing of the cervix, or cervical incompetence—the inability of the cervix to hold a fetus within the uterus.

Keep in mind that there is a tremendous tendency in this country to overtreat HPV, considering that up to 70 percent of the time it goes away on its own. Removing the areas has not been shown to prevent lesions from occurring in other parts of the cervix or vagina.

OVARIAN CANCER'S TRUE RISK

Several years ago, the horror of undiagnosed ovarian cancer was brought to the public eye as we watched the popular comedian Gilda Radner fight a losing battle with the disease. Her long, painful illness and death caused something of a panic in the population. Suddenly, everyone was clamoring to be tested. Although there are only about twelve thousand new cases diagnosed every year, the panic was created by the fact that ovarian cancer is such a silent disease. There are no real symptoms in the early stages, and by the time a diagnosis is made the cancer is advanced. Only 38 percent of women with ovarian cancer survive for five years, and that hasn't changed in twenty years. Only 1 to 3 percent of women with ovarian cancer have a family history of the disease in a first-degree relative (mother or sister).

A family history of breast or colon cancer may also be associated with risk. Risk can be transmitted by the father as well as the mother. The incidence of ovarian cancer is 46 percent higher in Caucasian women and increases with age. Women who have had colon, breast, or uterine cancer are at risk for ovarian cancer.

The relationship of female hormones to ovarian cancer risk can be seen from some of the following associations:

Oral contraceptive use seems to decrease the long-term risk of contracting ovarian cancer by 30 percent, with increased benefits after five years of use.

The risk also appears to diminish with each pregnancy and a first pregnancy at an early age, as well as the time spent breast feeding. Otherwise, tubal ligations also seem to decrease the risk. Ovarian cancer has been associated with high-fat diets.

Some researchers also find a relationship between the use of talc in the genital area to increased risk of ovarian cancer. And two recent reports linked the use of fertility drugs to ovarian cancer. Given the growing use of these drugs, it is imperative that well-designed studies be conducted to test this association. We also need to know if the association holds true for women who do conceive this way and have full-term pregnancies. After all, the risk for ovarian cancer is reduced 15 to 20 percent for each full-term pregnancy.

OVARIAN CANCER RISK FACTORS

1. **Do you have an immediate family member who has had ovarian cancer?**
2. **Have you had breast, endometrial, or colon cancer?**
3. **Do you eat a high-fat diet?**
4. **Have you had no children? Have you never breast-fed your children?**
5. **Have you never used oral contraceptives?**

The Choice in Ovarian Screening

My regular physical examination includes a pelvic exam, which allows me to feel the organs and check for enlargement of the uterus. And I always think of ovarian cancer in women who have nonspecific bowel complaints.

Sometimes I can determine whether there are abnormalities in the region of the ovaries. However, the pelvic exam alone is not a very good way of picking up early problems. There are two other tests used to evaluate ovaries for cancer—the ultrasound and the CA125 blood test, which is a tumor marker sometimes found in the blood of women who have certain types of ovarian cancer. The problem with the CA125 test is that the marker also shows up when there are other pelvic problems, like pelvic inflammatory disease, endometriosis, or other infections or tumors. It also shows up in pregnant women and in nonpregnant healthy women. There's a high false positive rate that increases further if you're under fifty. Combined with a pelvic exam and an ultrasound, the test is more accurate. But the real question is: Do all women benefit from this screening?

The value of screening tests is based on their cost, accuracy, personal risks, and the prevalence of the disease in the population. In view of this, CA125 and ultrasound tests may not be appropriate for everyone. I only perform them for select patients—those who have abnormal pelvic exams, nonspecific abdominal complaints, or who are at increased risk for ovarian cancer because of family history or personal history of breast or colon cancer. Gilda Radner had a strong family history of ovarian cancer, so her case is not necessarily a strong argument for across-the-board screening. But used in the right setting, a combination of pelvic exam, CA125, and ultrasound can be an effective screening trio—especially in young women who have two or more first-degree relatives with ovarian cancer, as Gilda Radner did.

A friend of mine recently asked me if I thought she should have a CA125, which her gynecologist had recommended. I asked if he had also recommended sigmoidoscopy and she was quite surprised. "He never mentioned colon cancer," she said. "You mean, I have to worry about that, too?" I assured her she didn't necessarily have to "worry" about it, but her statistical chances of colon cancer were much higher than of ovarian cancer, and that should be considered in ordering tests.

Ultrasound presents another type of screening problem. Many of these tests are being done as part of a routine checkup, especially for women on hormone replacement therapy. What we're learning is that the postmenopausal ovary is not inert. It has the capability of forming cysts, just as it does in younger women. But traditional teaching says that cysts found after menopause must be removed to rule out cancer. This scare of cancer is bringing women into operating rooms for surgery on benign conditions. The question is, how do we differentiate benign from cancerous cysts? It's the same problem we have in evaluating breast lumps. My concern is that surgeons are removing too many ovaries with benign cysts, assuming that women don't need their ovaries after menopause. The error of this premise is discussed further in Chapter 11.

There's another reason why unnecessary surgeries are dangerous. The common logic about cysts goes something like, "It might not be cancer, it's probably not cancer, but why take a chance?" I'll tell you why. I recently saw a woman in her late fifties whose routine ultrasound picked up a cyst. Her doctor told her she needed a hysterectomy and to have her ovaries taken out. She had the cyst removed, as well as everything else, and was in bed for a week. That week of bed rest took a big toll on this woman's overall health. With her degenerative nerve condition, it has taken her months to recover her musculoskeletal strength. In addition, she developed a severe case of antibiotic-induced diarrhea, which kept her out of work and cost a lot of money to treat. We have to ask, what are the seldom discussed risks of surgery and bed rest as opposed to the potential of cancer? In my opinion, gynecologists find it too easy to recommend the treatments they are trained to perform, especially in the malpractice climate that discourages conservative treatment plans. Doctors have also been too content with the total hysterectomy as the answer to a "questionable ovary." Methods are needed to better distinguish cysts from cancers. And new ways of detecting disease beyond the ovary are needed to slow the rush to remove all of the reproductive organs. Transvaginal ultrasound has been a refinement on transabdominal ultrasound, and is an excellent way to pick up ovarian masses. When combined with Doppler imagery, some ovarian cancers can be distinguished from ovarian cysts.

ENDOMETRIAL CANCER: COMMON AND CORRECTABLE

Endometrial cancer is cancer of the uterine lining. It's the most common but least lethal reproductive cancer. Its incidence rises with age, especially between ages forty-five and sixty-four, and then declines. It rarely occurs in women under forty. Older Caucasian women have worse survival rates, as do African-American women of all ages.

Endometrial cancer can often be found in association with a premalignant condition called atypical endometrial hyperplasia. Early detection and treatment with progesterone or hysterectomy if necessary can be lifesaving.

The role of estrogen therapy in the risk of endometrial cancer continues to be debated. It is true that incidences rise with the dosage and duration of estrogen therapy, when estrogen is used alone. Hormone replacement that combines estrogen with progesterone seems to minimize the risk. The use of oral contraceptives and Depo-Provera decreases risk.

Unopposed estrogen is thought to be the reason that women who fail to ovulate regularly have an increased risk of endometrial cancer. Tamoxifen, which is used to treat breast cancer because of its "anti-estrogenic" effect on the breast, can increase the risk for endometrial cancer because of its "proestrogenic" activity on the uterus. Women on tamoxifen may be screened with transvaginal ultrasounds and/or endometrial sampling yearly, but recent studies show that these tests are best used for women with symptoms, such as

---

ENDOMETRIAL CANCER RISK FACTORS

1. Are you postmenopausal?
2. Are you overweight?
3. Do you have hypertension?
4. Are you diabetic?
5. Do you have a family history of the disease?
6. Are you infertile?
7. Do you have a history of menstrual irregularities or failure to ovulate?
8. Do you have polycystic ovarian syndrome?
9. Have you ever had breast, ovarian, or colon cancer?
10. Have you taken unopposed estrogen or tamoxifen?

---

abnormal bleeding. Women with a family history of uterine, breast, or colon cancer are also at high risk.

Endometrial cancer can often be totally cured by surgery alone. In severe cases when the tumor has invaded the wall of the uterus, radiation therapy is used to decrease the risk of recurrence, and these patients must then be screened carefully for colon cancer. Irradiated patients may have other problems as well, such as radiation colitis (bowel inflammation) or cystitis (bladder inflammation). Worse, they can develop vaginal stenosis, which can make intercourse painful if not impossible. Dilators are used to expand the vagina, and lubrication is a must to counteract vaginal dryness.

What is worse is that hormone replacement therapy is often withheld. It used to be thought that HRT was ruled out forever. Now we know it is safe after a period of time, depending on the nature of the tumor. Eighty-three percent of gynecological oncologists surveyed said they would use estrogen replacement in women whose endometrial cancers were the lowest stage and grade. The Society of Gynecological Oncologists says that ". . . selection of appropriate candidates should be based on prognostic indications and the risk the patient is willing to assume. If the patient is free of tumors, ERT cannot result in recurrence."

Getting Screened

If you have abnormal vaginal bleeding, this might be a sign of endometrial cancer, although not necessarily. Endometrial cancer is rare in women under forty, whose abnormal bleeding may be caused by benign fibroids or hormonal imbalance. However, any abnormal bleeding pattern, especially if you are postmenopausal, requires a tissue sample to rule out cancer, since 20 percent of postmenopausal bleeding represents endometrial cancer. Pap tests in women with abnormal bleeding can pick up endometrial cancer 25 percent of the time. Some doctors prefer to use endometrial sampling for high-risk patients, but it is most useful to evaluate abnormal bleeding rather than as a screening test for asymptomatic women. In this test, a narrow tube with a sharp edge is inserted through the cervix and into the uterus where scrapings are sucked into the tube. This is usually painless, although some women may require pain control. A new non-invasive procedure finding its way into use for cancer screening is transvaginal ultrasound, which measures the thickness of the endometrial lining (the lining that is built up and shed during the menstrual cycle). Although the ultrasound has not yet become the standard of care for abnormal bleeding, early studies show a high rate of accuracy in ruling out endometrial cancer if the lining is less than five millimeters thick. If fluid is present inside the uterine cavity or if the lining is more than five millimeters, a full D&C should be done. If noninvasive tests are not enough to detect the source of bleeding, a D&C is performed for removal of the entire uterine lining so it can be examined under a microscope. Gynecologists are now using the hysteroscope, a device that visualizes the uterine cavity, before doing a D&C, so that treatment can be more definitive.

OTHER REPRODUCTIVE CANCERS

Other reproductive cancers are rare, except in certain high-risk women. Vaginal cancer is hardly seen, except in women who were exposed to the drug DES in the uterus. These women should be screened regularly. Vulvar cancer has been linked to HPV. Its incidence in the United States has risen 460 percent over the last fifteen years. If we don't become more serious about preventing sexually transmitted diseases, vulvar cancer may cease to become the rare cancer it has historically been. Women who have had their uteri removed for cervical cancer still need Pap tests of the vagina and inspection of the vulva for HPV-induced cancer. Women who have had their uteri removed for benign bleeding do not need ongoing Pap tests but should have their vulvas inspected. HPV can also cause cancer of the anus, especially in women who engage in rectal intercourse. Tumors can also arise from placental tissues formed during pregnancy. (See Chapter 12.)

SKIN CANCER: THE UNREPORTED EPIDEMIC

A tanned body seems to glow with health, and most women like the way they look with a summer tan. But we now know that too much exposure to the sun is the leading cause of skin cancer and premature skin aging. Every year, more than half a million Americans develop skin cancer, and 9,100 die from it. The "healthy glow" is a facade.

There's no way to safely tan your body. If you're lying in the sun or using a tanning salon, you're getting too much exposure to ultraviolet rays. To prevent damage to the skin from sunburn, skin cancer, or the aging effects of sun, always use a sunscreen with a sun protective factor (SPF) of fifteen or more. Stay out of the midday sun, which is the most intense of the day, and avoid tanning parlors completely.

Early skin cancer can look like a tiny brown or black mole or a small bleeding blister. It doesn't necessarily appear ominous. Your best detection

---

ARE YOU AT RISK FOR SKIN CANCER?

▶ **Do you have regular, unprotected exposure to ultraviolet rays from the sun?**
▶ **Do you use a sun lamp?**
▶ **Do you use a tanning booth?**
▶ **Do you have fair skin that freckles or burns easily?**
▶ **Do you live in the South or Southwest U.S.—areas of the country with higher levels of UV radiation?**
▶ **Do you work outdoors?**
▶ **Did you experience severe sunburns as a child?**
▶ **Do you have a family history of skin cancer?**
▶ **Do you have a higher-than-average number of moles?**

method is to become familiar with the normal moles and freckles on your body so you can catch the appearance of a new one. If you are concerned about an unusual mark on your body, a dermatologist can examine the mark and take a biopsy to detect cancer.

There are three kinds of skin cancer: basal cell and squamous cell, which are nonmelanoma cancers, and malignant melanoma. Basal cell and squamous cell cancers are the most common kind, and they are usually detected easily. Basal cell cancer commonly appears as a translucent nodule with rolled borders and ulcerations. Squamous cell cancer presents as a scaly red plaque with a fuzzy border, or as a lesion with rounded borders and ulcerations (making it seem similar to basal cell). Basal cell cancer grows very slowly and rarely spreads, although it can be disfiguring and destroy bone and cartilage if it's left untreated. Squamous cell cancer spreads more rapidly, but because it is easy to detect, it is curable.

Malignant melanoma is much rarer, although rates are on the increase among young women. It is the most common cancer seen in women aged twenty-five to twenty-nine, and second most common in those aged thirty to thirty-four. It is the most deadly form of skin cancer, although women have better survival rates than men. If it remains untreated, it will spread throughout your body; treated early it has a 95 percent cure rate. There are conflicting reports about hormones and melanoma, including some data that tamoxifen may be useful in its treatment.

Screening for Skin Cancer Makes a Difference

There are two types of screening indicated—self-examination and regular examination by a physician. Since 1985, The American Academy of Dermatology has been conducting an annual screening and public education program, with free skin cancer screening performed by volunteer dermatologists at hospitals, health centers, and community events across the country. This is a start. The next step is for all primary care doctors to include routine skin cancer screening in their examinations. This includes visual inspection of the entire body, beginning with the head and scalp and working down, especially looking at the labia, where melanoma can appear. Although skin cancer usually appears in sun-exposed areas, it can occur anywhere, so a good exam will include areas hidden from exposure. Your doctor will also be looking for signs of chronic sun damage, such as excessive wrinkling and hyperpigmentation, that indicate your risk might be higher.

At home, you are encouraged to perform regular self-examination. The American Academy of Dermatology recommends the following method:

1. **Examine your body front and back in a mirror, then your left and right sides with arms raised.**
2. **Bend your elbows and look carefully at your forearms, upper underarms, and palms.**
3. **Look at the backs of your legs and feet, including the spaces between your toes and the soles of your feet.**
4. **With the help of a hand mirror, examine the back of your neck and your scalp. Part your hair or use a blow dryer for a closer look. Look for asymmetry, border irregularities, color irregularities, and a mole greater than one-fourth inch.**
5. **Using a hand mirror, check your back and buttocks.**

Make note of changes in moles or freckles, unusual skin discolorations, new growths, and sores that don't heal. Look for ABCs: Asymmetry, border irregularities, color irregularities, and size greater than one-fourth millimeter.

COMPLICATIONS OF CANCER TREATMENT

For a woman, the major complication of being treated for any type of cancer is infertility. This is especially true for young women treated for Hodgkin's disease and other lymphomas. Sometimes the result is premature menopause which, if unaddressed, raises the risk for early CAD, osteoporosis, and other conditions of estrogen deficiency. Women with brain tumors who receive radiation to the brain can become infertile as a result of problems caused by a dysfunction of the hypothalamus; they can also develop other endocrine disorders. So, preventive health care in young survivors of cancer depends on an awareness of the risk of premature ovarian failure. For women who want to preserve fertility, cryopreservation of eggs is now available for future in-vitro fertilization.

Cancer treatment, whether it's chemotherapy or radiation, can put you at risk for second malignancies. Hodgkin's patients can go on to develop breast cancer or cancer of any of the other organs caught in the field of radiation. Breast cancer patients treated with chemotherapy can go on to develop leukemia. Women who receive radiation therapy for uterine cancer can go on to develop colon cancer.

Sometimes cancer treatments can be toxic to certain organs and cause organ failure. For example, heart failure has occurred in some breast cancer patients treated with high doses of Adriamycin; This deadly complication has been somewhat reduced by careful monitoring of dosages. A toxicity blocker has been shown to be effective in clinical trials. We are also seeing an increase in both benign thyroid disease and thyroid cancer in women receiving radiation to the neck. It is obvious to me that all women cancer patients need good preventive care by a trained woman's health specialist—someone who understands the complications of various treatments.

FOUR WAYS TO LOWER YOUR CANCER RISKS

As we head toward the twenty-first century, we still have a long way to go in the fight to prevent cancer. But as women, we have one important tool that we did not have one hundred or even thirty years ago. That is, our increased awareness that the decisions we make every day affect our health. While we have not achieved the ultimate power, which would be to eliminate the cancers that are killing us, we do have the power to make changes that are known to benefit our health. We have the power to use our knowledge of screening technologies to assist doctors in catching precancerous conditions. And we have the power to fight our way through a system that is resistant but must, of necessity, pay attention to our needs.

In the imperfect medical environment in which you must operate, there is nothing you do that carries a certain guarantee for avoiding cancer. But if I were to head you in the right direction, I would offer these four suggestions:

1. Stop Smoking

If I sound like a broken record on this subject, it's because, tobacco industry protests to the contrary, we are growing more certain every day of the harmful effects of smoking. As you are learning, women who smoke risk not only cancer but also heart disease, osteoporosis, pregnancy complications including stillbirth, infertility, early menopause, strokes, thyroid disease—the list goes on. Smoking may not kill you in a swift and sure way through lung cancer, but it will damage your quality of life and that of your children. Unfortunately, smoking is an especially hard habit for women to break, not only because of the nicotine addiction but also because they use smoking to relieve stress and control their weight. Women have often told me that their biggest worry in stopping is that they'll gain weight. This is a sad commentary on the way our society values being thin and the extremes to which women will go to meet the false ideal.

I try to help women smokers put the issue into perspective—to make a connection in the mind that overrides their emotions and irrational thinking on the subject. The key is deciding to do something good for yourself, to take control in an area where you have power. After all, you can't control air pollution or food contamination, but if you smoke, you are self-administering one of the most toxic substances there is.

Once the realization clicks and the decision is made to quit smoking, any one of the available aids, such as behavior modification groups or the transdermal nicotine patch, will work. In Chapter 17, you'll find many good suggestions about how you can quit smoking.

2. Eat Nutritionally

Current data suggest that as many as 40 percent of cancer deaths in this country (including cancer of the colon, pancreas, breast, ovary, and endometrium) are associated with nutrition.

The popular literature is filled with news about the relationship between cancer and diet. Sometimes it may seem confusing, especially since there is a preponderance of scare items about the carcinogenic effects of certain foods. The bottom line is far less confusing than the literature might suggest. For prevention of breast and colon cancer, in particular, evidence is building that high-fat, low-fiber diets increase the risk factors. Currently under investigation are the potential protective effects of certain vitamins and minerals—such as beta carotene for lung and breast cancer prevention. When researchers at Harvard University examined the eating habits of almost ninety thousand women and followed their health for eight years, they found that women whose diets were inclusive of vitamin A-rich foods every day were less likely to develop breast tumors. These foods are spinach, carrots, sweet potatoes, cantaloupe, and yellow squash.

Diets high in beta carotene (a vitamin A derivative) are associated with reduced risk of lung cancer. Smoking or inhaling secondhand smoke can deplete your body of vitamin C. This places you at greater risk because vitamin C counters certain cancer causing chemicals. Smokers or women inhaling secondhand smoke need to supplement their vitamin C intake. Adding these foods may only be protective if your current diet is deficient in them, not by eating excessive amounts. For now, the bottom line is this: Eat a well-balanced diet that includes adequate calories and a healthy mix of nutrients. You might also want to limit your alcohol consumption. The Nurses Health Study showed that women who consumed three to nine alcoholic drinks a week were 30 percent more likely to develop breast cancer. Other studies support this link.

Specific studies are currently under way which test the role of soy protein in the prevention of breast cancer. There are convincing long-term studies that link high-fat diets to breast cancer. Calcium may also reduce the risk of colon cancer. While it is unwise at this point to isolate certain nutrients to the exclusion of others (remember, a well-rounded diet is important), these promising early studies show just how powerful nutrition's role is in the prevention of disease.

What nutritionists often recommend is the "ideal" diet. However, an "optimal" diet is closer to what most people follow—that is, the diet that is realistically achievable given cultural behavior and taste. The ideal diet would have less than 25 percent of total calories coming from fat and more than 25 grams of fiber per day, divided between soluble and insoluble fibers. Also, eating smaller amounts of food at more frequent intervals seems to lower cholesterol, decrease weight, and reduce the risk of colon cancer. Eating five to nine servings a day of fruits and vegetables should provide anticancer micronutrients.

3. Get Regular Screening

I hope you are beginning to see the importance of good screening in the reduction of cancer risks. Review the screening recommendations from each section of this chapter and create a personal chart to help you keep track of your own screening schedule, depending on your risk factors.

4. Be Your Own Advocate

Resist the temptation to let fear guide your choices. Remember that science is inexact, and there is much that is not known about cancer. When evidence is clear (such as smoking and dietary factors), decrease your risks by paying careful attention to your habits. But in muddier areas, like estrogen replacement, become an aggressive investigator of the pros and cons. Ask informed questions, get more than one opinion, and never assume that your doctor is going to tell you everything you need to know.

COMMON QUESTIONS ABOUT CANCER

Does an abnormal Pap smear mean cancer?

No. For most women, an abnormal Pap smear does not mean cancer. Sometimes it's the result of an inadequate sampling. Other times, abnormal cells are detected, but even these aren't necessarily cancer. If you have an abnormal Pap smear, be sure to have it repeated within three to six months.

Should I avoid getting pregnant if I've had breast cancer?

There is no evidence that past breast cancer negatively affects a normal pregnancy. Even breast-feeding is okay, and it might even protect you from a recurrence of cancer.

I read that taking aspirin every day will protect me against colon cancer. Is this true?

Animal and some human studies suggest that deaths from colon cancer might be decreased by as much as one-half in people who take aspirin sixteen or more times a month. Nonsteroidal anti-inflammatory drugs, like ibuprofen, have also been found to decrease the growth of colon polyps. But the initial studies don't account fully for other factors. It's too soon to tell.

Are women exposed to carcinogens less than men because of differences in occupation?

There has always been a myth that women's work is safe. But the statistics show otherwise. For example, studies of nurses exposed to certain anticancer drugs show incidences of spontaneous abortions, leukemia, and bladder cancer. Unusual levels of esophageal and pancreatic cancers have been observed in women who worked for ten years or more in the dry-cleaning industry. Female agricultural workers, sales workers, electrical manufacturing workers, and seamstresses have increased risks for brain cancer. Women living on farms have been known to have increased incidences of non-Hodgkins lymphoma, especially if they were using water from a hand-dug well.

What are antioxidants?

Vitamins C and E and beta carotene are antioxidant biochemicals that mop up cancer-causing chemicals produced in the body. Cruciferous vegetables can actually detoxify cancer-causing chemicals. So can green and black teas and selenium. Soy proteins may inhibit the growth of cells already transformed.

Are lesbians at higher or lower risk for cancer?

There are two important factors affecting lesbian health: Ignorance on the part of the physician, and discomfort on the part of the patient. Often doctors fail to ask about sexual orientation, or they assume that a lesbian woman has never been pregnant. When the patient is a lesbian, doctors sometimes fail to ask about prior heterosexual activity, thereby ignoring an important risk factor for sexually transmitted diseases and cervical cancer. All women should have Pap smears regardless of sexual orientation, and doctors should not fail to ask lesbian women about their childbirth history since multiple full-term pregnancies decrease their risks for breast and ovarian cancer.

Does colon surgery mean I'll have a colostomy?

Not necessarily. It's more common for surgeons to reconnect parts of the large intestine after the cancer is removed. If you do have a colostomy, you can still lead a normal life. See the resource recommendations at the end of this chapter for a booklet on "Sex and the Female Ostomate."

Do bigger breasts have more chance of developing breast cancer?

No. Breast cancer is not a volume problem. Bigger breasts are at no more risk than small breasts for becoming cancerous.

Do I need chemotherapy after a lumpectomy if all my lymph nodes test negative for cancer?

Chemotherapy is toxic. It makes you feel unwell, has side effects, and can predispose you to second malignancies. So its use should never be casual or automatic. Since only 30 to 40 percent of breast cancers recur when lymph nodes are negative, it's worth discussing your relative risks with your medical team.

To figure out who needs chemotherapy, we try to look at each tumor individually and make educated guesses about its prognosis based on a set of diagnostic standards. In addition, we now know that women who carry the p53 gene have a worse prognosis.

RESORCES

ORGANIZATIONS
American Cancer Society
1599 Clifton Road NE
Atlanta, GA 30329-4251
800-ACS-2345

American Institute for Cancer Research
Nutrition Hotline
1759 R Street NW
Washington, DC 20009
800-843-8114

Breast Cancer Hotline
Physicians Committee for Responsible Medicine
P.O. Box 6322
Washington, DC 20015
800-875-4837

Cancer Information Service
Office of Cancer Communications
Building 31, Room 10A24
Bethesda, MD 20892
800-4-CANCER

National Cancer Institute
9000 Rockville Pike, Suite 414
Bethesda, MD 20892
800-422-6237

Y-Me Breast Cancer Support Program
18220 Harwood Ave.
Homewood, IL 60430
800-221-2141
708-799-8228

PUBLICATIONS
The American Cancer Society Cancer Book
by Arthur Holleb, M.D.
Doubleday & Company, 1986

The Breast Cancer Digest: A Guide to Medical Care, Emotional Support,
    Educational Programs, and Resources
National Cancer Institute
9000 Rockville Pike, Suite 414
Bethesda, MD 20892
800-422-6237

Cancer Facts For People Over 50
The National Institute on Aging
P.O. Box 8057
Gaithersburg, MD 20898

Dr. Susan Love's Breast Book
by Susan M. Love, M.D.
Addison-Wesley, 1990

Sex and the Female Ostomate
The United Ostomy Association
36 Executive Park, Suite 120
Irvine, CA 92714
800-826-0826/714-660-8624

What You Need to Know About Cancer
The Cancer Information Service
Office of Cancer Communications
Building 31, Room 10A24
Bethesda, MD 20892
800-4-CANCER

7

DIABETES MATTERS

It's the Invisible Health Crisis

~~~~~~~~

"I have to do something about my weight," forty-six-year-old Judith told me when she came to my office. "I'm desperate." She told me that her weight had hovered between 190 and 220 pounds since she had been a teenager, in spite of her many efforts at dieting. It had been a constant source of unhappiness for her, but now she had more reason to worry. Two years earlier, Judith had been diagnosed as being "moderately diabetic," and her doctor told her the reason was her weight.

I listened closely as Judith talked, because I knew from experience how issues related to weight and diet hit close to home with women. I was curious to know why Judith had waited two years to seek further medical treatment, especially since her previous doctor had warned her about the dangers of diabetes. Indeed, adult diabetes frequently accompanies obesity, and Judith fit all the classic risk factors. When I asked her about it, she shrugged guiltily. "I don't know . . . I guess it was because this doctor was so irritated with me. His attitude was, 'Get it together, lady, or you'll be sorry.' He gave me a printed diet and I tried to follow it. I was embarrassed to go back to him until I lost some weight." She sighed. "So, here I am, still at square one."

Judith told me that what propelled her to do something now was an article she had read about how diabetic women have a high risk of heart disease. "My previous doctor never mentioned that," she said. "He didn't explain what diabetes was, or that it was so dangerous. When I read that article, suddenly it clicked. I don't want to be sick or die of a heart attack. Now I'm ready to do something."

It turned out that Judith was seriously diabetic; given her age, she was a walking time bomb for heart disease, hypertension, and other problems. Once again, I was discouraged by how little attention we give to women's risk of diabetes. I was frustrated that Judith had been so poorly served by the health care system. Instead of addressing the medical consequences, her previous doctor had skipped straight to a guilt-producing lecture about her weight. The result: Judith missed two years of vital care because she was ashamed about not losing weight.

I guess I shouldn't have been surprised. Even though diabetes is the third highest factor in female mortality, it has been given scant attention as a life-threatening illness for women. Few of my patients are able to describe their risks or explain the difference between childhood and adult diabetes. Diabetes is one of those topics that seems to make people's eyes glaze over. And I believe it isn't taken seriously enough because adult diabetes usually attacks women like Judith, who are obese. Obese women are subjected to subtle and not-so-subtle forms of contempt. They are told, "Just stop eating so much," and sent on their way without receiving real help.

But we must be clear that diabetes is a life-threatening disease that affects nearly every organ of the body. It is a special issue for women because, for reasons we don't fully understand, diabetes cancels the protective benefits of estrogen and leaves women vulnerable to coronary artery disease. In the Framingham Heart Study, diabetic women were more obese, hypertensive, and had substantially lower HDL cholesterol levels. Their relative risk factors are far greater than those of diabetic men. Remember, as we discussed in Chapter 5, diabetes is the link in the deadly quartet.

What Is Diabetes?

To better understand diabetes, let's examine how your body metabolizes food. Before your cells can use nutrients, they must first be processed. Carbohydrates are converted to a simple sugar, glucose, which is then sent to your cells for use as energy or converted to fat and stored. Protein and fat are also converted into smaller components to be used by the cells.

When you eat, your pancreas releases insulin into the bloodstream that helps to absorb and utilize glucose, fatty acids, and amino acids. If your pancreas does not produce insulin, or if your body can't properly use it, the foods you eat can't be metabolized. Instead of being used for energy or stored, glucose collects in the blood—which is why diabetics are said to have high blood sugar. If there is too much glucose in the blood, it can't be processed by the kidneys, and glucose is excreted in the urine. The proper term for the disease, diabetes mellitus, means literally "flowing with honey," referring to the amount of sugar excreted in the urine.

Diabetes is really two different diseases. Type I diabetes, also known as juvenile or insulin-dependent diabetes, occurs when the pancreas ceases to produce insulin. Type I diabetes usually begins in childhood and lasts throughout a diabetic's life. It can only be controlled by injected insulin and daily food monitoring. Although this is the most familiar type of diabetes, it accounts for only about 10 percent of all cases.

More common is Type II, also known as adult or noninsulin-dependent diabetes. It is most often seen in obese people over forty. Type II diabetes is more prevalent in women, especially those who gain the most weight after age twenty. It is particularly common in African-American and Mexican-American women. One in four African-American women over age fifty-four is diabetic, and the rate of diabetes is three times as great in Mexican-American women. This might be due to greater overall fatness and specifically more abdominal fat.

In Type II diabetes, the pancreas produces insulin but the body fails to use it properly. This is called insulin resistance.

Type II diabetes can usually be controlled by diet, weight loss, and exercise, but this presents a special challenge to women, since most women gain weight with age. Treatment is also complicated by the arbitrary standards set for weight. Most women don't know what constitutes obese, or what kind of fat places them at risk. We have been culturally conditioned to believe that all body fat is bad, and that being "too fat" might mean being as little as ten or twenty pounds overweight. In reality, a normal woman has between 20 and 25 percent of her body weight as fat. Obesity is a clinical definition that involves two factors: total body fat above 32 percent, and a predominance of abdominal fat (in ratio to hip, thigh, and buttock fat). High abdominal fat is a predictor of diabetes and is associated with insulin resistance.

A third type of diabetes, known as gestational diabetes, is a temporary condition that afflicts between 2 and 6 percent of pregnant women. It normally appears between the sixth and seventh month and disappears after delivery. The condition is most common among women who have a family history of diabetes, or who have previously given birth to babies weighing more than nine pounds. Gestational diabetes is thought to be caused by a combination of increased weight and the rising level of hormones, which antagonize the action of insulin.

Gestational diabetes presents problems for both mother and infant. If it is not controlled, it can mean intrauterine death and a high risk of neonatal mortality. It also increases the risk of hypertension during pregnancy, the need for Caesarian section, and establishes a lifetime risk factor for diabetes. Up to 25 percent of women with gestational diabetes will get permanent diabetes within ten years. Women who have gestational diabetes in one pregnancy have a 50 percent chance of recurrence in future pregnancies. This so-called temporary condition is not really so temporary when you consider the lasting impact on the woman and her offspring.

WHO'S AT RISK?

Scientists still don't know exactly what causes diabetes, but there is strong evidence that the tendency to develop the disorder is genetic—particularly Type II. Family studies have demonstrated that if there is Type II diabetes in your family (especially if your parents or siblings have it), your own risk of contracting it is between 20 and 25 percent. Type I has a slimmer hereditary connection—only 6 percent. That's because Type I diabetes seems to be caused by an autoimmune reaction that attacks the cells that make insulin in the pancreas. It is possible that childhood diabetes is triggered by a virus.

On the other hand, Type II diabetes seems to be associated with obesity and the way the body uses insulin. Many people have the misconception that diabetes is the result of eating too much sugar. Actually, epidemiological studies have shown that obese people eat less sugar than thin people. The real issue is the way your body converts the food you eat—especially carbohydrates. And when it comes to obesity, high-fat, low-fiber diets are the real culprits, not too much refined sugar.

Family studies have shown that nondiabetic offspring of diabetics have higher fasting glucose levels, which is a result of insulin resistance. These studies also show that if a woman has a family history of diabetes or hypertension, she is more likely to develop higher insulin levels when she reaches middle age—again, a possible predictor of the future development of diabetes.

A sedentary lifestyle also increases your risk for diabetes. Studies done with men show that exercise lowers diabetes risk independent of high blood pressure or percentage of body fat. The more frequent the exercise, the lower the risk. A study done with women also shows that the least active women also had the highest insulin levels. Increased activity improves the efficiency of how your insulin works. This effect is probably affected by weight. Exercise is also known to lower a diabetic's need for insulin. That's important because, as we learned, insulin is atherogenic (enhancing the process of heart disease) and we want to minimize its levels.

Multiparity (having more than one pregnancy) can also increase your risk of Type II diabetes, independent of age, body mass index, or fat distribution. A positive family history of diabetes doubles the risk of multiparous women becoming diabetic.

Smoking accelerates the complications of diabetes. It is a particularly strong risk factor for CAD in women aged thirty to fifty-five even if they are not diabetic. It also accelerates the progression of blocked arteries in the legs.

RISK FACTORS FOR ADULT DIABETES

Family history
Obesity
Sedentary lifestyle
High-fat/low-fiber diet
Multiparity

DIABETES AS A DISEASE TIME BOMB

What makes diabetes so dangerous for women is the secondary risks for which it sets you up. These are the most severe:

CORONARY ARTERY DISEASE: CAD is the leading cause of death among people with diabetes. The risk of having a heart attack is 150 percent greater in diabetic women, whether it's Type I or Type II. In one study, Type I diabetics were followed for twenty to forty years, and nearly 25 percent of them died from CAD. The higher risk may be due in part to the countereffect diabetes has on estrogen and the high insulin levels that contribute to elevated triglycerides, low HDL cholesterol, and hypertension. Diabetics have been shown to have higher blood pressure levels. In African-American women with diabetes, hypertension is even more widespread, affecting between 63 and 70 percent of them.

When diabetics get CAD, it is more severe, with more heart attacks and more in-hospital deaths than occur with nondiabetics. Diabetic women have three times the risk of complications from CAD that diabetic men have. The risk of dying within one to five years following heart attacks is worse in diabetic women than virtually any other group. Diabetic women also have the highest risk of heart failure not caused by CAD. It often appears before any atherosclerosis develops and is called diabetic cardiomyopathy. Aspirin has been shown to reduce the risk of heart attacks in diabetic men, but its benefits are less clear for women. What's worse is that diabetics often get silent (painless) heart attacks, thereby increasing the risk of ignoring CAD.

ENDOMETRIAL CANCER: Both Type I and Type II diabetic women have a greater risk of endometrial cancer. This is thought to be due to the failure of the ovary to ovulate (anovulatory cycles), leading to constant estrogen exposure without progesterone—or "unopposed estrogen." Insulin affects ovarian function. One interesting study showed higher estrogen levels in postmenopausal women using insulin, independent of body weight. It is unclear whether this risk is associated with high insulin levels alone or is related to high body weight.

CIRCULATION PROBLEMS: Elderly diabetics tend to have severe circulation problems caused by impaired blood flow through small arteries. Diabetes is the cause of some forty thousand leg and foot amputations a year in older men and women. Diabetic women lose the pulses in their feet at twice the rate of men. These women are at even higher risk for stroke or CAD.

BLINDNESS: Over time, diabetes can cause bleeding from the tiny capillaries in the retina. Untreated, this condition can lead to blindness. Oral contraceptives may decrease the severity of retinal changes in diabetics.

KIDNEY FAILURE: This is the complication of diabetes that carries the greatest risk of death. Gender bias in access to kidney dialysis makes it even more severe for women.

REPRODUCTIVE DYSFUNCTION: Type I diabetics tend to have shorter fertile periods and more menstrual disturbances. High insulin levels are associated with excess androgen levels and these interfere with ovarian function and ovulation. Type I diabetics may make antibodies to their ovaries which may cause premature menopause.

HYPERTENSION: More than half of diabetic patients over age forty-five also have high blood presssure, especially women. Together, diabetes and hypertension drastically elevate the risk of CAD.

ENDOCRINE DISORDERS: Type I diabetic women have a higher risk of autoimmune disorders, which are common even in nondiabetic women. Frequently, these disorders affect other glands besides the pancreas, including the thyroid, ovary, and adrenal glands. Frequently, antibodies are made against cells lining the stomach that make a protein needed to absorb vitamin B_{12}; this can lead to pernicious anemia. Premature menopause caused by ovarian disorders is more common in Type I diabetics, so they need to be screened for this and for other autoimmune disorders during regular checkups.

EATING DISORDERS: There is a clear link between diabetes and eating disorders. By its nature, this disease involves an ongoing preoccupation with food. Most Type II diabetics already have eating disorders; many have struggled for most of their lives with being overweight or obese.

DIABETES IS A RISK FACTOR FOR . . .

Coronary artery disease
Hypertension
Menstrual irregularities
Thyroid disease
Endometrial cancer
Vaginitis
Premature ovarian failure
Blindness
Kidney disease
Amputations
Eating disorders
Depression

Type I diabetics have a unique pathway to eating disorders. A young Type I diabetic normally presents as underweight, not overweight, since most of her excess calories are lost in the urine. She may get in the habit of eating large amounts of food without gaining weight. But once insulin controls her diabetes, she will experience weight gain. At an age when girls are highly sensitive to their weight, the gain associated with insulin can be traumatic. A number of studies have found that insulin dependent diabetics—especially young women—quickly learn to manipulate insulin doses when they want to lose weight. In one study, between 30 and 40 percent of young diabetic women reported doing this regularly.

DIABETES SCREENING

Although people with Type I diabetes almost always suspect they are ill, Type II diabetes can develop gradually over a period of months or years without a person realizing there's anything seriously wrong.

Typical symptoms include increased thirst and hunger, frequent urination, unexplained weight loss, blurred vision, recurrent urinary tract infections, and vaginal infections. Any woman over age forty who is obese, has hypertension, or who has a family history of diabetes should get regular blood sugar tests—whether she is experiencing symptoms or not.

WHO SHOULD BE SCREENED FOR DIABETES?

The American Diabetes Association recommends screening for any woman over forty who has one or more of the following risk factors:

▶ Family history of diabetes (parents or siblings)—especially Type II
▶ Obesity—20 percent or more above recommended body weight
▶ Racial or ethnic risk—especially among Native Americans, Latinas, and African-Americans
▶ Previous experience of glucose intolerance
▶ Hypertension or significant hyperlipidemia
▶ History of gestational diabetes or delivery of infants weighing more than nine pounds

The basic screening method for diabetes is the fasting blood glucose test, which measures the amount of glucose in your blood before you have eaten. The normal range is between 70 and 100 milligrams per deciliter (mg/dl). A blood sample is taken in the morning before any food is eaten. If the test shows a glucose level above 140 mg/dl, it is a sure indication of diabetes. However, a reading between 115 and 140 mg/dl will require further testing in the form of a glucose tolerance test. A glucose tolerance test should be done any time fasting blood sugar is more than 115 mg/dl, or postprandial (after eating) glucose is over 160 mg/dl. A glucose tolerance test takes several hours. You are given a sugary liquid to swallow that temporarily produces high blood sugar. Then, blood samples are taken at intervals of thirty minutes, one hour, two hours, and three hours, and the glucose level is measured in each sample. This tells how quickly your body is able to bring the blood sugar level back down to normal. More recently, fasting blood glucose determinations and glycohemoglobin levels are done instead of three-hour glucose tolerance tests. A glycohemoglobin measures glucose levels over time when sugar gets attached to hemoglobin in the blood.

Should all pregnant women be screened? Although gestational diabetes affects a relatively small percentage of women, the consequences can be so devastating, that I think screening by the last trimester is called for. If you are African-American, Latina, or Asian, ask your doctor about recent studies that suggest you might need a different cutoff value than 140 mg/dl in your pregnancy screening.

If you've ever had gestational diabetes, be sure to start regular screening for Type II diabetes after age forty.

TAKING CONTROL OF DIABETES

Diabetes is a good example of the way many diseases hit women harder and more diversely than men. When it is not tightly controlled, Type I diabetes can have a direct negative effect on a woman's reproductive life. In the days before injectable insulin was available, young diabetic girls never menstruated. Now, diabetic girls do start menstruating, but at a later age. At least 30 percent suffer from menstrual irregularities and the attendant diminished fertility throughout their lives. This is especially true if the diabetes is poorly controlled.

It takes an incredible amount of effort, day after day, for a Type I diabetic to maintain control of her blood glucose level, and it's especially tough for young girls who desperately want to avoid being labeled "different" from their peers. If you are the mother of a diabetic daughter, you have to be sensitive to the social implications and find ways to positively encourage her. Be on the lookout for depression or rebellion against taking insulin, and let her know you understand her frustration and are proud of how hard she works to stay healthy.

Whether you have Type I or Type II diabetes, it is an illness that requires the maximum amount of patient involvement. You can't be passive about it. You have to take charge and focus on yourself, on your eating, on your wellness, on your lifestyle habits, on going to the doctor. It's a very intensive, self-directed activity. And that's difficult for women because we tend not to take care of ourselves. We're the last ones on the list, unaccustomed to asking for support, even from husbands, lovers, and families. Being self-directed doesn't come naturally, but if you're diabetic, you have to keep reminding yourself that it's going to keep you healthy.

Becky was a forty-three-year-old woman who had suffered from adult diabetes for several years, although she tried to ignore it and rarely visited the doctor. She paid some attention to her diet and took pills to keep her diabetes under control. When she first came to see me as a patient, I spent a good deal of time educating Becky about the long-term complications of diabetes. I succeeded only in scaring her off; she didn't return for two years. When she came back, twenty-five pounds heavier, Becky admitted that she was worried. She had reason to be. Even though she was taking the highest dose of oral medication available, her blood sugars were still out of sight.

Becky agreed to enter a medically supervised weight-loss program, and she lost a few pounds. However, her need for insulin increased, and the endocrinologist who supervised the program urged her to start injecting insulin—a prospect she had always dreaded. It could not be avoided any longer.

Even though Becky was fully aware of the dangers of her disease, she didn't change her eating habits and paid little attention to monitoring her sugar levels. I was quite concerned about what might be getting in Becky's way, and I referred her to a psychotherapist hoping she could get past whatever was keeping her from taking charge of her health. But she only saw the psychotherapist now and then, and I watched her with a growing sense of alarm. I was convinced that disaster was not far away.

Finally, while on a trip to Florida, Becky developed chest pains. Remembering what I had told her about the risks of coronary artery disease for diabetic women, she went to a hospital emergency room. There, it was discovered that one of her coronary arteries was in the process of closing. She was whisked to the catheterization lab where a cardiac catheterization revealed that all of her coronary arteries had some blockages. A balloon angioplasty was performed to open the arteries.

Back in New York, Becky returned to my office, now scared to death. Tearfully, she told me that she had just become engaged to be married and couldn't believe she had almost had a heart attack. Unfortunately, within a few weeks she was experiencing pain again, and needed another angioplasty. She managed to get through her wedding and honeymoon, but then she sank into a deep depression. Today, despite antidepressants and twice-weekly psychotherapy, Becky continues to gain weight. It's hard to be a woman, I think, but even harder to be a diabetic woman.

An important recent study of Type I diabetes has clearly shown that tight control of blood sugar levels means fewer complications. We can assume that this is also true of Type II diabetes. Tight control means intense self care: frequent blood glucose testing, careful diet and exercise habits, and regular adjustment of insulin dosages. Good self-care is best achieved by a team: you, your doctor, nutritionist, nurse educator, and psychotherapist. As you can see, being a diabetic is not easy. Here are some practical suggestions for staying healthy.

1. Eat for Balance

The American Diabetes Association recommends these general guidelines for diet control and weight management:

1. **Maintain a diet high in complex carbohydrates, such as starchy vegetables, whole grains, and fruits—approximately 50 to 60 percent of your daily intake.**
2. **Increase your intake of fiber, found in foods like oats, barley, lentils, beans, vegetables, and whole grains. Studies show that high-fiber diets can help to reduce blood sugar levels by slowing down the rate of sugar absorption.**
3. **Decrease your intake of high-fat foods to no more than 25 percent of daily calories. Of those calories, only about 10 percent should come from saturated fat. It is important to be aware of new studies showing that low-fat, high-carbohydrate diets in patients with Type II diabetes may actually**

raise triglyceride, glucose, and insulin levels—just what we don't want! When researchers substituted monounsaturated fats (olive, safflower, sunflower, and peanut oils, and avocados and nuts) for about 15 percent of the carbohydrates (in a 55 percent carbohydrate diet) they found that this effect did not occur. The assumption that low fat always means healthy is not necessarily true for diabetics.

4. Limit your daily cholesterol intake to about 300 milligrams.
5. Limit your consumption of foods made with refined or processed sugar.
6. Decrease your intake of salt and foods with a high sodium content.
7. Regulate your food schedule, eating the same amount of foods at the same times every day. It's best to spread out food consumption throughout the day.

The American Diabetes Association also distributes a food exchange system for meal planning that helps diabetics control their food intake. The system is comprised of six lists, each containing foods that are similar in calories and nutrient content. Many women find it a useful method.

2. Keep Track of Your Sugar Levels

It is often recommended that both Type I and Type II diabetics regularly test their sugar levels. There are several home tests that can help you do this. The most effective is a finger stick test with a home glucose meter that measures your sugar levels from a drop of blood. You might be squeamish about pricking your finger, or worry that repeated pricking will cause scars, but most diabetics who have mastered home tests have found them to be relatively painless and not at all disfiguring. Although self-monitoring requires discipline and commitment, many diabetics feel empowered by the sense of control it gives them. Also, home testing might be even more accurate than the tests you get in the doctor's office. Research has shown that there's a phenomenon of "white coat hyperglycemia," similar to "white coat hypertension." For some people, the anxiety produced by a visit to the doctor makes blood sugar levels rise.

3. Exercise for Low Blood Sugar

Diabetics are encouraged to adopt a regular program of exercise. Studies show that exercise can lower blood sugar in Type II diabetics, even in the absence of weight loss. We already know exercise reduces risk factors associated with CAD, the most life-threatening outcome of diabetes. Regular low-intensity exercise (such as walking) has a proven benefit, resulting in better cardiovascular conditioning, lower blood pressure, and improved lipid levels.

I understand that starting an exercise program can be difficult if you are heavy—not because you lack discipline or motivation, but because your choices may be somewhat limited. Aerobics and other exercises classes can be intimidating if you're overweight, since the pace is often fast, and there's little time spent on instruction. I think the best way for a normally sedentary, overweight woman to get started on exercise is to begin taking a twenty- to thirty-minute walk at least three times a week. Enlist a friend to join you, or use it as well-deserved private time. Exercise is a good way to lower your stress levels—and experts say that high stress makes diabetes worse. So figure that your exercise program is helping you in two important ways. Gradually, you can increase the time and duration of your program. You'll know when you're ready. Talk to your doctor about whether or not you should receive a stress-echo test before you begin your exercise program. Silent ischemia (the lack of blood flow to the heart muscle) is a risk for diabetic women.

4. Manage Your Stress

You've probably heard about the importance of diet and exercise, but you may not realize that stress management is equally important. That's because a part of the stress response involves the elevation of hormones like epinephrine, cortisol, and growth hormones. These are known as counter-regulatory hormones; they counter the effects of insulin and make glucose available. This is part of the fight-or-flight protective response. When you experience stress, your body gets a signal that there's danger and makes more glucose available to give you energy. If your stress state is chronic, your body continues to adjust by raising insulin levels. There are a number of ways to reduce stress, including yoga, meditation, and physical exercise. Also keep in mind that a good doctor-patient relationship, in which open communication exists, has been shown to correlate with better control of blood glucose.

5. Plan Your Pregnancies

If you are diabetic, you cannot afford to have an unplanned pregnancy that might arrive at a time when you have poor control of your diabetes.

Under the right conditions, a diabetic woman can have a successful pregnancy, but many complications have been associated with poorly controlled diabetes. The Centers for Disease Control and the American Diabetes Association strongly urge diabetic women to plan their pregnancies carefully, get counseling prior to becoming pregnant, and make sure they have access to regular care throughout the pregnancy. Screening for gestational diabetes in the third trimester should be done for all women, but especially for those with family histories of diabetes, obese women, and women over age thirty-five.

6. Be Aware of Your Cycle

Remember that diabetes is not an isolated illness. Nor does it manifest itself in a consistent way. Most important, it is affected by your monthly cycle. High levels of estrogens counter the action of insulin. Your energy expenditure (metabolism) also varies and is higher premenstrually. This is associated with higher food intake because of the sugar craving many women experience premenstrually. So watch out because good diabetic control can be lost at this time of the month. As diabetic women become menopausal, insulin requirements often decline and glucose levels are lowered.

If you take insulin, you may need to adjust your dosage depending on where you are in the cycle. For instance, you may need to take slightly more insulin premenstrually. Find your own cyclical levels by tracking your cycle and noting changes in your energy level, urination, hunger, thirst, etc., as they occur during the month.

COMMON QUESTIONS ABOUT DIABETES

Should I take estrogen replacement at menopause if I'm diabetic?

I wish I could give you a clear-cut answer to this question. I normally inform menopausal women about estrogen because of its clear benefits in protecting against heart disease and preventing osteoporosis. However, it appears that diabetics don't receive the same benefits from their own estrogen before menopause, which is why their CAD risk is so much greater. Furthermore, osteoporosis isn't as great a threat since Type II diabetics have more androgen activity to keep bones dense. Since diabetics have an increased risk for endometrial cancer, one would think estrogen replacement alone would not be recommended. Progesterone is a must.

MONTHLY CYCLE JOURNAL

The following chart will help you keep track of your diabetes during the course of your monthly cycle. Using a home test kit, check your fasting blood sugar (before eating), then your postprandial (after meal) levels. Also note if you have unusual hunger and thirst or other symptoms.

DAY OF CYCLE	FASTING BLOOD SUGAR	AFTER-MEAL BLOOD SUGAR	HUNGER/THIRST LEVELS	OTHER*

*Includes changes in urinary habits, energy levels, mood, or other notable symptoms.

On the other hand, some early studies show a decrease in Type II diabetes with estrogen replacement. And one might rationalize that by becoming menopausal, diabetic women take on an extra CAD risk. Why not try to decrease it? I hope further research will be able to assess the impact of HRT.

With menopause, the normal fluctuations in blood sugar are lost unless you take a combined cyclic hormone therapy. Some studies show that insulin requirements decrease at menopause. Hormone therapy may prevent the abdominal weight gain that accompanies menopause, a point in its favor since android fat contributes to the deadly quartet of diabetes, high triglycerides, low HDL, and hypertension.

When considering hormone replacement, diabetics may fare better with transdermal patches instead of pills, because of slow stomach emptying and problems absorbing estrogen. Also, diabetics have a high incidence of gallstones, which can be worsened by oral estrogen.

Why can't insulin-dependent diabetics just take insulin pills instead of injections?

When you swallow a pill, your body treats it like any other food and breaks it down in your digestive system. An insulin pill wouldn't be able to perform the action of the pancreas. However, since people with Type II diabetes have working pancreases, sometimes they can take pills that increase insulin release and utilization.

I've heard that women who eat the wrong foods sometimes get hypoglycemia.

Hypoglycemia is a condition that involves lower than normal levels of blood glucose. It is not related to diabetes. In recent years, diagnosing hypoglycemia in overweight women has become a popular diet gimmick. Proponents of this approach tell women that they are "allergic" to sweets, and that's why they are overweight. This is a myth that has cost many fad dieters plenty of money on expensive blood sugar tests. In fact, if your blood sugar level is too low—and it's debatable what that level might be—you can easily deal with it by eating well balanced, regularly scheduled meals. Having a brisk release of insulin in response to an ingested sugar load is a normal physiologic response in young women. Most glucose tolerance tests done to rule out hypoglycemia show little correlation between blood sugar and symptoms. And even when they do, this is not a "disease." It is your variation, and it serves as a signal that you should avoid refined sugar and eat in a more balanced way. For example, if your pattern is coffee and a donut for breakfast and a candy bar for an afternoon snack, you'll want to rethink your diet.

Do Type II diabetics ever need insulin injections?

Approximately 20 percent of Type II diabetics have conditions severe enough to require insulin. In addition, women with uncontrolled gestational diabetes are sometimes given temporary insulin injections.

Can I take birth control pills if I'm diabetic?

Although there is a slight risk of a stroke with oral contraceptives, most diabetic women under age thirty-five can safely take them. This is a case where the risk of an unplanned pregnancy far outweighs any potential risks of taking the pill. The lowest dose combination pills should be taken, as these have negligible effects on glucose levels. If glucose levels do rise, the condition is completely reversable by stopping the pill. However, because of the high risk of an unplanned pregnancy, oral contraceptives are the contraceptive of choice for diabetics. An IUD may also be used without worry; studies show that diabetics are not more prone to uterine infections or pelvic inflammatory disease.

Can diabetes be cured?

Once you have diabetes, you are never cured of it. However, most diabetics who have good control can lead normal lives.

Are there doctors that specialize in the treatment of diabetes?

Generally, diabetes is treated by internists and endocrinologists. Some of these, who have specialties in diabetes, are called diabetologists. If you are pregnant and diabetic, your obstetrician should work closely with your diabetes team—doctor, nutritionist, and nurse educator. Diabetes is a disease that requires more than just a woman's health specialist. The fine-tuning of diabetes management requires a multidisciplinary approach.

My husband is a diabetic and he can't get an erection. Do women with diabetes also have problems with sex?

There is an overabundance of literature on impotence in male diabetics, but very little research has been done with women. Diabetes can affect the nerves going to the genital area and decrease lubrication as well as orgasm. Diabetic women also suffer from recurrent and severe candidal infections of the vagina which cause itching and painful intercourse. When it is out of control, diabetes can affect libido through its impact on mood.

How does diabetes affect my mood?

Glucose fluctuations are associated with changes in mood. Low sugar is clearly related to irritability, combativeness, and the symptoms related to the release of adrenalin—tremulousness, palpitations, anxiety, and sweating. Occasionally, low blood sugar can lead to inactivity and becoming withdrawn. High sugar levels can be associated with positive mood states, but for those who associate good mood with high glucose levels, there is a risk of poor control in order to feel good.

RESOURCES

ORGANIZATIONS
American Diabetes Association
149 Madison Avenue
New York, NY 10016
212-725-4925

Juvenile Diabetes Foundation
60 Madison Avenue
New York, NY 10010
800-223-1138

National Diabetes Information Clearing House
Box NDIC
Bethesda, MD 20892
301-654-3327

PUBLICATIONS
The American Diabetes Association and American Dietetic Association's
    Family Cookbook
Published by Prentice Hall, 1980, 1984

Diabetes Self-Management
A bimonthly magazine published by R. A. Rapaport
    Publishing Company
150 West 22nd Street
New York, NY 10011

Health-O-Gram
A newsletter published by the Sugarfree Center
P.O. Box 114
Van Nuys, CA 91408

A free report describing the most current research in diabetes is available
from the Joslin Diabetes Center, One Joslin Place, Boston, MA 02215.

8

PREVENTING OSTEOPOROSIS

Don't Become a Little Old Lady

~~~

Martha came into my office, walking slowly and struggling to keep her balance. She appeared frail and sickly, and I was surprised to learn that she was only sixty-four. She seemed much older than her years. Martha's complaint was an unexplained pain that radiated up from her left foot. She said, "I don't know what's wrong. Suddenly, I can barely stand to walk on this leg." She was fearful that some mysterious ailment was crippling her or that she might have bone cancer. I examined Martha and ordered X rays, which showed that she had suffered a bone fracture.

Martha was astonished. "I can't understand it," she said. "I don't remember slipping or banging my leg or anything that would have caused this." She thought it over carefully, and the only unusual incident she could recall was stepping out of bed one morning and coming down a little too sharply on her left foot. "But that was nothing," she said.

Martha was wrong—as further bone density tests showed. Her bones were so brittle that the smallest stress was capable of causing a fracture.

How easily we accept the idea that older people are weak and frail. But how does it happen? When does a strong, healthy woman cross the line into "old age?" What is it that goes into making a little old lady? It's not just the loss of height. There's something else that happens. Her gait changes. She's a little more wobbly and unsure on her feet. She can't walk as fast. She tends to fall more. She experiences a functional decline, and some of it is related to the natural process of aging. But what we are learning now is that much of what makes an elderly woman frail is not natural at all.

Osteoporosis—the disease that weakens the bones and leads to frailty and fracture in older women—may seem very distant to you. Young and even middle-aged women often don't relate to it, and I think this is because we, as a society, have so much trouble relating to our elderly. If something is perceived as a problem of the elderly, we ignore it. If you're reasonably educated about good health, you probably know that osteoporosis is a women's health issue. But unless you have an elderly mother or relative who has fractured her hip or spine and is frail, you probably don't realize how severe an impact osteoporosis can have on your life. Simply put, it's going to be the difference between being free living and independent and being weak and dependent in your older years.

You might also have trouble taking osteoporosis as seriously as you might another disease, such as CAD, because the process of osteoporosis is long and insidious whereas heart disease seems to be more dramatic and acute. If you have a heart attack, it's a tangible event that gets your attention. There are no such warning moments in the development of osteoporosis until it's already too late. The most common first sign of osteoporosis is a serious fracture in a woman who has already lost up to 50 percent of her bone density. Today, between fifteen and twenty million American women suffer from osteoporosis; statistically, 25 percent of Caucasian women over age sixty will break a bone because of it.

We have to start reorienting our perspective about this disease and make it a priority from adolescence on. Most women reach peak bone mass between the ages of twenty-five and thirty, then begin a slow decline at the rate of about 1 percent a year. At menopause, the rate of bone loss speeds up to about 5 percent a year over a period of around five years before slowing down again. Bone loss is not an overnight event.

WHAT IS OSTEOPOROSIS?

Your bones are not static. They are living cells that are constantly in the process of breaking down and repairing. For much of your life, this process is so efficient that you don't even know it's going on. With osteoporosis, the calcium that keeps bones strong is lost and new bone formation stops occurring to repair bone loss. The result is that your skeleton becomes fragile and your bones grow thin and brittle. Bone loss happens over time, accelerating with age and menopause. To some extent, every person, male and female, experiences a degree of bone loss with age. But it's a far less severe problem for men since they have about 30 percent more bone mass than women and tend to lose it more slowly. It's also less severe in African-American and dark-skinned women, who have about 10 percent more bone mass than Caucasian or light-skinned women.

If you have osteoporosis, you can fracture your spine without even falling because your vertebrae get so weak that they collapse amongst themselves. That's the reason elderly women grow shorter. While this is painful and deforming, it is not necessarily life-threatening. Hip fractures, on the other hand, are very dangerous. Another factor contributes to hip fractures besides low bone mass, and that is falling. Compare the way a younger and an older woman fall. When you're young, your gait is faster. Say you trip and fall. Most likely, you're going to fall forward, extending your arm to break the fall. Maybe you'll fracture your wrist, although you might not even do that if your bones are strong.

If an elderly person is walking, she will be slower and unsteadier on her feet. If she trips, she will most likely fall to the side or backward because she's lost the reflex of falling forward and stretching out her arm. The result is that she breaks her hip. Certainly, the overmedication of our elderly contributes to the danger of falling.

Hip fractures among elderly women can be considered a costly and devastating epidemic in this country. Osteoporosis carries a 7-billion-dollar annual medical price tag every year, and 5 billion dollars of that is attributable to hip fractures. Aside from the cost, hip fractures are associated with high morbidity and mortality. Falling down is the leading cause of death among people over age seventy-five—most of whom are women. All patients with hip fractures require hospitalization, and between 12 and 20 percent die during the first year. Of those who survive, 50 percent will never walk independently again.

Hip fracture is the single most important factor that leads to a woman's fragility—to her never being able to walk on her two legs again without a cane or a walker. It puts her at risk for being in the hospital, requiring bed rest, becoming more frail, getting pneumonia or pulmonary embolism, or other complications, and perhaps never being free-living again. More than three hundred thousand women suffer hip fractures every year. Of these, thirty thousand die and another one hundred thousand require long-term care.

Hospital or bed rest presents an additional, seldom discussed, threat for older women. Each day of bed rest is equivalent to a year of sedentary living in terms of its impact on a woman's functional status. The effects are so damaging that some experts are calling for bone strengthening programs for older people before they enter the hospital so they spend less time in bed.

I've seen the ill effects of bed rest even with young, healthy people. A woman in her thirties may be in the hospital for minor surgery or a broken bone. After a week, she's lost some cardiovascular conditioning. She feels light-headed and dizzy when she gets up. She can't maintain her blood pressure. Her pulse rate is faster. Bed rest causes you to lose conditioning very quickly, whether it's cardiovascular or musculoskeletal.

The irony is, our tendency is usually to coddle the elderly. If an older woman has a fall or gets sick, we discourage her from going out or getting exercise—the very things that might help restore her conditioning and aid her recovery.

I believe that osteoporosis has been growing as a problem. Its prominence seems to parallel the rise of industrialism and sedentary living. Along with industrialization came particular notions about the way people are supposed to behave after a certain age. The fight against osteoporosis and frailty in older women must be waged culturally as well as medically. We encourage people to retire when they reach their mid-sixties, and urge them to begin living more sedentary lifestyles—even though a sixty-five-year-old woman can no longer be considered elderly. It is my hope that the mandatory physical and social retirement of women in their sixties will change somewhat as the masses of the baby-boom generation grow older. We don't necessarily want to retire when we're sixty-five; we plan on living longer, more active lives.

EVALUATE YOUR RISK

To some extent, bone density is controlled genetically since you inherit your body type and bone structure. If you are a larger person with larger bones and your mother and grandmother do not have osteoporosis, there's a good chance you won't have it either. We also know that African-American women have much denser bones than Caucasian women and are at less risk.

Although age-adjusted rates of hip fracture in African-American women are half those in Caucasian women, the rates of mortality and disability after hip fractures are higher among African-American women. The protective factors in African-American women are not clear, although increased bone and body mass may be a partial explanation. I would caution, however, that we shouldn't ignore the issue of osteoporosis for African-American women, wrongly believing they are not at risk.

There are no specific data on Latinas, although bone density does seem to be greater in darker-skinned women and women with greater body mass. Osteoporosis also appears to be more prevalent in intemperate climates than in the tropics. The highest resported incidence of osteoporosis in the world is in Rochester, Minnesota.

There are new studies that show a relationship to pregnancy and child-bearing and the development of osteoporosis. Pregnant and breast-feeding women benefit from additional surges of estrogen that accompany pregnancy and follow breast-feeding—especially if they consume a nutritional diet during

---

ARE YOU AT RISK?

Does your mother have osteoporosis?
Are you thin and small?
Are you Caucasian or Asian?
Do you lead a sedentary lifestyle?
Do you smoke?
Do you drink caffeine or alcohol to excess?
Do you consume inadequate dietary calcium?
Do you have an endocrine disorder?
Do you have an eating disorder?
Do you have a high-protein diet?
Do you exercise excessively?
Do you have low muscle mass?
Do you take calcium-depleting medications?
Have you had a premenopause hysterectomy?
Have you had an early surgical menopause?
Did you have an early menopause?
Are you menopausal now?

those periods. But these benefits don't apply to very young mothers whose own bones are not fully developed. Teenage pregnancy is a risk factor for osteoporosis, especially if the young woman is not receiving adequate dietary calcium. The RDAs recommend at least 1,200 milligrams of calcium for pregnant and lactating women. Some experts recommend more—as much as 1,500 to 2,000 milligrams—especially for teenage mothers whose own bones are still developing.

Beyond these factors, there are no firm predictors for who is going to become a rapid bone loser at menopause. You can best evaluate your own risk and protect yourself by avoiding the behaviors that seem to contribute to the development of osteoporosis, and by taking positive action to prevent bone loss.

THE CALCIUM CONNECTION

Calcium is a mineral essential for building bones and teeth and for maintaining bone strength. Your bones and teeth contain 99 percent of the body's calcium stores. When your bones don't contain enough calcium, they weaken. It sounds like a simple problem to fix and, indeed, there has been a rush on calcium supplements during the past few years. But the calcium connection is really more complex than it seems. Osteoporosis is not merely caused by a calcium deficiency that can be overcome by consuming large amounts of calcium-rich foods or supplements. This assumption is lucrative for many manufacturers (sales of calcium supplements total about 200 million dollars a year), but not necessarily helpful. Your body's ability to absorb calcium is influenced by the form in which it is consumed, its interaction with other nutrients, and the way it is absorbed into and eliminated from your body.

Certain nutrients have a direct effect on calcium absorption. Vitamin D, which is converted to a hormone called calcitriol, regulates the transport of calcium from the digestive tract to the bloodstream and into the bones. However, that doesn't mean you should consume large amounts of vitamin D, which can be toxic in high doses. Normal amounts of vitamin D (5 to 10 micrograms a day), which you get primarily from the sun and by consuming fortified foods, are sufficient to do the job. If you are not regularly exposed to sunlight—for example, during winter months—you might need a little more dietary vitamin D; otherwise, most people get enough. (Elderly women who have difficulty getting out in the sun also need more vitamin D.)

People with lactose intolerance, especially Asian women, avoid dairy products and are at risk for osteoporosis. Excessive use of caffeine and alcohol also worsen osteoporosis, especially when a diet is low in calcium.

Phosphorus is another mineral that has an effect on bone density. Too much or too little phosphorus in the body can harm bone formation. Most Americans probably consume too much phosphorus, since it's present in red meats, colas, baked goods, and many processed foods. Likewise, too much sodium in your diet can increase the amount of calcium excreted in urine.

Magnesium is important for the body's utilization of calcium and vitamin D. However, there is a common myth that you must take magnesium in proportion to calcium to retain the right balance, and many health food stores sell tablets that combine the two. Just the opposite is true. You should never take calcium and magnesium together for the simple reason that magnesium competes with calcium for absorption. If you do use magnesium supplements, take them at a different time.

Protein is vital to the formation of bones, but too much protein can increase the amount of calcium lost in the urine. High-protein diets have been another side effect of industrialization. In addition, some weight-loss programs encourage high protein intake. Americans eat far too much protein, which also accounts for the high percentage of saturated fat in our diet. Dietary guidelines suggest we consume only about 0.8 of a gram of protein for every kilogram (2.2 pounds) of body weight. For a 130-pound woman that would translate to 188 calories a day. However, the average American diet includes two or three times that amount. Excessive protein has a negative effect on calcium. When protein breaks down in the body it produces organic acids, and the body pulls calcium carbonate out of the bones to act as a buffer. Acid-base imbalance itself can lead to a progressive decline in bone mass with age. But an interesting new study has shown that buffering blood acidity with daily supplements of potassium bicarbonate in postmenopausal women can slow down loss of bone mass. So although too little protein can damage your bones, too much can weaken them.

Certain medications can also leach calcium from your system. For example, thyroid hormone encourages bone turnover, so women taking thyroid medication must use special care and make sure they're not taking too much. This is a major issue for women because of the high incidence of thyroid disease and the abuse of thyroid medication for the alleged purpose of losing weight. Also, as we get older, our need for thyroid hormone declines, so women on thyroid replacement need to check and see if their dosages should be lowered. (See Chapter 10 for more details.)

Other medical treatments that can deplete calcium include cortisone, used for asthma and certain immune disorders; chemotherapy; long-term lithium therapy; anticonvulsants; and long-term use of phosphate-binding antacids.

Endocrine disorders can also contribute to osteoporosis. These include hyperthyroidism, hyperparathyroidism, Cushing's syndrome, and Type I diabetes.

THE RECOMMENDED DIETARY ALLOWANCE (RDA) FOR CALCIUM

The RDAs are based on the evaluation of scientists regarding daily intake of important nutrients. They are updated periodically to reflect new knowledge. In 1985, a National Institutes of Health committee on osteoporosis noted that American women consumed only about half the recommended allowance of calcium. Given the importance of calcium, the committee suggested that the RDA for adult women be increased to between 1200 and 1500 milligrams a day. While this recommendation has not yet been formally accepted, there is strong evidence that adult women should be taking more calcium. The current recommendations suggest that women consume at least this much calcium per day:

AGE	MILLIGRAMS OF CALCIUM
0–10	800
11–24	1200
25 and older	1000
Pregnant	1200
Lactating	1200
Postmenopausal	1500

AN ESTROGEN-DRIVEN EVENT

The most dangerous time for bone loss in women is in the first years after menopause when estrogen levels are rapidly changing. Estrogen keeps calcium in your bones in three ways: It helps your intestines absorb more calcium from the foods you eat; it slows the process of calcium loss from the bones; and it helps your kidneys save more calcium and excrete less in the urine.

Estrogen is such a critical factor in the prevention of bone loss that if you have a high risk profile, you may not be able to retard further bone loss without the use of estrogen after menopause. Taking calcium helps, but it's not as effective as estrogen.

A number of studies support this conclusion. In one conducted by Kaiser Permanente in California, eighty-three postmenopausal women were placed on three separate regimens for a year. One group received estrogen and calcium supplements. A second group received estrogen but no calcium supplements. A third group received calcium supplements but no estrogen. When researchers compared bone densities at the end of the year, they found that women in the first two groups suffered no bone loss, while those in the third group suffered substantial bone loss.

When you're considering estrogen replacement, you should know that low-dose formulas do not seem to be as effective against osteoporosis. Unfortunately, our profession is not yet very sophisticated about measuring the appropriate dosages. Doctors sometimes assume that a standard dose works the same for every woman. But each person absorbs and metabolizes estrogen differently.

There is some early research suggesting that it's not just estrogen that determines bone density, but also progesterone. Women with a luteal-phase deficiency—which means their bodies don't make enough progesterone in the second half of their menstrual cycles—have lower bone density. Some early research suggests that women runners might have this deficiency. If that is so, it could negate some of the bone strengthening effects of running. However, I must stress that research regarding the role of progesterone in bone density has not yet shown a definitive connection.

Like all important decisions you make about your body, estrogen replacement must be weighed in the context of other factors. I have found, however, that women who truly understand the debilitating effects of osteoporosis are eager to do anything they can to prevent it. A recent experience brought this home to me.

Vivian was fifty-six when she began coming to me for checkups and treatment. A lovely, active woman with a busy professional and family life, she was very careful about getting regular checkups. Her mother had died of breast cancer some years earlier, and Vivian was in a high-risk category for this disease. Because of that, she had written off any idea of taking estrogen replacement until we began a discussion of relative risks. Her mammograms continued to show no problems and I was concerned about the greater risks she might be inviting. But Vivian was staunch in her refusal to take estrogen, and wouldn't even discuss the matter. Finally, worried about bone loss, I asked Vivian to have a bone density test. It showed significant bone loss—more than 50 percent.

Suddenly, Vivian woke up. It was as though the proverbial scales had fallen from her eyes. For the first time, she began to pepper me with questions about osteoporosis and estrogen. "I know I have a breast cancer risk," she said fervently, "but I also know that I can't stand the idea of becoming a bent little old lady!"

I sent Vivian to an osteoporosis specialist who could work with her and give her the range of hormonal and nonhormonal treatments and who might be able to enroll her in a clinical study.

What struck me about this incident was how strongly Vivian believed she had no choice—that a risk of breast cancer automatically meant no estrogen. But good women's medicine is all about choices, about weighing risks and benefits and deciding what will improve quality of life the most.

SCREENING FOR OSTEOPOROSIS

I discuss osteoporosis with all of my women patients, not just those who are approaching menopause, since it's best prevented when women start being bone conscious early in life. My discussion is more serious with a menopausal woman or a woman who has had a premenopausal ovary removal. For this woman, I will first perform a nutritional assessment to determine whether or not she is consuming enough calcium. Then, since we know that the body loses bone density very rapidly during the first five years of menopause, I will educate her about estrogen replacement therapy.

Low bone density is a risk for fracture in the same way that cholesterol is a risk for heart attack or high blood pressure is a risk for stroke. However, although clinical history is a potent predictor for risk in CAD, it is not sufficient to determine the risk of fracture. The only real predictor is a measurement of bone density.

However, normally, I won't ask for bone density tests unless there are other reasons to be concerned about bone loss aside from normal menopause, or when a woman needs more information to help her evaluate the comparative risks of estrogen replacement therapy. I might recommend it for a woman with vertebral abnormalities, someone who is receiving long-term steroid treatment, or a woman taking medication for thyroid disorders requiring high doses to suppress thyroid activity. I would also add bone density screening for women receiving chemotherapy or radiation treatments, since they can lead to premature menopause.

Ordinary X rays don't detect early bone loss and are not specific enough for screening. The technique used is bone densitometry, and the most precise and least costly method is the DEXA scan, which can measure bone density levels at various sites in the body, and which exposes women to very little radiation.

Where DEXA scans are not available, quantitative CAT scans are done— although these deliver more radiation, are more costly, and are limited to examining the spine. Osteoporosis can also be diagnosed on lateral chest X rays, but by the time it shows up on routine X rays, at least 30 percent of bone has been lost.

PROTECT YOURSELF—NOW AND FOR LIFE

Here are five ways to protect yourself from osteoporosis:

1. Don't Smoke

Smoking is a very big factor in the development of osteoporosis, and it's probably underreported in the scientific literature. Smokers begin to lose bone density at a rapid rate even before menopause. When I have conducted bone density tests on premenopausal women because they have other risks, I have found that virtually all the women who have had significant bone loss have been smokers.

In addition, women who smoke tend to have earlier menopause, which is an osteoporosis risk factor. Smoking is also believed to hamper the body's metabolism of estrogen prior to menopause and can negate the benefits of estrogen replacement after menopause.

2. Get Enough Calcium

The best way to get calcium is by eating highly absorbable calcium-rich foods and receiving adequate vitamin D to help absorb them. However, few women consume enough calcium in their diets, and supplements have become an essential part of our calcium intake. There are several forms of supplementary calcium, but not all of them contain enough absorbable calcium to be effective. Calcium found in supplements isn't pure, since it's bound with other chemicals. Most women prefer calcium carbonate that contains 40 percent calcium and is easily found in powdered form, tablets, or in the antacid Tums. But one study showed better effects on all bone sites from calcium citrate.

Many health food stores sell chelated calcium under the guise of its being more effective when just the opposite is true. A chelator is an agent that securely binds an element like calcium. You cannot disassociate the calcium and absorb it separately from the chelating agent. You have to be careful when you shop in a health food store because you might just be spending your money for nothing. Also avoid bone meal or dolomite, substances that may be contaminated with lead or other toxic metals.

An acidic environment aids the absorption of calcium, especially in older women, so it's best to take calcium with meals when the stomach is producing acid. Calcium citrate is good because it provides its own acidic environment. Some experts recommend taking calcium supplements with the evening meal, since there's more bone turnover when you're in bed at night.

There are four primary dietary sources of calcium: leafy green vegetables, dairy products, salmon and sardines with soft bones, and soy products.

Although several vegetables are high in calcium, some nutritionists question their absorption rate. Scientists at Creighton University Hard Tissue Research Center in Nebraska and at the Department of Foods and Nutrition at Purdue University in Indiana gave a group of people spinach and traced the route its calcium took inside their bodies. They found that only about 5 percent of the calcium was absorbed. Other studies, however, indicate that spinach might be the exception and other leafy green vegetables, such as kale, have calcium absorption rates as good as that of milk. The best rule of thumb when considering a balanced diet is to eat a healthy variety of foods.

Dairy products are excellent sources of dietary calcium, but they are also high in fat so many women avoid them altogether. But you derive just as much calcium from nonfat dairy products as from high fat.

What if you are lactose intolerant? That means your body does not contain an enzyme that helps you digest dairy products. Many lactose intolerant people can consume small quantities of dairy products, but lactose-free milk is now available, as are tablets that contain the missing enzyme. Nearly 70 percent of African-Americans and Asians are lactose intolerant, although African-Americans have more natural protection because of higher bone density. In Asian cultures, people rarely consume milk or other dairy products. They get their calcium from soy products. Tofu, made from soy milk with a mineral binder, is widely available in America and is an excellent source of calcium.

Canned salmon or sardines with the bone are excellent sources of calcium, although their caloric and fat content make them less practical as a constant dietary source.

3. Maintain a Healthy Body Weight

Thin women have less bone mass than larger women, and this can be added to the dangers of anorexia. A heavier person will have higher bone density, since maintaining a certain degree of weight puts pressure on the bones and also provides you with more estrogen around and after menopause. Weight on bones helps them to produce more bone tissue, and fat stores on the hips, thighs, and buttocks (not the abdomen) help maintain estrogen stores.

Anorexia nervosa also causes amenorrhea (loss of menstruation). Amenorrhea depletes estrogen levels and halts the production of progesterone. Anorexics begin to lose bone mass at the same rapid rate as menopausal women.

4. Exercise Regularly

Regular exercise provides many different kinds of benefits, and the right kind of exercise can be a crucial protection for your bones. Not every type of exercise strengthens the bones. It must be what is called weight-bearing exercise—in other words, exercise that makes your body work against gravity. Swimming, for example, may build muscle and aid cardiovascular conditioning, but it won't have a direct effect on your bones. Here's a good illustration. No one would question that astronauts have fine conditioning, but if you put an astronaut in space where he or she is weightless, osteoporosis will develop. Our bones need to feel the effect of gravity to remain strong.

Upper body exercise is very important for women because, between osteoporosis and gravity, the natural tendency is for us to stoop over.

Exercising with hand weights helps to strengthen the back extensor muscles which pull us upright. Note that in one study, women who took aerobic classes still showed bone loss in the upper body until hand weights were added. Weight training is not limited to the young. Studies have shown that weight training can prevent bone loss even in elderly women.

Let me add a cautionary note about exercise. Although it is essential to building and maintaining bone strength, women who overdo it may risk a reverse effect. Intense physical activity can cause menstrual dysfunction, and athletes who have amenorrhea have much less bone density than athletes with normal cycles. Furthermore, one study showed that ovulatory disturbances occurred in 29 percent of women, whether they were marathon runners, joggers, or just normally active.

THE BEST BONE-BUILDING EXERCISES

► **Walking**
► **Jogging**
► **Wearing wrist and ankle weights while walking or jogging**
► **Jumping rope**
► **Upper body weight lifting**
► **Low-impact aerobics**

---

5. Take Estrogen Replacement at Menopause

Since bone loss begins to happen very rapidly with estrogen depletion, the number-one risk factor is menopause. That includes the surgical removal of ovaries. A fifty-year-old woman who had her ovaries removed at age thirty has a bone density comparable to a seventy-year-old woman who reached menopause at fifty.

Some doctors prescribe estrogen replacement therapy for ten to fifteen years, then discontinue it. Although temporary ERT is certainly better than none, as soon as you stop taking it, you'll start losing bone again, just as you would have had you not taken hormones after menopause.

If you can't take estrogen, you'll need to be especially aggressive in your approach to osteoporosis prevention. That means watching your daily calcium intake, not smoking, and performing regular weight-bearing exercise. You should also ask your doctor about some of the new treatments that appear to have bone-strengthening effects.

One promising new treatment is the drug editronate, which has been found to reverse some of the bone damage to the spine caused by osteoporosis. There is no evidence that editronate will reverse bone damage in other parts of the skeleton.

Calcitonin injections promote the absorption of calcium, and some doctors recommend them for women who cannot take replacement hormones. However, this is an extremely demanding form of therapy, since the injections must be administered every day. (A nasal spray form of this drug is in the future.)

If you are considering any of these treatments, you need to weigh the risks and benefits with your doctor. And never assume that drug treatment will replace a bone-strengthening nutrition and exercise program.

Fortunately, aside from some relatively rare genetic factors, osteoporosis is a completely preventable disease affected by lifestyle factors. If we can be educated about risks and make the necessary adjustments, we could nearly erase it from the map of ailments that afflict elderly women. You and your daughters would not grow into frail little old ladies, but maintain your strength and independence long into life. That's a goal worth striving for!

COMMON QUESTIONS ABOUT OSTEOPOROSIS

I'm fifty. Is it too late to start protecting myself against osteoporosis?

You can't rebuild the bone mass you've already lost, but you can halt further bone loss. Since you're only fifty, you may be premenopausal or have just started menopause. If you begin estrogen replacement therapy within five years of menopause, you can halt rapid bone loss, and even have some bone gain. If you don't smoke, estrogen replacement therapy, in combination with sufficient dietary or supplemental calcium and regular weight-bearing exercises, will keep your bones strong. Incidentally, it is never too late to start estrogen replacement. Even if you are seventy-five years old, it can have a beneficial bone strengthening effect.

Should every woman get a bone density test at menopause?

If a woman does not have prominent risk factors and she is taking estrogen after menopause, I normally don't prescribe a bone density test. It's not particularly cost-effective for every woman to be screened, especially since current tests don't indicate the likelihood and rate of future bone loss. For women who start ERT for documented osteoporosis, I usually get a follow-up scan at one year to assess the efficacy of the treatment.

I have been advised to do weight-bearing exercises to prevent osteoporosis, but I have also heard they're not safe. What's the answer?

Weight-bearing exercise helps keep your bones dense, but certain types of weight-bearing exercise can be harmful to women who have osteoporosis. For example, carrying heavy bags of groceries or other weights can place too much pressure on the spine, causing spinal compression fractures. If your bone density is already compromised by osteoporosis, many otherwise safe activities can fracture your ribs. Even a very tight hug or being in the missionary position during sex can be harmful.

Is osteoarthritis the same as osteoporosis?

It's similar in the sense that it afflicts older women and impairs function. But it's a very different disease. Osteoarthritis is a chronic noninflammatory deterioration of the bone cartilage. It is more common in women than in men. A generalized form of osteoarthritis can occur acutely in women at menopause, and it is believed to be affected by estrogen levels. You see it most often in women's hands, especially knobby knuckles, but also in the knees, hips, feet, and vertebrae. The signs of osteoarthritis are very clear; you'll feel pain, aching joints, and morning stiffness. The temptation is to remain sedentary, but the best thing you can do for this condition is to stay active.

Does the estrogen patch protect your bones as much as the estrogen pill?

Yes. This has been clearly shown, even when the patch delivers minimum levels of estrogen.

Calcium supplements constipate me and give me gas. What can I do?

Try a different formulation—like changing from calcium carbonate to calcium citrate. Or try to get your requirements through diet alone. If you are lactose intolerant, drink lactose-free milk or take lactose tablets. Or try drinking soy milk or eating soy products.

Should anorexic women take estrogen?

Yes. Women with eating disorders who fail to menstruate are in danger of osteoporosis. Oral contraceptives are a recommended treatment for those who are unable to gain weight.

I take diuretics (water pills) for high blood pressure. Do I need to worry about osteoporosis?

Thiazide diuretics are associated with decreased urinary loss of calcium and increased bone density, especially among Caucasian women. A recent study did not show this to be true for African-American women. However, the results might be due to increased body mass, not diuretic use. The data are not yet clear.

RESOURCES

National Osteoporosis Foundation
1150 17th Street, NW, Suite 500
Washington, DC 20036
202-223-2226

9

SENSITIVE BLADDERS
The Unspoken Complaints

~~~

By the time Barbara made her way to my office, she had run the gamut of medical specialists and was at her wit's end. Her problem was creating havoc in her life, yet no one had been able to identify the cause—much less recommend a solution. I listened carefully as this forty-five-year-old woman described her symptoms in high-pitched agitation.

"I urinate about thirty times a day," she said. "Actually, day and night. I wake up several times. And it hurts so much—like I'm getting cut open. At first, I thought it was a urinary infection, which I've had before. I went to my doctor figuring he'd prescribe an antibiotic and that would be that. But he couldn't find any sign of infection. He sent me to a urologist and he couldn't find anything. He said maybe it was caused by stress. I never knew stress could cause something like this, but I tried relaxation exercises just to see if it would help. To tell you the truth, my worst stress was what was happening to my body."

Barbara went on to describe weeks of spiraling frustration, pain, and physical exhaustion. "My husband was sympathetic at first, but he's losing patience," she said. "He thinks I'm imagining it or bringing it on myself, and I should just stop. Our sex life is nil, he's hostile, I'm on edge. What a mess.

If only I knew what was wrong, I think I could deal with it. The problem is not knowing."

As I listened to Barbara, I could feel the depth of her unhappiness and confusion. Her symptoms were very real; she was not imagining the constant need to urinate, nor the pain. Based on her symptoms, I immediately considered interstitial cystitis, a poorly understood bladder condition suffered mostly by women that often remains undiagnosed. I told Barbara, "I know you don't believe that what you're experiencing is all in your head. Neither do I. Let's take it step by step and eliminate the possibility of an infection or other cause. If we do this, we can investigate what it might be." I explained to her that some bladder conditions don't have visible causes, and she might have one of them. She looked so relieved to hear this that she almost cried. Finally, she was being taken seriously.

Bladder problems are one of the great unmentionables among women's ailments. One reason is our embarrassment and reluctance to talk about symptoms that are associated with sexual activity or bladder functions. Another reason is that the medical profession has been slow to identify and treat what has become a crippling problem for so many women. Women who report bladder problems are often not taken seriously. When doctors fail to find a specific bacterial source, they readily blame stress or psychological problems. This attitude drives women away. It only makes sense that you would be reluctant to complain about symptoms if you think you're going to be told their basis is psychosomatic. The fact is, while bladder diseases may be made worse by stress, they are never caused by stress.

I've seen women who had recurring bouts of cystitis throughout their adult life, and their dominant attitude was one of resignation: "This is my cross to bear. Nothing can be done. I have to accept it."

Bladder related diseases afflict women thirty times as often as men, and that may be why there has been such a silence about them. Again, if the medical norm were based on women, there's little doubt that we would have made a major effort to address and educate the public long ago. It's hard to imagine hundreds of thousands of men suffering in silence from afflictions that cause so much pain, inconvenience, and embarrassment.

THE NORMAL BLADDER

Unlike your bowel or vagina where bacteria live normally, the bladder is a sterile environment that contains no bacteria. The flushing that occurs several times a day with urination helps maintain a healthy, sterile bladder. Bladder infections occur when bacteria enter the bladder and are not fought off by its defenses. However, there are also bladder complaints that are not related to bacteria. These have typically been the most difficult to diagnose and treat. Even when bacteria are found, there is no clear explanation for why some women have recurrent infections, while others do not.

The wide range of complaints related to the bladder have commonly been grouped together in a broad category known as cystitis. But bladder problems are not always urinary tract infections caused by bacteria; they differ in character and cause. The following are the most common.

BACTERIAL CYSTITIS: A PERSISTENT PROBLEM

Bacterial cystitis, a term meaning bladder infections, is one of the most common afflictions women suffer. By some measures, one of every five women will suffer from bacterial cystitis during her life. And many of those women will live with bacterial cystitis as an ongoing ailment, constantly treated only to reappear months or years later. It is terribly disheartening to these women, since nothing seems to end the cycle. They feel stuck with it for life.

What causes bacterial cystitis? Essentially, it is the result of bacteria getting into the bladder. The primary causes seem to be sexual activity and hygiene. Postmenopausal changes can weaken the bladder's ability to keep bacteria out.

You may have heard of "honeymoon cystitis," an inaccurate term used to describe an infection of the bladder that sometimes accompanies sexual activity. It has been found that cystitis often follows the beginning of sexual activity, a change in partners, or frequent intercourse. In fact, one study showed that cystitis was 12.8 times more common in the general population than it was among nuns who were assumed to be celibate.

The explanation is simple. During intercourse, bacteria that normally live in the vagina can be pushed into the bladder through the urethral opening, which is just in front of the vagina. The problem seems to be greatly enhanced if you use a diaphragm during intercourse because it puts pressure on the urethra and changes the angle between the bladder and urethra, obstructing the flow. Bacteria, which can easily enter the bladder, are quickly eliminated during urination. However, sometimes they "stick" to the inside of the bladder and cause infection.

A urinary infection is different from a vaginal infection although the two conditions can be related. Vaginal infections can cause urethral irritation and produce symptoms like painful urination. But in these cases, the urine itself contains no bacteria. By the same token, common treatments for urinary infections can lead to vaginal infections. Some antibiotics that kill bacteria in the urinary tract and bladder can also kill "good" bacteria living in the vagina, predisposing you to a vaginal yeast infection. These "good" bacteria keep the vagina acidic and prevent the overgrowth of yeast.

Pregnant women are often susceptible to cystitis because of hormonal changes that affect the kidney and bladder. Often this cystitis is silent—only detected through urine tests. A urine test is a standard part of every prenatal visit to rule out an infection that might cause more serious problems for both the mother and the fetus, such as premature labor.

Bacterial cystitis can also occur without sexual activity when the normal bacteria that live in the bowel and the vagina invade the bladder. This happens if stool matter gets into the vagina. The issue here is hygiene, although it can happen to even the most scrupulous person. In fact, *E.* coli (*Escherichia* coli) bacteria, the most common bowel bacteria, are said to be the cause of most bladder infections.

SYMPTOMS OF BACTERIAL CYSTITIS

▶ **Painful, frequent urination of small amounts**
▶ **Sensation of pulling or pressure in the pelvis**
▶ **Low-back pain (accompanied by other symptoms)**
▶ **Low-grade fever (accompanied by other symptoms)**

Diagnosing Bacterial Cystitis

Sometimes a woman will experience painful, frequent urination, the doctor will do a test and discover bacteria in the urine, an antibiotic will be prescribed, and that will be the end of it. But large numbers of women experience cystitis as a recurring syndrome. If you're among them, you have an entire history related to your problem. Therefore, before you see a doctor, take time to write down your history. In particular, you should document:

▶ The number, dates, symptoms, and duration of previous infections.

▶ How were they treated? Did the treatment work?

▶ What medications have you taken that were specifically related to bladder infections, and what other medications are you currently taking?

▶ If you are sexually active, the frequency of sex, the number of partners, whether you have a new partner, and your method of contraception.

▶ Incidences of cystitis during pregnancy.

▶ Surgeries—especially pelvic surgery or hysterectomy.

When I see a woman who has symptoms of cystitis, I'll normally perform a urinalysis, looking for the presence of white blood cells, but sometimes I treat cystitis empirically, based on symptoms, without incurring the cost of a urinalysis. Then, if the symptoms don't resolve, I will do a culture and urinalysis to see if there are bacteria present that are not sensitive to the antibiotic, or if there's another cause for the symptoms.

Recurrent cystitis is actually quite normal in a young, sexually active woman. Cystitis is also a problem for postmenopausal women. The urethra and vagina depend on estrogen to grow thick and healthy tissues. Without estrogen, they thin out and become more vulnerable to infection. Recent studies have shown that hormone treatment (even in the form of estrogen cream applied to the vagina) is helpful in eliminating recurrent postmeno-pausal cystitis.

Taking Control of Bacterial Cystitis

For an isolated case of cystitis, antibiotics usually resolve the problem. Be aware, however, that antibiotics are no longer prescribed for a ten-day course. Three days are usually enough to resolve the problem, and you don't need the extra cost and exposure to antibiotics—especially if you're sensitive to yeast infections. If you know you get yeast infections every time you take antibiotics, take acidophilus in pill form or by eating yogurt, or use anti-yeast creams in the vagina simultaneously.

If, in spite of antibiotic treatment, you have recurring bouts of cystitis, there are several things you can do to take preventive measures.

1. **Adjust Your Sexual Activity.** Sometimes intercourse or clitoral stimulation by a partner or yourself pushes bacteria into the urethra. Try to void urine after sexual activity to flush out any bacteria introduced during

intercourse. Women with recurrent infections sometimes take an antibiotic tablet before or after sex and find that this helps control the problem.

Whether you're susceptible to bladder infections or not, never follow anal intercourse with vaginal penetration, since that gives bacteria a clear pathway.

If you use a diaphragm for contraception, try another method. Early evidence suggests, for example, that the cervical cap does not carry the same infectious risk.

2. **Use Rigorous Hygiene.** After a bowel movement, always wipe from front to back to reduce the chance that bacteria will be pushed into the vagina.

Change tampons and sanitary pads frequently to discourage bacterial growth.

3. **Watch Your Fluids.** Drink plenty of fluids, especially water, to dilute the urine and lower its bacterial count. It's unknown whether drinking cranberry juice helps to fight infections. If it works for you, go ahead. But it doesn't work for everyone.

Mechanical flushing of the bladder is very helpful to preventing infections, and this can be accomplished by drinking large amounts of any fluid. Also, take time to fully empty your bladder; don't leave behind small amounts of urine in which bacteria can grow.

The Hypersensitive or Painful Bladder

Many women get bladder symptoms that seem like bacterial cystitis but do not show any bacteria. They are often given antibiotics, which do little to relieve their symptoms. Some women notice increased symptoms if they eat or drink certain substances—alcohol, spicy foods, coffee, or citrus drinks. Other women report increased symptoms after sexual intercourse. These women have "hypersensitive bladders" or "painful bladder symdrome." Since there is no single treatment that works for all women, you must experiment to find out what works best for you. Try the following:

▶ Increase your fluid intake to dilute your urine.
▶ Take a urinary anesthetic like Pyridium.
▶ Take hot baths or place a heating pad on your bladder area.
▶ Use nonsteroidal anti-inflammatory drugs like ibuprofen.
▶ Practice bladder training—forcing yourself not to urinate when you feel like it.

Women with bacterial cystitis or hypersensitive bladders have often been told they have a narrow urethra and they are subjected to a procedure called urethral dilation which stretches the urethra with increasingly larger metal rods. This procedure is commonly practiced, even though it does not even appear in urology texts and has no clinical basis. It has been called "the rape of the female urethra." If you are told you have a small urethra and need this procedure, find another doctor!

INTERSTITIAL CYSTITIS: A DOUBLE CRISIS

Like Barbara, the patient I described earlier in the chapter, many women suffer the double whammy of interstitial cystitis (IC)—an extreme form of hypersensitive bladder. Not only do they experience ongoing pain and a complete disruption of their normal lives, but they are frequently blamed for causing the problem or imagining it. Indeed, only in the last decade did the standard urology textbooks stop describing IC as a hysterical female condition. Even today, many doctors will discount the symptoms when they fail to find a bacterial association. The fact that IC afflicts women instead of men 90 percent of the time has made it easier to dismiss. This problem can occur at any age. Infections might be caused by organisms that don't easily show up in cultures—such as chlamydia, mycoplasmas, and ureaplasma. One clue to their presence is when white blood cells appear in the urinalysis but the culture fails to show bacteria. These organisms require special cultures but may be treated with certain antibiotics while the cultures are being tested.

The greatest breakthrough in addressing interstitial cystitis as a valid medical complaint came in 1987 when the Urban Institute, a Washington, D.C., social research organization, conducted a survey. U.I. sent a random questionnaire to 400 urologists and some of their patients and concluded from the results that there were as many as ninety thousand diagnosed cases in the United States—a figure that could be quadrupled if one considers how infrequently the problem has been accurately diagnosed. The U.I. found that the average person with IC symptoms saw two to five doctors over a period of more than four years before they were diagnosed.

The Urban Institute went on to produce some startling statistics that powerfully contradict any lingering suspicion that IC might be a nonexistent disease. Of those diagnosed:

— 50 percent reported having pain while riding in a car
— 63 percent reported painful intercourse
— 50 percent were unable to work full-time
— people with IC rated the quality of their lives lower than did people on kidney dialysis

---

SYMPTOMS OF INTERSTITIAL CYSTITIS

▶ A constant awareness of the bladder
▶ Urgency to urinate
▶ Frequent daytime and nocturnal urination
▶ Pain in the bladder, urethra, or vagina
▶ Pressure or pain in the area over the pubic bone, relieved by voiding
▶ Painful intercourse, or increase in symptoms following intercourse
▶ Difficulty emptying the bladder
▶ Difficulty in starting to urinate

Diagnosing IC

There is no known cause of IC; a commitment to research is a clear mandate. In the meantime, you must be your own advocate: If you're experiencing the symptoms common to IC, make sure that your doctor considers it as a diagnosis. Physician failure to consider this clinical entity is the chief reason for a misdiagnosis. So if your doctor doesn't mention it, you should. If your doctor dismisses it, find another doctor.

Prepare for your doctor's visit by making a complete record of your symptoms, their duration and the times during the day or night when they occur. A daily record might include the following notations:

▶ The times you felt the urge to urinate.
▶ The times you urinated and the quantity of the flow (light, medium, heavy).
▶ A description of pain and when it was greatest—for example, constant pain, burning with urination, pain relieved by urination, painful sexual intercourse.

Also, compile a history of other bladder problems you've had, including previous instances of bacterial cystitis or other complaints.

Ultimately, the only sure way to diagnose IC is with a cystoscopy and bladder distension, performed under general anesthesia. These reveal tiny hemorrhages in the bladder lining that are otherwise invisible and are considered diagnostic of IC.

Sometimes the distension of the bladder under anesthesia relieves the symptoms of IC. If it doesn't, the next standard treatment is injecting a solution of hydrocortisone and dimethylsulfoxide (DMSO) into the bladder on a weekly basis for about eight weeks. Other treatments include amitryptyline and biofeedback for pelvic floor relaxation. A patient-organized group, the Interstitial Cystitis Association, offers local support groups, funds research, and provides information.

INCONTINENCE: THE SHAMEFUL SECRET

Fifty-year-old Lee came in for a checkup after a friend recommended that she see me. She was a well dressed, elegant woman who was very composed as she gave her medical history. I learned that she'd had a hysterectomy two years earlier, but was taking estrogen and experiencing no problems. Lee admitted that she had recently felt worn out and "a little depressed," but she shrugged it off as the pressures of work. When I examined her, I noticed no overt irregularities, but I could sense by Lee's demeanor that something was troubling her. After the examination, we sat in my office and talked. "So, what's happening in your life?" I asked—a question I address to all of my patients. Lee told me that she was doing well except for the tiredness and feeling a little depressed. Then she paused and looked away. "There's one thing," she said, her face flaming with embarrassment. "Maybe you could tell me . . ."

"Of course. What's up?" Noticing the sudden shift in her mood, I tried to sound casual.

"Well," she stumbled. "I have these, uh, accidents. Not often, just once in a while, but it bothers me."

I tried to soothe her embarrassment. "I'm very glad you mentioned this," I said. "It's important, and it sounds as if it's creating a problem for you. Let's talk this through and see if we can find out what's wrong."

Lee relaxed visibly when I said this, and I knew how hard it must have been for her to admit to a problem that she found so humiliating. I imagined the torment she had been feeling, wondering if a doctor would just dismiss this piece of information as "nothing," or worse still, tell her it was normal after a hysterectomy and she'd just have to live with it.

Incontinence is accompanied by so much shame that it often goes undiagnosed simply because patients can't bear to mention it. They carry their humiliating secrets as an ever present burden, never knowing when an accident might happen. Surveys show that only one person in twelve seeks help for incontinence—and those who do seek help wait an average of nine years before doing so.

The social stigma of incontinence is accompanied by a sense that it only happens if you're old or infirm. As one of my patients put it, "I thought accidents only happen to babies and senior citizens." In fact, although it is more common among the elderly, incontinence can be caused by a variety of factors and can afflict the thirty-year-old woman as well as the seventy-year-old.

Incontinence isn't necessarily a daily experience. Many people have leakage only once a month or a few times a year. On the face of it, this might not seem very serious. But I think it's always serious if it is disrupting your life, causing you to make significant changes in your patterns "just in case," or always hanging over your head as a possibility at work or in social situations. As Dr. Katherine Jeter, editor of the HIP (Help for Incontinent People) Report points out, "Some health professionals refer to a person as being 'slightly incontinent.' That is like being 'a little pregnant.' The unexpected loss of urine in any amount, on a regular basis, in an inconvenient place is incontinence."

The major risk factor for incontinence is vaginal delivery. Since the

---

SYMPTOMS OF INCONTINENCE

▶ The urge to urinate, followed by leakage before you can make it to the bathroom.
▶ Urinary leakage caused by coughing, sneezing, laughing, or exercising.
▶ Nocturnal wetting.
▶ Leakage at unpredictable times.

beginning of recorded medical history, vaginal delivery has been known to damage the pelvic floor, causing bladder and bowel incontinence. Over time, we have learned to intervene before prolonged pressure of the fetal head on the pelvic floor destroys the area. Even when a rupture of the anal sphincter is repaired, women can go on to have incontinence of stool and gas. Forty-four percent of women who gave birth multiple times without suffering overt ruptures of their anal sphincters have some disruption of the sphincter. Little research has been done on how the effects of age or disease might complicate childbirth damage.

A number of things may trigger an episode of incontinence. You might leak urine when you laugh, sneeze, or cough. It might happen when you're nervous. You might suddenly feel the urge to urinate and leak before you can make it to the bathroom. But why do these triggers affect some people and not others? What exactly is incontinence and what causes it? There are four basic types of incontinence:

▶ Stress Incontinence—the leakage of urine during exertion, coughing, sneezing, laughing, sports, or other activities that place stress on the bladder. This is caused by a weakness in the pelvic floor muscles and tissue that support the urethra and bladder when there is increased abdominal pressure. All the abdominal force comes down on top of the bladder instead of around it because the bladder is lower than it should be. This often happens after vaginal deliveries or with physical changes associated with aging. It is not caused by "emotional stress"—a common myth.

▶ Urge Incontinence—the inability to hold urine long enough to reach the toilet. This is increasingly common as women grow older, and it is often found in people with conditions like stroke, Parkinson's disease, and multiple sclerosis. Bed-wetting often occurs in these conditions. Urge incontinence is also known as unstable bladder because the bladder spasms and pushes out the urine at unexpected moments.

▶ Overflow Incontinence—the leakage of small amounts of urine from a bladder that is always full because the bladder muscle is too weak to push the urine out; often, there is no sense of having a full bladder. Overflow incontinence is relatively uncommon, usually occurring in people with diabetes.

▶ Functional Incontinence—a condition of disabled or elderly people who have normal bladder control but because of arthritis or other crippling disorders have trouble reaching the toilet in time.

There are two basic underlying causes of incontinence that manifests itself in the first three conditions. One is the failure of your bladder to properly store urine. The other is the failure of your bladder to properly empty urine.

Stress and urge incontinence can sometimes overlap, and tests may not accurately determine which group a patient falls into.

It's important to get an accurate diagnosis of your condition—and to make sure the cause is treated, not just the symptoms. Treatments will vary depending on the type of problem you have.

Diagnosing Incontinence

Since I became aware of incontinence, it has become routine for me to include questions about it. It's been an eye-opener! I admit I have been shocked to see how many women have problems with incontinence, and how many women dismiss it as not being worthy of discussion or treatment.

If you are a woman who has this problem, I urge you to be open about it. There's nothing shameful (or futile!) about incontinence. Tell your doctor.

Prepare for your doctor's visit by compiling the following information:

▶ A description of when your incontinence occurs, frequency, amount, and what you're doing when it happens.
▶ An account of other bladder-related problems.
▶ The medications you're taking.
▶ Other conditions, such as diabetes, multiple sclerosis, Parkinson's disease, or stroke that might influence your condition.
▶ Childbirth history.
▶ Surgical history.

A full examination of the pelvis is important. Does the bladder drop down when you are asked to bear down? Is there prolapse (falling down) of the pelvic organs pressing on the bladder? Does the vagina look thinned out due to estrogen loss?

If an infection is present, often treating the infection will eliminate the incontinence. Vaginal atrophy can be treated with estrogen replacement, although it takes a while to restore the tissue. Incontinence unresponsive to simple measures should be referred to a urologist specializing in female bladder disorders.

Managing Incontinence

Often, urinary incontinence is manageable and responds well to behavioral, medical, or surgical treatment. Since most urologists and gynecologists are trained in surgical approaches to these problems, they will often fail to recommend nonsurgical remedies or will tell women that they are ineffective. If you have incontinence, there are several effective nonsurgical ways to reduce its impact on your life—and potentially eliminate it.

1. Practice Pelvic Exercises

Here's an exercise program that has been shown to be very effective for both stress and urge incontinence. It is adapted from the Pelvic Training Manual, produced by HIP.

STEP 1: Identify the two different muscle groups: the muscles around your anus, and the muscles around your vagina and urethra.

Muscles Around the Anus: Tighten the area around your anus as if you are trying to stop a bowel movement. The muscles working are the ring of muscles around your anus.

Muscles Around the Vagina and Urethra: Tighten the muscles around the vagina and urethra, as if you were trying to stop the flow of urine. (If you're not sure which muscles these are, practice while you're actually urinating, stopping and starting the flow.)

STEP 2: Lie comfortably on the floor or bed, breathing steadily and deeply. Place one hand on your lower abdomen; it should remain still while you are doing the exercises, since contracting the abdominal muscles will make leakage worse.

Tighten the anal muscles, pulling inward and upward. Hold tightly while counting slowly to ten. Relax. Be sure you're not just contracting the muscles in your buttocks.

Tighten the vaginal muscles, pulling inward and upward. Hold tightly while counting slowly to ten. Relax.

Repeat a series of twenty, five times a day, to a total of one hundred. Be patient. It takes at least three months to tell if it works.

2. Practice Biofeedback

This is a learning technique that can help you exert better control over urine storage and release. It utilizes visual or audio aids to give you moment-by-moment information on how well you are controlling your muscles. Over time, you learn to better control your muscles automatically. Biofeedback has been shown to produce complete control of incontinence in 20 to 25 percent of patients and to provide substantial improvement for an additional 30 percent.

3. Retrain Your Bladder

Bladder retraining is a process that sets defined intervals for urination, in effect reducing the frequency of stress and urge incontinence. What you are doing is scheduling your daily urination at regular short intervals, then gradually extending the intervals until you have established a new pattern. Obviously this method takes a great deal of planning and schedule flexibility, so it might be impractical for many people.

4. Use Postmenopausal Estrogen Replacement

Estrogen can be a productive element in incontinence treatment for postmenopausal women. Estrogen affects the female continence mechanism because the vagina and urethra both depend on estrogen to maintain proper functioning. Although estrogen has not been shown to be effective in reducing stress incontinence, it is very effective in reducing urge incontinence. However, it takes at least one month to see a response, and up to one year for the lining of the urethra and vagina to fully restore themselves.

Certain medicines can control involuntary bladder spasms and urge incontinence. Stress incontinence can sometimes be helped with over-the-counter medicines commonly used as decongestants, which tighten the urethra. The only treatment for overflow incontinence is self-catherization, a process where a tube is placed inside the bladder at fixed intervals to drain the urine.

While you are in the process of getting urinary incontinence managed, it may be necessary to wear absorbent pads. But never consider absorbent pads as a permanent solution. If your doctor hasn't been helpful in dealing with your incontinence, find a urologist who specializes in female bladder problems.

When Is Surgery Appropriate?

Stress incontinence is not usually a well-defined state. There is a wide spectrum of profiles ranging from a seventeen-year-old gymnast who experiences mild leakage when she hits the mat, to the older woman who experiences copious leakage when she clears her throat. Conservative therapies should always be tried first, but if these don't work a woman should never be told, "It's normal. Learn to live with it."

These are some things you should know about surgery:

▶ Surgery relieves only stress incontinence, not other urinary disorders.
▶ Surgery sometimes produces new voiding problems. This occurs in between 5 and 15 percent of surgery patients.
▶ Stress incontinence often coexists with pelvic organ prolapse. This should be ascertained prior to surgery so that all organs can be repaired during one operation.
▶ Stress incontinence is caused by either poor urethral support or poor urinary sphincter function. Surgery must be tailored to the specific cause.
▶ Hysterectomy is not a standard part of this surgery and is indicated only if there is a uterine disease.

Managing Your Social Life

If you have pain, the constant need to urinate, or incontinence, it is going to have some impact on your social life. You may feel restricted from enjoying sports and other physical activities, resist going to parties, restaurants, or the theater, avoid long trips, or stop inviting friends to visit. Every decision about your day may become framed around whether there is a convenient bathroom, or if you dare to wear certain styles or colors of clothing. Your bladder may become your obsession.

The most dramatic arena affected is your sex life. The dread surrounding sex is based on a relentless barrage of worries:

▶ What if I wet the bed?
▶ I want sex, but it hurts too much.
▶ How can I relax about sex when it might cause an infection?
▶ I don't feel very sexy.
▶ What if I have to keep getting up to go to the bathroom?

▶ How do I explain my condition to a new partner?
▶ Won't my partner be turned off?
▶ I don't feel very good about myself right now.

Unfortunately, our cultural ideals about sex have made it very difficult for people with any kind of physical disabilities to be fully sexual. It helps enormously to have a sensitive partner who doesn't hold your disability against you. If you do not have a partner, and worry that no one will ever be interested in you, you might find support from one of the organizations listed at the end of this chapter. The most important point, however, is that you know you're not less worthy because you have an infirmity that life dealt you. Bladder problems (even incontinence) don't have to run your life.

COMMON QUESTIONS ABOUT BLADDER PROBLEMS

I occasionally leak a little urine while playing tennis. Does that mean I'm incontinent?

I imagine most women leak urine at one time or another, especially if they haven't emptied their bladders fully during urination. It's not uncommon for this to happen while you're exercising. I suggest you practice the pelvic exercises described in this chapter. You might also take an over-the-counter decongestant (like Sudafed) that will act to keep the urethra closed. Make sure it's okay with your doctor and, if so, try taking it one hour before exercising.

Is incontinence reversible?

It is more accurate to say that incontinence is controllable. To a great extent, the prognosis depends on the reason for your incontinence. If it is the result of prolapse, you may need a surgical solution. If the cause is weak pelvic floor muscles, exercise can help. Doctors have also found that very small doses of antispasmodics or antidepressants that also have antispasmodic effects can be effective for treating urge incontinence.

I am already taking oral estrogen, but I still have a problem with incontinence. What should I do?

Sometimes oral estrogen is not enough to have a full effect on the urogenital lining—either because you aren't absorbing enough or because the absorbed estrogen isn't getting into the vaginal area in sufficient amounts. I sometimes add estrogen vaginal cream for women who have persistent incontinence and vaginal atrophy while on oral therapy, and I consider other avenues of treatment if that doesn't work.

RESOURCES

ORGANIZATIONS
Help for Incontinent People (HIP) Inc.
P.O. Box 544
Union, SC 29379
Publishes the *HIP Report.*

Interstitial Cystitis Association
P.O. Box 1553
Madison Square Station
New York, NY 10159
Publishes the *ICA Update.*
212-979-6057

PUBLICATIONS
Overcoming Bladder Disorders: Compassionate, Authoritative Medical and Self-Help Solutions for Incontinence, Cystitis, Interstitial Cystitis, Prostate Problems, Bladder Cancer
by Rebecca Chalker and Kristene E. Whitmore, M.D.
HarperPerennial, 1990.

Overcoming Cystitis: A Practical Self-Help Guide for Women
by Wendy Smith
Bantam Books, 1987.

10
THE FATIGUED WOMAN
Mysteries of the Immune System

~~~

The most frequent complaint I see in my practice is fatigue. I am no different from other doctors in that respect. In fact, one out of four complaints to primary care practitioners is fatigue. But fatigue is not just one clearly defined complaint. For some women, it is physical tiredness, for others mental exhaustion, and for others irresistible sleepiness. Sometimes fatigue follows on the heels of a viral illness or a body injury. Often it comes at a time of stress, and it's frequently associated with depression. It can accompany a feeling of achiness and abnormal sleep patterns. Some women experience waxing and waning sore throats, swollen glands, and low-grade fevers. The patient group is very diverse and the medical literature is very muddy. What strikes me as most interesting, though, is that fatigue sufferers are overwhelmingly female, usually white, and on average in their thirties. This profile is so similar to the diagnosis of neurasthenia of one hundred years ago that it makes me wonder if we are living in another one of those times when women resort to this type of sick behavior to extricate themselves from unhappy lives.

What do we know about the causes of fatigue? Some experts think the source is a viral illness that tickles the immune system into prolonged activity, and the fatigue symptoms are secondary. Others believe that altered neurochemistry associated with depression can cause sleep abnormalities, lower pain threshold, and depress immune function. Still other experts are convinced that all fatigue-related symptoms stem from a primary sleep disturbance that causes an alteration of the immune system, irritability, and muscle pain.

An interesting study evaluated men and women who were referred to a sleep clinic because of snoring. The classic snorer shows altered breathing patterns during sleep, daytime sleepiness, and fatigue; the syndrome is most commonly seen in men. However, when snoring women were evaluated, a different clinical picture emerged. Women had more fatigue, headache, and trouble getting to sleep, and fewer of the male-defined symptoms like altered breathing pattern during sleep. This may be another case in which female patterns go unrecognized.

There is some evidence that progesterone is implicated in fatigue and may be an important modulator of the stress hormone called cortisol. Some fatigue sufferers seem to show abnormal progesterone levels.

What seems clear to me is that fatigue is a final common pathway to many disorders, and physicians must validate the experiences of patients who complain about it.

Depression, pain, and fatigue often overlap, and it is not up to the physician to make a value judgment about what is worthy of consideration and what is not. Physicians need to be good detectives in finding aspects of the illness that are treatable, and to be advocates in helping their patients go on with their lives. In particular, doctors need to be wary of prescribing a "rest cure" for a woman who complains of fatigue. Although rest might seem to be the perfect antidote for tiredness, it has been well documented that chronic pain, fatigue, injury, or illness can initiate a cycle that causes deconditioning—a state where aerobic capacity is reduced, and the heart works harder at rest and at lower levels of exertion.

There is no objective marker or simple blood test to aid a diagnosis. However, there are two distinct types of fatigue syndromes. The first is called fibromyalgia, a disorder accompanied by multiple sore spots on the body that exist in the context of disturbed sleep, fatigue, and depression. Exercise reduces fatigue, and low doses of certain antidepressants can quite effectively eliminate all the symptoms. Some researchers find that women with fibromyalgia are "hypervigilant"—more aware of sensations, especially pain.

Jennifer presented a typical profile of fibromyalgia. When I first met her, I was impressed by what a dynamo she was. She was a physician and a mother. Her energy level was high, she exercised regularly, and it seemed there was nothing she couldn't do.

Jennifer started having severe muscle aches when she was forty. She would feel stiff in the morning, gradually loosening up as the day went on. However, she couldn't shake the feeling of being fatigued, except when she was jogging. At night, she tossed and turned in bed, unable to find a comfortable position. As time went on, Jennifer grew irritable and depressed. Nothing seemed to help. She finally came to see me and spilled out her misery.

Working with a rheumatologist, we did a complete immune workup and found nothing. We began treating Jennifer's muscle soreness with anti-inflammatory drugs, and her pain lessened somewhat, but her fatigue, sleeplessness, and depression remained unchanged. I had read the studies concerning the potential of low-dose tricyclic antidepressants to treat fibro-myalgia. We started Jennifer on this medication and a miracle ensued. Not only did she feel better, she was able to discontinue the anti-inflammatory medication and just stay on tricyclics. It was a real success story.

The other type of fatigue pattern, called Chronic Fatigue Syndrome, is more complex, and I suspect that it has been overused as a label by patients and doctors. The best criterion for CFS is that of the Centers for Disease Control, which identifies CFS as persistent fatigue lasting six months or more, not linked to any other medical or psychiatric disorder. Symptoms of CFS include chills, sore throat, muscle weakness, painful lymph glands, fatigue, headache, and sleep disturbance.

Rita was a classic case of CFS. A vibrant, healthy woman all of her life, she got sick last summer with a fever of 103 degrees Fahrenheit, a mild sore throat, and a headache. Because she spent a lot of time on Fire Island, an area with endemic Lyme disease, I took the precaution of treating her even when her Lyme antibody test came back negative.

Rita's fever went away, but nearly a year later, she still has profound fatigue, trouble concentrating, and recurrent episodes of sore throat, swollen glands, and achiness. Every time she exerts herself, she winds up in bed for three days, and she has taken a leave of absence from her job as a film editor.

Recently, I have been talking to Rita about the possibility of her trying Prozac, which is a serotonin-enhancing drug. Serotonin is a neurotransmitter responsible for certain mood-related functions. Studies had indicated that low serotonin levels are often found in sleep disorders, chronic pain, and depression, and sometimes Prozac helps people with CFS. Rita has been hesitant to use Prozac. Like many women, she is rightly afraid of having her real symptoms dismissed as unreal or irrational. Being diagnosed with a viral illness feels acceptable to her, but having a psychiatric one is not. So, we go round and round on the discussion of the mind-body connection. I feel for Rita because both her illness and her fears are legitimate. I hope we can find a way to help her get the relief she needs.

CHECK IT OUT

If you relate to the descriptions I have given of fatigue, I urge you to have your symptoms checked out with a physical exam. Your doctor should be thorough in getting a good history: Did your fatigue start abruptly following a flu-like illness, or was it insidious? What is your mood, stress level, and social support? Have you had any acutely stressful events, like a loss of some kind? Are you overextended in your responsibilities and activities? Do you take any medication that can cause fatigue, like antihistamines, antihypertensives, sedatives, or cardiac medications? High risk behavior for HIV infection should be asked about, as well as other health behavior. Poor nutrition, smoking, alcohol, caffeine, opiates, and cocaine use can compromise your immune system. When was your last period, and have you had unprotected intercourse? Could you be pregnant, or menopausal? Sometimes menopause starts with a flare in multiple joint pains, known as generalized osteoarthritis, and chronic pain can lead to sleep disturbances and altered mood.

Associated symptoms should be detailed; make a list in preparation for your doctor's visit. The list might include night sweats, weight loss or gain, temperature intolerance, change in bowel habits, excessive thirst, and chest discomfort or shortness of breath. Headaches and a history of head trauma can be an important clue in older women who might suffer fatigue and irritability as a sign of a brain bleeding called a subdural hematoma. Skin changes or rashes might signal autoimmune disorders. Sleep patterns should be investigated, including difficulty in getting to or staying asleep, snoring, and daytime sleepiness.

When a patient comes to me complaining of fatigue, I order a number of tests to rule out specific conditions—thyroid test, blood count, liver and kidney chemistries, autoimmune markers, pregnancy, or menopause tests, and tests for infections when they're appropriate.

The Female Immune System

Fatigue is also a prominent symptom in autoimmune diseases, another women's health issue. The immune system differs in men and women because it is in part regulated by sex hormones. There is an intimate connection between the ovary, the thymus (a gland crucial to immune system development and functioning), and the trio of glands known as the HPA axis—hypothalamic, pituitary, and adrenal. All work in concert to regulate many of the body's functions. Immune cells fluctuate during menstruation and pregnancy. Estrogen receptors have been found on T cells, especially suppressor T cells, and these have been found in ovarian follicular fluid, suggesting that immune cells may play a role in follicle maturation.

By our very nature, women have a unique set of hormonal activities that complicate the job of our immune systems. Estrogen depresses immunity, including cancer immune surveillance. Progesterone encourages the growth of T-helper cells, which is why women have higher levels of antibodies than men. Women also have higher levels of autoantibodies—antibodies made against their own tissues.

Autoantibodies are normal to some extent, but when they hyperactivate and begin destroying an organ, that's pathological. A good example is insulin-dependent diabetes where the immune system literally destroys the pancreas. Or systemic lupus erythematosus (known as lupus) where antibodies float around in the bloodstream and settle in locations designed to collect them. They go on to disrupt those organs by inciting an inflammatory response. For example, if these complexes settle in joints, the result is arthritis; if they settle in the walls of the blood vessels, vasculitis—and so on.

Although the immune system is designed to fight foreign elements, a successful pregnancy depends on the body's ability to recognize and tolerate the presence of male antigens, and to allow a fetus to live and grow without being rejected. So, pregnancy requires a temporary suppression of the immune system. (In fact, a woman who is given a skin graft or other transplant while she's pregnant is less likely to reject it.)

Stress Plays a Role

Joan's husband had been dead for three months when she developed a persistent cold she couldn't shake. When she came in for treatment, she said, "I guess my resistance is low." People often half-seriously explain their colds and flus this way, noticing that infections seem to occur following times of exceptional stress and hard work. They probably don't realize just how direct the connection is. In Joan's case, I was sure she was right. Bereavement studies have borne out the theory that following the death of a spouse and an intense period of mourning, people's immune systems are weaker.

There is convincing evidence that stress has a direct impact on the immune system. From a clinical standpoint, stress represents the reaction of your body to stimuli that disrupt its normal equilibrium—often with deleterious effects. We are used to thinking of stress as a mental problem. But stress is not all in the head. There's a chain reaction when you're experiencing stress. Regardless of the trigger—divorce, a death in the family, overwork, job loss, sexual abuse or discrimination, or general unhappiness—stress releases chemicals from the brain. These neurotransmitters are under the influence of sex steroids, and therefore differ for men and women. They go on to affect the adrenal gland that produces adrenalin and cortisol, the stress hormone. This discharge of neurotransmitters can affect immune function, cortisol being immunosuppressive. The reverse is also true—immune cells can affect the brain.

Many studies have demonstrated a relationship between the inability to handle stress and the body's inability to kill viruses and cancers. The length of survival of people with cancer and certain other infectious diseases, including AIDS, has been correlated with psychosocial factors like depression and social isolation.

Countless studies demonstrate the relationship between immune function and stress. An examination of seventy-five first-year medical students found that those who received high scores on stressful life events displayed significantly lower levels of immune "killer cell" activity. Another study of women who had undergone major life changes showed them to have poorer immune function than women who had fewer changes. In addition, women who experienced long-term stress—such as those who were caretakers for loved ones with Alzheimer's—showed lower immune function.

It was also found that people who experienced extreme stress were more likely to turn to drugs, alcohol, or smoking for relief—activities that further compromised their immune systems. Depression in itself is immunosuppressive, and recovery from depression returns the immune system to its prior normal state.

A strong connection has also been shown between stress levels and the occurrence of insulin-dependent diabetes mellitus. In one study, 46 percent of those diagnosed reported a disturbing life event six months prior to the diagnosis.

Studies demonstrate that a type of inner hardiness is characteristic in people who have healthy immune systems. This hardiness is manifested in a strong commitment to self, an attitude of vigorousness toward one's environment, a sense of personal meaningfulness, and a feeling of being in control. It transcends the actual situations in which people find themselves.

It is fascinating to note that people whose immune systems are most capable of fighting off "bad" elements seem to have a corresponding psychological defense mechanism that allows them to fight off emotional trauma.

To date, the most extensive research in this area has been conducted on two autoimmune disorders that primarily affect women—systemic lupus erythematosus and rheumatoid arthritis.

Lupus is an inflammatory immune disease that is characterized by excessive production of autoantibodies directed against the body's own tissues. It is nine times more common in women than men, and more common still among African-American, Latina, and Asian women. It classically strikes after puberty and before menopause. Lupus is also related to abnormalities in the metabolism of estrogen, progesterone, and androgens.

In addition to symptoms such as fever, skin rash, anemia, photosensitivity, and arthritis, people with lupus often display dramatic psychiatric manifestations. In fact, psychiatric disorders are often diagnosed prior to a diagnosis of lupus.

Rheumatoid arthritis is a debilitating arthritis of multiple joints that affects three times as many women as men. It can occur at any age. RA leads to significant pain and disability and carries a decrease in life expectancy comparable to that of triple-vessel CAD. Symptoms vary with the menstrual cycle and improve with oral contraceptive use, hormone replacement therapy, and pregnancy. Studies have shown a low incidence of RA among oral contraceptive users. When women with rheumatoid arthritis get pregnant, the disease can go into remission, although it can flare up again when the pregnancy is ended. There is also some indication that estrogen replacement in postmenopausal women improves the condition.

Evaluations of women suffering from rheumatoid arthritis have defined certain personality characteristics that are common among them. They appear to be self-sacrificing, compliant, prone to denial of hostility, and depressed. They often have histories of nervousness, tension, and are considered "high strung." Women with this disease who are depressed or who have poor coping mechanisms have a more rapidly progressive course, are more incapacitated, and respond less well to treatment. In fact, physically healthy relatives of RA patients, who themselves have the RA factor present in their blood, appear to be psychologically healthier than those who express the disease.

You've probably heard it said that a positive attitude helps fight disease. In a profound sense, that seems to be true. The way you live your life and the way you feel about yourself and others is a signal to your immune system. We must also be aware that the health care system often focuses on women's weaknesses and risks—biological, physical, and psychological. Women's resilience is rarely considered. Resilience is the ability to mobilize our individual and social resources in response to risk or threat. Contrary to the assumption that women are weak, we often struggle with adversity, defy the odds, and not only survive but thrive. Women who are resilient not only bounce back after illness or insult, they also get a "value added" effect that brings them to an even better place than they were before.

THE THYROID-IMMUNE SYSTEM CONNECTION

Faith got sick while she was on vacation in the country. She had been vomiting for an entire day, and she grew so weak and dehydrated that her husband insisted she go to the emergency room of a small hospital nearby. Faith had a fever, and although they couldn't find evidence of infection, the doctors treated her with antibiotics. It didn't help much. Faith still felt very sick, and she vomited everything she ate.

In desperation, Faith and her husband returned to the city, where she came to see me. She was a forty-seven-year-old woman who had an enlarged thyroid that up until now had been functioning normally. My assessment was that Faith was thyrotoxic (having an extreme excess of thyroid hormone), and I admitted her to the hospital. Her thyroid hormone blood levels were off the wall. Instead of the usual symptoms of palpitations, anxiety, weight loss, excessive sweating, and frequent bowel movements, she presented with fever, vomiting, and heart failure.

Since the thyroid sets the metabolic rate and regulates the function of hormones, it plays a central role in the operation of all parts of your body.

Thyroid disorders like Faith's are sometimes hard to pinpoint. That's not because we don't have good diagnostic tests. It's because thyroid disease isn't considered, even though it's the most common autoimmune disease in women.

The thyroid is a gland that sits in front of the windpipe and works with the pituitary gland to regulate the body's metabolism. It does this through the hormone thyroxine. Thyroxine synthesis depends on having an adequate amount of iodine in the diet (found mostly in seafoods and iodized salt). When iodine is low, a goiter is formed and thyroxine production may fail.

When there is a deficiency of thyroxine, the pituitary gland senses the deficit and produces a stimulating hormone called TSH, which makes the thyroid grow and work harder to keep thyroxine production going. This hormone can now be measured with high accuracy to diagnose thyroid disorders.

Hyperthyroidism, the most common thyroid disease, is the result of too much thyroxine being made by the thyroid gland. The signs of hyperthyroidism are relatively clear when they appear in young women. A good physical exam and blood test can usually pinpoint them. Overproduction of the thyroid hormone causes a speedup of the metabolism, leading to weight loss, excessive hunger, palpitations and racing heart, heavy sweating, frequent bowel movements, and menstrual disorders. In some cases, bulging eyeballs will result from the swelling of tissue behind the eyes.

Hyperthyroidism can be caused by an overactive area of the gland, known as a nodule or adenoma. Or it can be caused by an autoimmune condition known as Graves' disease.

A few years ago, the public became more aware of Graves' disease when First Lady Barbara Bush was diagnosed with the condition. In Mrs. Bush's case, the condition was severe enough that her thyroid gland needed to be destroyed with radioactive iodine. This is a definitive treatment not given to women of childbearing age. Young women are treated with medications that cause the thyroid gland to stop making thyroxine, but it takes a long period of time. Pregnancy can occur while on low dosages of these medications, and sometimes hyperthyroidism can be passed on to the fetus, fortunately without lasting effect.

Hyperthyroidism may be more difficult to recognize in older women. They might lack many of the usual symptoms such as goiter and weight loss, but present with heart palpitations, arrhythmia, or gastrointestinal problems.

The opposite of hyperthyroidism is hypothyroidism, which is an underproduction of thyroxine. Its occurrence increases with age; up to 45 percent of thyroids in women over sixty show some sign of thyroid inflammation called thyroiditis. Many common symptoms of hypothyroidism can be passed off as signs of aging—cold intolerance, constipation, sluggishness, gait problems, fatigue, fluid retention, slow heartbeat, anemia, and high cholesterol.

But again, a thorough physical exam and a simple blood test to measure the TSH levels can easily diagnose hypothyroidism.

Hypothyroidism is almost always an autoimmune disease where antibodies are made to a woman's own thyroid gland. Treatment is easy, with synthetic thyroxine replacing what the body is missing.

TELLTALE SIGNS OF THYROID DISORDERS

HYPERTHYROIDISM	HYPOTHYROIDISM
Excessive thyroid hormone production	**Inadequate thyroid hormone production**
❖	❖
—Weight loss	—Weight gain
—Excessive hunger	—Hair loss
—Heavy sweating	—Dry skin
—Palpitations	—Fluid retention
—Racing heart	—Muscle weakness and aching
—Frequent stooling	—Gait problems
—Bulging eyeballs	—Cold intolerance
—Goiter	—Constipation
—Menstrual abnormalities	—Sluggishness
—Heat intolerance	—Fatigue
	—Menstrual abnormalities

STRESS AND THYROID DISEASE

A clear link has been found between thyroid disease and stress. The most dramatic example was a study of the Danish population during the 1941–45 German occupation that showed a very high incidence of hyperthyroidism in the population, compared with that of the previous 100 years. A recent study of 116 women with Graves' disease found that most of them experienced stressful events immediately prior to their diagnoses.

Depression is associated with hypothyroidism, and subclinical hypothyroidism is common in depressed women. Adding small doses of thyroid hormone can sometimes be very effective in treating the depression. On the other hand, aggressive thyroid replacement in hypothyroid women can induce mania in some.

We can also see a relationship between thyroid disease and depression in that lithium, a drug used to treat manic depression, often causes hypothyroidism. Somehow lithium stimulates the production of antibodies that didn't exist before and these attack the thyroid, and this effect is ten times more common in women lithium-takers. Lithium itself has effects on the immune system. If you have a family history of autoimmune disease and develop manic depressive illness, be sure you stay alert to symptoms when taking lithium.

I often see hypothyroidism in women who have just had babies. Postpartum thyroiditis occurs in between 4 and 6 percent of women. Women will come dragging into my office complaining of extreme fatigue. They're a little embarrassed to be worried about it. I might simply shrug it off to the understandable exhaustion in new mothers. They say, "Of course, I'm tired. My baby isn't sleeping that much at night . . ." and so on.

Diane was typical. A thirty-eight-year-old woman who had delivered a baby four months earlier, she came in for a routine physical. She told me she'd been having trouble sleeping, had lost weight, and was very tense. "I guess I'm just a nervous new mother," she laughed.

My examination showed that Diane's thyroid was swollen, although she had not experienced any pain. This so-called silent thyroiditis occurs 50 percent of the time in recently pregnant women. It is believed to have an autoimmune component related to the activity of the immune system during pregnancy. Although it is usually a transient condition that is treated symptomatically, women with postpartum thyroiditis should be followed because up to 50 percent of them will later develop hypothyroidism.

Thyroid disease affects ovarian function, and if a woman has hyperthyroidism or hypothyroidism she is likely to have menstrual irregularities, including irregular bleeding and infertility. Unfortunately, the connection is not fully understood, but there is plenty of evidence that shows premature menopause and other ovarian problems in women with thyroid disease.

Thyroid disease is another place where abuse exists. Thyroid medications are sometimes prescribed by doctors as a diet aid. The medication speeds up metabolism and causes quick weight loss. I have seen instances where doctors gave thyroid medication to fourteen- and fifteen-year-old girls for weight-loss purposes. Some women are always on the lookout for easy solutions to their weight problems, and they're happy to go along with a doctor who says, "The reason you're overweight is that you have a slow metabolism caused by hypothyroidism. Take this medication." But hypothyroidism is rarely a cause of being fat, and medication should never be used for the purpose of speeding up the metabolism. The usual reason for slow metabolism in women is yo-yo dieting and frequent cycles of weight loss and weight gain.

Overall, I caution you to be careful when you seek care for an immune related disorder—be it CFS or a thyroid problem. It's an area in medicine where many mysteries remain, and the potential for misinformation and quackery is abundant.

COMMON QUESTIONS ABOUT AUTOIMMUNITY

How does a breast implant affect the immune system?

For many years, few problems with silicone breast implants were reported, which led to the assumption that they were safe. Now it turns out that many women have experienced problems—among them, immune system disorders. Many reported cases involve a disorder that looks like scleroderma, a disease associated with toxic chemicals and silica dust. Others have suffered more typical immune diseases such as rheumatoid arthritis and lupus. A recent review of reported cases showed no association between silicone implants and RA, SLE, gout, or muscle pain syndromes. However, more cases of scleroderma occurred in implant users than among the general population of women.

Are there other endocrine problems that are common to women?

Many women have what is known as polyglandular syndromes, where two or more conditions exist simultaneously. It is fairly common, for example, for a woman to present with a thyroid problem and diabetes. Other autoimmune endocrine disorders involve the adrenal gland and the ovary, causing adrenal insufficiency and premature menopause. These disorders are also associated with autoantibodies to other sites, leading to pernicious anemia, myasthenia gravis, and other syndromes.

I have long-standing fatigue. Should I be tested for Epstein-Barr virus?

All of us have been exposed to the Epstein-Barr virus, and whenever the immune system is stimulated, antibody levels to many viruses go up. High levels of EBV are a secondary phenomenon, not a cause. Performing these tests generates income for laboratories and are a way to label patients as having a disease.

Every time I get a cold, I feel wiped out for weeks afterward. Is something wrong with my immune system?

If you are under a great deal of stress, viruses are hard to ward off. Once you have a virus, it can further weaken your immune system, making you vulnerable to further attacks by other viruses. On the other hand, fatigue is a perfectly natural outcome of a virus. Once an infection gets started in your system, your immune system spills out substances that travel to the brain and make you feel fatigued. Your fatigue might well be a sign that your immune system is functioning perfectly.

Do I have to worry about taking too much thyroid hormone?

Yes. When you take too much thyroid hormone, you'll experience symptoms of hyperthyroidism—anxiety, palpitations, extensive sweating, and weight loss. Too much thyroid hormone can also mobilize calcium away from your bones worsening osteoporosis. That's why all women taking thyroid hormone need to keep the dosage in check. And older women need to be very cautious about starting thyroid replacement therapy if they have underactive thyroids. Too much all at once can precipitate angina.

RESOURCES

Lupus Foundation of America
4 Research Place, Suite 180
Rockville, MD 20850
800-558-0121

Myasthenia Gravis Foundation
53 West Jackson Boulevard, Suite 660
Chicago, IL 60604
800-541-5454

National Multiple Sclerosis Society
733 Third Avenue
New York, NY 10017
800-344-4867

American Sleep Disorders Association
1610 14th Street N.W., Suite 300
Rochester, MN 55901-2200
507-287-6006

Arthritis Foundation Information Line
P.O. Box 19000
Atlanta, GA 30326
800-283-7800
404-872-7100 in Georgia
9:00 A.M. to 7:00 P.M. (Eastern Time) Monday–Friday
Provides local physician referrals and information concerning local
chapters of the Arthritis Foundation. Free brochures and other literature
available upon request.

THREE

WOMEN'S LIFE CYCLES

11

PERIODS

The Patterns in Women's Lives

~~~

Evelyn called me complaining about episodes of diarrhea that she was convinced were related to a menstrual problem. I asked her why she thought so. "Well," she replied, "I've been getting diarrhea before my period, and sometimes during my period. I also get it in the week after my period."

As I listened to Evelyn's account of the various times that she experienced diarrhea, I realized that she was describing random episodes that occurred throughout the month. But in her mind, the diarrhea was linked to her menstrual cycle because she charted the episodes in relationship to her period.

I've seen this phenomenon very often in women. Their menstrual cycles are such timekeepers for them that they tend to describe all other events according to where they fall in the cycle. Most of us do this unconsciously. Our periods mark points on our personal calendars. Consider how often you've heard women say—or have said yourself—"It happened the week before my period." Or, "I remember because it was right after my period."

There are many things that mark the distinctive characteristics of a woman apart from her menstrual cycle. But menstruation is the visible sign of life that makes you different as a female. That's not the same as saying you are defined by your menstrual cycle. In the past, scientists believed that

199

women were controlled by their reproductive organs and that there was a direct link between ovaries, uterus, and brain. We saw the demeaning outcome of that thinking in the paternalistic practices of a hundred years ago—ranging from bias to butchery. Regardless of a woman's medical complaint—be it pain, heart palpitations, headaches, depression, fatigue, or seizures—it was diagnosed as an illness of the reproductive organs. Today, when I say that your cycle is the visible sign that makes you different, I am not saying that it controls you, or is the determining factor that makes you who you are. In fact, what is most remarkable to me is that in spite of the fluctuations, discomforts, and inconveniences of menstruation, for the majority of women life goes on. We do our jobs, we take care of our families, we function as productive members of society. Menstruation may be uncomfortable, but it is not, as our predecessors believed, dysfunctional. It is a distinguishing feature of the female physiology, but it does not define you as a woman.

IF WOMEN WERE THE NORM

In 1978, Gloria Steinem wrote a tongue-in-cheek piece entitled, "If Men Could Menstruate." In it, she posited what might occur if by magic it were men who menstruated instead of women. "Clearly," she wrote, "menstruation would become an enviable, boastworthy, masculine event.

"Men would brag about how long and how much.

"Young boys would talk about it as the envied beginning of manhood. Gifts, religious ceremonies, family dinners and stag parties would mark the day . . .

"Generals, right-wing politicians and religious fundamentalists would cite menstruation ('men-struation') as proof that only men could serve God and country in combat ('You have to give blood to take blood') . . ."

And so on. Steinem's premise is amusing, yet our laughter is not without a tinge of bitterness—for it is yet another reminder of how relentlessly the physiological norm is defined from the male perspective.

Imagine how our social institutions and lifestyles might differ if the female experience were used as the norm. Perhaps there would be a rotating three-week work cycle to accommodate women's menstrual cycles. Childbearing would be incorporated as a natural process of life—not the interruption of hard-won career goals. Career tracks would not necessarily be established in the twenties and proceed in a straight, uninterrupted line, but would develop throughout adult life. Support systems would be available for the caretaking roles women perform—be it raising children or nursing elderly parents. Family obligations would be shared equally by men and women. The Social Security system would pay women to be home-based caretakers, allow them to work longer given their later entry into the workforce, and credit their years of caretaking service toward retirement benefits—an advance that has been made in some European countries. Women don't necessarily want to retire at sixty-five. That's when many of them are riding the crest of performance in the workplace.

As it is, women are constantly made to feel as though their very beings are an insult to the smooth operations of society. Bosses worry about hiring women for fear that training will be wasted on someone who might leave to have children. Women are afraid to even mention menstrual irregularities because they don't want to be marked as too temperamental or sickly for serious consideration. (The pejorative remark, "She's on the rag," has been made by more than a few men to insinuate dysfunction.) The normal processes of womanhood are kept a shameful secret, from the time menstruation begins until the time it ends in the most shameful event of all—menopause. Within the male-dominated culture, the most successful women are those who best sublimate their femaleness. They minimize monthly fluctuations, discomforts, flashes, and cramps.

Each woman comes to the issue of menstruation already burdened by centuries of taboos, secretiveness, shame, and misinformation. As I listen to women talk about their periods, I find that most of the focus is on finding ways to make them disappear or not be a problem—or to avoid discussing them because they are an embarrassment. Women are saddled with practical worries every month that never touch men's lives: The woman who sits in a lengthy meeting and prays her tampon won't soak through her skirt; the woman who plans a trip to accommodate her period; the woman who worries because her period is late. Our cycles are a real part of our lives, yet we struggle to make them (and often ourselves) invisible to the world. In doing so, we unconsciously continue the bias that our natural functions make us sick, crazy, or an embarrassment.

It's not at all hard to understand where these attitudes come from. Throughout the centuries, taboos regarding menstruation have been reinforced by religious and cultural practices. The common reference to menstruation as "the Curse" originated with the notion that it was inflicted upon Eve because of her sin, to be passed on to women for all time. The taboo and stigmatization accompanying menstruation has been seen in virtually every religious and cultural tradition.

While many ancient taboos and attitudes have disappeared in this century, the cultural stigma runs so deep that even today, we are influenced by its lengthy history. "Hormonal influences" make an easy scapegoat for dismissing the opinions and actions of women—even when those women are powerful and well regarded. In 1982, during a debate at the United Nations on Great Britain's attack on the Falkland Islands, one diplomat stated that "Prime Minister Margaret Thatcher's actions had to be understood in the context of the glandular system of women."

A woman's relationship to having periods depends on both the cultural standards and the level of education and comfort she feels at the start of menstruation.

Recently, a friend told me of the traumatic reaction her young daughter had to getting her first period. My friend had prepared her daughter for the event—talking to her about it long in advance, giving her books to read, telling her it was a cause for celebration. "I thought I had prepared her pretty well," my friend said wryly. "But when it happened, she was horrified. She thought it was disgusting and she refused to leave her room. She begged me not to tell anyone, especially her father. What I had planned as a celebrative event turned into a catastrophe."

This mother was surprised that her daughter's reaction was so negative, since she had taken great pains to prepare her. But preparation needs to include more than a physiological description of the process. Misconception and confusion abound on the specific details of what it's like to have a period. In one study, college women asked to recall their experiences of menarche, reported that although they were intellectually prepared for menstruation, they hadn't known how much bleeding to expect, that a range of colors from dark red to brown was normal, or that there would be a smell. They were not prepared for the logistics of menstruation—for example, the need to plan for it or have access to a bathroom.

And it's probably impossible to prepare young women for the insults, teasing, and prejudice that are the norm in a society that denigrates women's natures. But in spite of these prejudices, which continue today, I feel very strongly that we must not be afraid to describe ourselves for what we are out of fear that our "difference" will be held against us. As long as we avoid a true delineation of the difference, women will be in collusion with the very system that forces on us a male model of normalcy.

Furthermore, rather than buying into the view that women's hormonal changes make them moody, less competent and sickly, I urge you to see the power in your menstrual cycle, and to acknowledge your competence in the midst of the cyclical changes you encounter every month. It is remarkable that given the multitude of physiologic changes that occur in the course of a menstrual cycle, women maintain such a constancy. I liken it to an orchestra where the sounds of individual instruments rise and fall, shift in melody and volume while the music remains a harmonious whole. Each instrument, separately and in tandem, adds to the richness and texture of the music.

YOUR PERIOD: WHAT'S NORMAL?

Nearly every woman asks, at one time or another, "Am I normal?" Without a point of reference from which to describe her experience, the issue of normalcy is often a great source of worry. We are not taught to define normalcy across a wide range of unique experiences. When a woman asks me if her cycle is normal, my first question is usually, "What is normal for you?" I look for the patterns of her own cycle.

Most women have learned that a normal cycle takes twenty-eight days. But in fact, there is a great variability in cycle length, regularity, and accompanying symptoms. Each woman has her own personal pattern of menses that remains constant for most of her adult life. So when you ask what is normal, the answer must be that there are many different experiences within the spectrum of normalcy. Some women experience few symptoms and only bleed a couple of days a month. Others find their bodies in a constant state of flux. Some women have little discomfort, while others struggle with fluid retention, cramping, moodiness, weight gain, breast tenderness, diarrhea, or constipation. The norm is very diverse, although most women lose about an ounce of blood and menstruate four to five days.

Your menstrual norm becomes established the first year after menarche—that is, when you start menstruating for the first time. The age and experience of menarche is controlled by a variety of factors. Family and twin studies give substantial evidence of a hereditary link to the age of menarche. It might surprise you to know that the link is not just with your mother, but with your father, too. Both parents' age of maturity are factors in the age when you reach menarche.

Another critical element is nutrition and energy expenditure. Girls who are undernourished because of poverty or anorexia nervosa, or who exercise to the point where they have little body fat (as athletes and ballet dancers do), may have delayed menarche. It is believed that this is related to our bodies' natural instincts for survival. When a woman does not have the fat reserves necessary to support and sustain new life, her body is programmed to prevent pregnancy.

Illnesses can also influence the timing of menarche. Diseases which negatively affect nutrient absorption—such as ulcerative colitis, cystic fibrosis, and diabetes mellitus—tend to delay menarche. Other diseases, especially those that involve bed rest or extended periods of inactivity, tend to accelerate the onset of menarche.

The average menstrual cycle takes approximately twenty-eight days, during which time your body's many systems work together. A typical menstrual cycle can be divided into four stages:

Stage 1 is menstruation, lasting about five days. Menstruation is the shedding of the endometrium (the lining of the uterus), a signal that an egg has not been fertilized during the cycle. At the time of menstruation, your female hormones, estrogen and progesterone, are at their lowest levels, a signal to your hypothalamus and pituitary glands to start secreting FSH and LH. FSH is the hormone that stimulates the development of the ovarian follicle, prompting the maturation of a new egg to be released at ovulation. LH stimulates the production of estrogen by the ovaries and is responsible for release of the egg (ovulation).

Stage 2 is approximately days six through eleven, during which time the LH and estrogen levels continue to rise.

Stage 3 begins about day twelve with a surge of estrogen and LH, followed by a decline in estrogen production and a rise in FSH. On about day fourteen (or within thirty-six hours of the LH surge), the follicle releases the mature egg and ovulation takes place. This is the time when fertilization occurs if a sperm unites with a mature egg.

Stage 4 comprises the second half of the cycle. The ruptured follicle that has produced the mature egg undergoes a change called luteinization, which allows it to produce progesterone. Progesterone is the hormone that prepares the uterine lining for pregnancy. During this stage of the cycle, LH and FSH levels drop while progesterone continues to rise, thickening the inner layer of the uterus in preparation for pregnancy. If the egg has not been fertilized, the endometrial lining will break up and loosen, finally being shed at menstruation. And the cycle will begin anew.

The pre-ovulatory phase is known as "follicular." The post-ovulatory phase is referred to as "luteal."

CHART YOUR MENSTRUAL CYCLE

There are two advantages to keeping a chart of your menstrual cycle. One, the chart will give you a level of comfort with what is normal for you. You'll know the length and characteristics of your average cycle, which will alert you to any changes that could signal problems, enable decisions about birth control, and help you plan pregnancies. Two, the chart will help you identify changes that typically occur during the month so you can accommodate them in some way. For example, if your record shows that you typically feel bloated in the week prior to the onset of menstruation, you can limit your salt intake during that time or take a diuretic.

MENSTRUAL RECORD

Month _____

DAY	MENSTRUAL ACTIVITY	SYMPTOMS

PMS: Myth and Truth

"What can I do about my PMS?" Julie asked when she visited me for a checkup. I asked her to describe her experience, and she said, "I never had any real problem before, but the last few months I've noticed that I'm so moody. I yell at my husband and daughter over nothing. I burst into tears. It's awful."

"So, what's going on in your life?" I asked.

Julie was surprised by my question, which seemed off the subject of her PMS, but she obligingly began to tell me about the upheaval of her family's move six months before from the city to a nearby suburban community. It had been very stressful, as such transitions usually are.

"Is it possible that you're just going through some extra stress?" I asked. "Since you say you've never had a problem with PMS in the past, your recent irritability and tension might not be related to your period at all."

Julie looked at me with widened eyes, "You know," she admitted, "I hadn't thought of that, but I guess it's true that I've been on edge lately. Actually, I didn't think of connecting it to my period until my husband said something last month. I was in a bad mood, and he told my daughter, 'Oh, your mother has PMS.' "

Like many women, Julie formed the idea of PMS, not because she was aware of experiencing premenstrual problems, but because someone else—her husband—suggested it as the cause of her irritability. As we talked further, I learned that Julie's real frustration wasn't hormonally based. She was feeling dissatisfied because she didn't think her husband was giving her enough support with the move. That was another issue entirely!

Some women do experience severe mood disturbances premenstrually. But it has been my experience—supported by some interesting research—that the PMS monster is nothing more than a mysogynist culture's way of making women's normal cycle dysfunctional. I think we have to be very careful that in our desire to be supportive about women's legitimate medical complaints, we don't give the message that normal equals sick. And we have to watch our context: Do we want to return to the era when every ailment was linked to the reproductive organs? We must be clear about describing PMS, since myths about menstrual impairment are historically given greater weight during times when women are making social advances. Premenstrual symptoms may exist for some women, but too often they are used as a convenient way to explain away real issues.

Comedian Lily Tomlin dramatized the point in a funny bit she did about a doctor's visit when she was told she had PMS:
"You're sure, Doctor?
Premenstrual syndrome?
I mean, I'm getting divorced.
My mother's getting divorced.
I'm raising twin boys.
I've got a lot of job pressure . . .
And you think it's my period and not my life?"

Premenstrual syndrome is almost impossible to define. Research in this area has been very difficult because the number and variety of symptoms women experience differ from one woman to another, and even with the same woman from one cycle to another. If you list all of the symptoms that have been connected with PMS, there are dozens—almost every known pathology. They include, among other things, acne, anxiety, depression, dizziness, fatigue, eating disorders, panic, swelling, rashes, nausea, weight gain, hives, breast swelling, irregular heartbeats, muscle pain, paranoia, and violence. It's a pretty daunting list, and so nonspecific that it's easy to see why PMS is difficult to study. Since the medical profession has been notably lacking in insight when it comes to women, how are we to say that most of the so-called symptoms of PMS are not really symptoms of other physical or psychosocial problems that are going unaddressed? Only about 5 percent of women have disabling premenstrual symptoms that interfere with work or relationships. New research points to a link with brain opioid (opiate-like) activity, PMS symptoms are thought to be similar to those observed in addicts who have stopped taking heroin. Regular aerobic exercise has been shown to help maintain opioid levels in the brain, and that's why jogging has been reported to lower PMS and contribute to a sense of well-being. Recent studies also indicate that drugs increasing brain serotonin levels (such as Prozac) may help to eliminate PMS.

All humans, male and female, experience mood fluctuations in the course of any given month. Cultural bias has led to the assumption that for women, these fluctuations are connected to the menstrual cycle. But a study conducted with male and female undergraduates at the University of Pennsylvania places a different perspective on the issue. In the study, eleven males and twenty-two females (half taking oral contraceptives) completed daily self-reports on moods, body awareness, pleasant activities, and stressful events. The results

FLUCTUATIONS ARE NORMAL

During your cycle, your body experiences many fluctuations—some slight to unnoticeable, others more definite. Become familiar with the fluctuations. They're a natural part of the miraculous adaptability of the female body.

During menstruation . . .
▶ Urinary and saliva flow increase
▶ There is more susceptibility to infections
▶ Alcohol tolerance is greater
▶ Allergies are strongest

In the week after menstruation . . .
▶ The five senses are sharper
▶ Arthritis conditions worsen
▶ REM sleep is better
▶ Body temperature is usually below 98.6 degrees

During and near ovulation . . .
▶ Cervical mucus changes and discharge becomes more runny and copious

After ovulation . . .
▶ Body temperature rises to 98.6 degrees
▶ Food intake and energy expenditure rise
▶ Craving for sweets increases

Premenstrually . . .
▶ The heart rate and blood pressure are higher
▶ Salt and water retention increases
▶ Tolerance for alcohol decreases
▶ Speech patterns are less fluent
▶ Breast tenderness increases
▶ Sleep patterns can be disrupted

showed that all participants, male and female, experienced mood fluctuations in the course of a month, with the men reporting more instances of less positive mood. While the women cited disturbances surrounding menstruation caused by bloating and other discomforts, their overall mood did not significantly change.

Stress causes changes in neurotransmitters that can lead to changes in cycle length or total absence of menses. Adrenal gland responses to stress are greater premenstrually than at midcycle. (Women using oral contraceptives don't have this fluctuation.) Women also report more stress during the luteal (or premenstrual) phase. Which comes first, the cycle or the stress?

The menstrual cycle is not the only rhythm in the universe. Men and women respond to a variety of cyclical influences, including the calendar, the seasons, and even the twenty-four-hour rhythm of the day. It helps to keep this in perspective when we're describing highs and lows that we think are related to the menstrual cycle alone.

SELF-HELP FOR PREMENSTRUAL SYMPTOMS

Breast Swelling	Wear a larger bra so you won't feel restricted and uncomfortable; take a soothing warm bath; avoid breast manipulation.
Bloating	Reduce sodium intake, increase potassium intake, and drink lots of fluids; wear roomier clothes. A mild diuretic may be helpful during the week before menses. Cucumber, parsley, and asparagus may also help.
Mood Swings	Perform relaxation exercises, yoga, or meditation; reduce caffeine and alcohol consumption. Regular aerobic activity throughout the month will reduce premenstrual mood swings.
Cramps	Take Non-Steroidal Anti-Inflammatory Drugs (NSAIDs) like ibuprofen to reduce uterine contractions; drink herbal teas such as raspberry leaf; apply a heating pad to your back or stomach.

Remember, too, we are not merely a set of unrelated body parts. The hormonal changes that are a constant in our lives have a direct impact on our other bodily functions. Menstruation is not just a reproductive event.

As women's cycles are dependent on the internal environment, they are also subject to changes in the external environment. The best example of this is the documented occurrences of menstrual synchrony. Over time, women who live together or work in interdependent environments adapt their cycles so they menstruate together. In one study, seventy-nine college women—among them close friends, neighbors, and random peers—were followed over a four-month period. The findings showed that among the close friends, the differences in the dates of menstruation grew smaller during that time, while they remained about the same among the neighbors and peers.

It is believed that there is a chemical phenomenon that causes menstrual synchrony. Pheromones, which are chemical substances given off by the body and perceived through the nose, drive the cycles. Researchers have studied the possibility that male scent might influence women's cycles. They have found that women who engage in regular sex with men tend to have more even cycles and are more fertile than women who are celibate or have infrequent sex. Perimenopausal women with regular weekly sexual activity have higher estrogen levels and a milder menopause.

In one study, underarm secretions were collected from men and women during a three-month period. The male secretions were combined with alcohol and applied to the upper lips of women who had abnormal cycles. In every case, the women's cycles became more normal. Although we aren't certain to what extent pheromones affect women's cycles, there are enough anecdotal and research data available to demonstrate a link between social environment and hormonal activity.

WHEN PERIODS ARE A PROBLEM

We count on our periods to tell us about our general well-being; a change is a red flag that warns us something might be wrong. Some women contend with problems their entire menstruating lives. Others develop problems in association with various life events, behaviors, or medical conditions. I have found that many women suffer silently, afraid to mention their concerns for fear they will be branded hypochondriacs or neurotics. But it's important to trust your instincts and experiences when you think something is wrong. Only you know what you're feeling. You know better than anyone what's normal for you and what isn't.

Problem periods fall into roughly three categories: painful periods, non-existent periods, and irregular periods.

Painful Periods

The most common menstrual disorder is dysmenorrhea, or painful periods. For many women, painful periods are the norm. Primary dysmenorrhea, defined as painful menses without any evidence of a physical abnormality, is present in all cultures. Historically, it was shrugged off as hypochondria or emotional imbalance. We now know there is a physical cause related to enhanced production of prostaglandins. This can sensitize pain fibers and also create stronger and more frequent uterine contractions. Women with dysmenorrhea have more forceful uterine contractions, which can be measured clinically. This condition can be treated with antiprostaglandin medication (like ibuprofen) or with oral contraceptives, which reduce prostaglandin production.

Other types of dysmenorrhea, commonly called secondary dysmenorrhea, are usually caused by identifiable anatomic abnormalities. If you experience pain, you should ask your doctor to check for one of the following sources:

► Pain caused by a congenital abnormality in the uterus: You have a normal cycle, but because the opening to the vagina is narrow or nonexistent, menstrual blood does not flow easily and the buildup can cause painful pressure. Surgery can correct this abnormality.

I once saw a young girl who was not menstruating and she was complaining of stomach pain. Her stomach was distended. She thought she was pregnant, even though she'd never had a sexual encounter. I discovered that she had an imperforate hymen (blocked vaginal opening) that was blocking her flow. She was menstruating, but the blood wasn't coming out. It was building up inside her and that's why her abdomen was distended.

► Pain caused by fibroids and endometrial polyps: Sometimes, the supply of blood to the uterine muscle is interrupted and it causes pain, excessive bleeding, or heavy clots in the blood.

► Pain caused by an IUD: An intrauterine device can cause pain and heavy bleeding because it stimulates endometrial prostaglandin levels. It is a foreign body and the uterus contracts trying to expel it. IUDs are also the culprit in many cases of pelvic inflammatory disease. A thorough examination is required. Sometimes ibuprofen relieves the pain, but if it doesn't, the IUD should be removed.

▶ Pain caused by endometriosis: Endometriosis is serious, since there seems to be a strong link with infertility and damage to other organs. It should be considered by a doctor whenever a woman has abdominal pain. It occurs when tissue from the lining of the uterus spreads to other organs in the pelvis, such as the fallopian tubes, ovaries, intestine, and bladder. One theory is based on the idea of retrograde menstruation; menstrual flow literally backs up the fallopian tubes in addition to going out the cervix. It can even migrate outside the abdominal cavity to distant sites, causing chest pain, collapsed lungs, or coughing up of blood; or it can travel to the nose where it causes nosebleeds.

Backaches, rectal pain with bowel movements, and painful intercourse can occur depending on where the endometrial tissue implants. There might also be irregular spotting, blood in the urine, and rectal bleeding.

Endometriosis is hard to diagnose. One major reason is the artificial "turf" separation that doctors have established when dealing with the abdominal cavity. Neither the gynecologist nor the internist will take full responsibility for the area. The abdomen and pelvis are one continuous cavity where intestines can reach down into the pelvis and form connections into the vagina (as in Crohn's disease), and endometrial tissue can creep up to the diaphragm and cause problems there. Yet, internists never adequately learn about endometriosis, and gynecologists have little training in bowel disease. The major stumbling block to swift and sure diagnosis of endometriosis is that doctors don't know enough about it.

The second problem is that there isn't a noninvasive way of diagnosing endometriosis without resorting to laparoscopy, and even a negative laparoscopy doesn't rule out endometriosis. The implants might be microscopic and not visible to the naked eye.

A variant of endometriosis that is even harder to diagnose is adenomyosis, when endometrial tissue lies within the uterine muscle causing severe menstrual pain. The diagnosis is usually not made until a hysterectomy is done for chronic pelvic pain, and the problem is found by a pathologist—although MRI (magnetic resonance imaging) appears promising as a way of predicting adenomyosis prior to surgery.

In mild cases, especially when fertility is not an issue, the best response might be to continue observation with no direct treatment except for ibuprofen to control the pain. Oral contraceptives with high progesterone levels can also help. In more serious cases, pharmaceutical or surgical treatment may be necessary.

Endometriosis is on the rise. This may be another example of how lifestyle affects biology. With fewer pregnancies and later pregnancies, women experience more menstrual cycles and therefore more opportunities for retrograde menstruation.

Absent Periods

I have seen it many times. A woman who spends most of her adult years grumbling about how much she hates her period, suddenly misses it one month. In a flash, she's in my office, panic stricken over the implications. If she's sexually active, she worries about an unplanned pregnancy. If she's on the cusp of forty, she wonders about early menopause. If she's neither pregnant or menopausal, she's scared to death that the absence of a period signals a health calamity.

It's actually not that unusual to miss a period occasionally, or to have a scant, barely traceable flow. We forget how intricately linked our cycles are to the other aspects of our lives—not just biological, but emotional and environmental as well. If you fail to start menstruating in the first place, genetic disorders or congenital absence of reproductive organs should be looked for. Primary amenorrhea is defined as the failure to menstruate by age fourteen along with the absence of secondary characteristics like breast and hair development, or just the failure to menstruate alone by age sixteen. Menstrual patterns run in families, so if a mother got her period late so might her daughter.

In addition to pregnancy and menopause (which should always be ruled out before anything else), some other causes are absolutely normal. For instance, following childbirth, you may not begin to menstruate again for several months. If you're taking birth control pills, your flow may become so light that you wonder if you've bled. (Some women fail to regain normal menses after stopping oral contraceptives, but most return to normal within six months.)

An increase or decrease in body fat may affect menstruation. But changes in body fat alone may be too simple a picture. Ballet dancers menstruate at times when they are not actively dancing and their weight is stable. And anorexics can fail to regain menses even when they gain weight.

Excessive athletic activity is often the cause of amenorrhea or abnormal periods. This effect is more prevalent in runners than in swimmers and is thought to be related to the endorphin surge that comes with running.

(Endorphins are our own brain's opiates.) It is more pronounced in winter and when running is done in the dark.

We've learned that stress can affect menstruation. A family crisis, an unusually heavy workload, a divorce or death in the family might all cause you to miss a period. So might rape or physical abuse.

Amenorrhea can also be a sign of possible endocrine system disorders; if the pituitary and hypothalamus areas of the brain abnormally produce hormones, your cycle can be interrupted. Thyroid dysfunction commonly causes menstrual irregularities. Other ailments that can interfere with normal hormonal interactions include chronic illnesses like diabetes.

Psychotropic drugs, anticonvulsants, chemotherapy, and antiestrogens like tamoxifen can also interfere with menstruation.

Diagnosing the cause of your amenorrhea requires that you become an investigator of your other symptoms. If a nipple discharge accompanies amenorrhea, the likely cause is a hormonal imbalance, which produces the

---

INVESTIGATE THE SOURCE OF YOUR AMENORRHEA

ABSENT PERIODS WITH ...	COULD BE CAUSED BY ...
weight gain	hypothyroidism. Check blood TSH levels.
fatigue	hypothyroidism. Check blood TSH levels.
nipple discharge	excess hormone made by the pituitary gland that produces lactation. Check prolactin levels.
hirsutism	excess male hormones. Check ovarian and adrenal levels: LH/FSH, DHEAS, free testosterone, and androstenedione.
virilization	a testosterone-producing tumor. Check blood testosterone levels.
hot flashes	menopause. Check blood for high FSH levels and low estradiol levels.
no symptoms	hypothalamic amenorrhea. Check blood for low FSH, LH, and estradiol levels.

same effects as lactation. This abnormality is responsible for as much as one-third of all amenorrhea. The usual diagnostic tool is a blood test that looks for an elevated prolactin level. This may be due to a growth in the pituitary gland. Although benign, high prolactin levels do have negative consequences, such as infertility and osteoporosis later in life.

If amenorrhea accompanies weight gain and fatigue, the cause might be hypothyroidism—easily checked by testing TSH levels (the thyroid stimulating hormone made by the pituitary gland when it senses that thyroid hormone is low).

Amenorrhea accompanied by hirsutism (excess facial and body hair, and sometimes acne and oily skin) implies a possible adrenal or ovarian disorder causing an excess of male hormones. An endocrine evaluation is needed, looking at both ovarian and adrenal hormones.

Amenorrhea in the setting of virilization (male-pattern hair growth, deepening voice, clitoral enlargement) can signal a testosterone-producing tumor that is picked up by finding high blood levels of testosterone.

Amenorrhea in athletes, anorexics, or women with severe stress may have no associated symptoms. Hormone testing is needed.

Irregular Periods

Some women have irregular periods all of their lives. Strictly speaking, irregularity can be defined as anything that deviates from the twenty-eight-day cycle. But if you've always been a little irregular, there's probably nothing to worry about; after all, each woman is unique and her cyclic activity is affected by many different variables. However, severe episodes of irregular bleeding should be addressed. There are several types of irregularities that fall within this category. The first is menorrhagia, which is increased flow. The normal menstrual flow is about two tablespoons; anything below five and a half tablespoons is within the acceptable range. Since that's a pretty wide range, your best clue that your bleeding is too heavy is, if it's heavy for you—if there are frequent blood clots, or if it lasts longer than seven days. The only clinical measure of excessive bleeding is a blood test that detects anemia.

Heavy bleeding might be caused by clotting abnormalities—perhaps caused by overuse of aspirin or other over-the-counter drugs and by genetic abnormalities. Uterine fibroids are a common cause of heavy flow.

Another type of abnormal bleeding is breakthrough bleeding—that is, blood flow that occurs randomly throughout the month. This can happen when estrogen and progesterone are not balanced, as in anovulatory (not ovulating) cycles or with certain oral contraceptives. Cervical polyps can also bleed at irregular times. Chronic infections causing cervical erosions, sexually transmitted diseases, and IUDs can all cause irregular bleeding. A forgotten tampon can cause an irritation and bleeding. And anything that causes amenorrhea can start off with irregular bleeding.

When a patient comes to me with irregular bleeding, the first thing I do is determine whether it is ovulatory or anovulatory. Menstrual irregularities associated with ovulation are most commonly caused by polyps, tumors, or fibroids. Ovulation can be documented by a rise in basal body temperature. Anovulatory irregularities are more frequent at menarche and menopause. They can be related to the causes of amenorrhea, or be caused by a fragile endometrium that sloughs off at different sites throughout the cycle—instead of all at once, which can happen with estrogen-progesterone imbalances.

Irregular periods are also associated with obesity. Fat cells can manufacture estrogen out of adrenal gland substances. With a steady level of estrogen, rather than the normal rise and fall, the hypothalamus isn't triggered to allow for ovulation. High insulin levels and greater production of male hormones that interfere with ovulation are also associated with obesity.

Irregular bleeding can often be controlled with hormones, especially oral contraceptives or a monthly five- to fifteen-day course of progesterone. Sometimes it can be controlled by anti-inflammatory over-the-counter medications like ibuprofen. If there is a visible abnormality, such as fibroids, a hysteroscopy (direct visualization of the uterine cavity) can detect and sometimes remove them. Only submucus fibroids—those close to the lining of the uterus—cause bleeding. Fibroids on the outside of the uterus don't.

Polycystic ovarian syndrome (PCOS) is a disorder of ovulation. Symptoms can be either amenorrhea or irregular bleeding. In this condition, a steady production of estrogen fails to allow for ovulation. Without ovulation progesterone is never made and the constant stimulation leads to multiple cysts. Many women with this condition are also obese. There is a link between obesity, anovulation, high androgen levels, and insulin resistance. This is also the picture of diabetes and CAD. In fact, 20 percent of obese women with PCOS have Type II diabetes; for them, weight loss can usually improve ovulatory function. This is also the profile for women at risk for uterine cancer.

There is some genetic predisposition to PCOS, and it is seen twice as often in Caribbean Hispanics. First-degree relatives are likely to have insulin resistance and are candidates for Type II diabetes.

The bottom line is that not ovulating, except when you're on oral contraceptives, is a health risk to the rest of your body. Besides causing infertility, it increases your risk for endometrial cancer threefold and breast cancer fourfold, as well as for diabetes and CAD. Therefore, anovulation needs to be treated not just to make you fertile, but to keep you healthy.

PROBLEM PERIODS: A CHECKLIST FOR SCREENING

1. **Check basal body temperature and keep menstrual charts; if there is no increase in temperature, there is no ovulation.**
2. **Make sure you get a full checkup, including a pelvic exam.**
3. **Tell your doctor relevant details about sexual activity, diet, exercise, current medications, family history, and recent or ongoing stresses.**
4. **Be sure your doctor knows about existing medical conditions, such as diabetes or thyroid disease.**
5. **In addition to a complete blood count (CBC), routine chemistries, and a pregnancy test, ask for a hormonal evaluation that includes prolactin, TSH, FSH, LH, and estradiol.**

THE LINK BETWEEN HORMONAL CYCLES AND DISEASE

If you already have a medical condition, be alert to changes that might occur in the course of your cycle. These are the most common:

Seizure Disorders

▶ Seizure disorders increase in frequency premenstrually and menstrually. They are rare before puberty or after menopause. Estrogen is epileptogenic—that is, it increases the sensitivity of the brain to seizures—while progesterone is an anticonvulsant, decreasing the sensitivity of the brain to seizures. Treatment can include a combined constant-dose oral contraceptive.

Migraines

▶ About one-fifth of all women have migraine headaches, with 60 percent of them occurring in the premenstrual phase of the cycle. It is believed that the arteries in the uterus constrict in response to estrogen withdrawal, and so might the cranial vessels. Estrogen is also thought to affect central neurotransmitters and endorphins, which may be related to occurrence of migraines. Standard antimigraine medication is often ineffective in premenstrual migraines, but they might be controlled with the twenty-eight-day use of monophasic or constant-dose oral contraceptives.

Rheumatoid Arthritis

▶ There is more morning stiffness and pain, joint swelling, and weakness during the early part of the cycle and less during the progesterone phase of the cycle—possibly because of the anti-inflammatory properties of progesterone. For this reason, the symptoms usually lessen or disappear during pregnancy, and might also be alleviated (and even prevented) with oral contraceptives.

Diabetes

▶ Diabetes is the hardest to control menstrually, when glucose tolerance is lowest. Insulin doses should be adjusted during the premenstrual and menstrual phase.

Asthma

▶ About one-third of all asthmatic women experience a premenstrual exacerbation of problems—in severe cases, they lead to hospitalization and even death. Women with premenstrual asthma (PMA) have more severe symptoms and higher hospitalization rates than other women with asthma. PMA is also associated with PMS and dysmenorrhea.

Acute Appendicitis

▶ Sex hormones may affect the inflammatory process, which signals acute appendicitis. In one study of menstruating women, 64 percent of appendectomies were performed in the luteal (post-ovulatory) phase, with evidence of inflammation in 84 percent of the cases. Conversely, those done in the pre-ovulatory phase were inflamed only 50 percent of the time, and most of those were perforated by the time they reached surgery. Therefore, appendicitis occurring during the first part of the cycle can have a more serious course.

Catamenial Pneumothorax

▶ Episodes of collapsed lung (spontaneous pneumothorax) can occur in a woman's thirties or forties and involve the right lung. They may be related to pleural or diaphragmatic endometriosis, which is literally a backup of menstrual flow into the lung or diaphragm.

It would be foolish to assume that we can separate out the pervasive activities of our sex hormones from other processes. But that is precisely what happens with the current fragmentation of medical care. How many respiratory specialists talk to women about their menstrual cycles when they're treating asthma? How often are oral contraceptives used to alleviate rheumatoid arthritis or control seizures? Fragmented knowledge leads to inadequate care for women. A women's health specialty is where all knowledge about women's health becomes integrated to repair this fragmentation. In the meantime, if you have any of the above conditions, it's time to have a talk with your doctor about your menstrual cycle.

You might wonder, what's really so bad about not having periods? In the short term, it may make you feel as if something is wrong—not a comfortable state in which to be. In the long term, the loss of sufficient estrogen leads to osteoporosis, earlier onset of CAD, and genital atrophy. With anovulatory cycles, the state of unopposed estrogen can place you at risk for endometrial cancer.

A Cautionary Word about Hysterectomies

Every year, three quarters of a million American women undergo hysterectomies. It's the second most common female surgery—Caesarian section being the first. In fact, the removal of the uterus (often accompanied by the removal of the ovaries) has become so common that many women believe it is normal and inevitable that they will undergo it at some time in their lives.

But increasingly, questions are being raised about the necessity of so many hysterectomies. Along with many of my female colleagues, I feel strongly that hysterectomies are overutilized, especially in African-Americans and those who have completed their childbearing. Frankly, many surgeons have the attitude, "If you don't need it, take it out. It's useless." The standard line is that when the uterus and ovaries are no longer needed for pregnancy, they are only risks for cancer. How interesting that a similar viewpoint isn't expressed regarding the male prostate! Especially since more than 165 thousand older men get prostate cancer every year.

During the 1950s and 1960s, hysterectomies were very popular among young women. At that time, most women had babies very young and were finished with childbearing by the time they were thirty. If they experienced heavy bleeding caused by fibroids or ovarian masses, or suffered chronic pelvic pain or abnormal bleeding, they would be advised to have hysterectomies, even when their conditions were benign. The doctors figured, why not? Why suffer the discomfort or take the risk (practically nonexistent) that the condition might lead to cancer? The result was that many young women were going through menopause years earlier than normal—and experiencing more severe bone loss and a higher risk for early coronary artery disease. Even today, hormone replacement isn't always prescribed following a hysterectomy, leaving women victims to health conditions caused by hormone depletion.

Furthermore, hysterectomies cause suffering in many other ways. Along with strong ligaments, the uterus is the center of the female pelvis that holds other organs in place. If you pull it out, there's a risk that other organs might descend into the vagina. Women who have had hysterectomies frequently complain of bladder problems (including incontinence), painful intercourse, inability to achieve orgasm, changes in the quality of orgasm, chronic pelvic pain, and other problems. It is far from being a benign course of treatment. A 1983 study by the American College of Obstetrics and Gynecology and the Department of Health and Human Services found "one-fourth to one-half of all women who undergo hysterectomies develop some morbidity, with fever and hemorrhage the most common type."

Nevertheless, the scare campaign continues. Women with fibroids, irregular bleeding, or chronic pelvic pain are regularly warned that removal of the uterus, the ovaries, or both is their only safe recourse. Doctors are still trained to perform hysterectomies as a preventive measure, rather than the treatment of last resort. For instance, compare the standard teaching about fibroids with the reality. Until recently, the standard teaching was that asymptomatic fibroids that grow rapidly over time or those that are over a certain size should come out for fear of cancer and the increased operative risks of removing large uteri. However, cancerous fibroids are as rare as hen's teeth—between 0.1 and 0.5 in postmenopausal women over fifty. Benign fibroids are one thousand times more common, especially in women under fifty, the bulk of the hysterectomized population. More important, the operative risk of hysterectomy done for benign conditions is up to 1.6 per one thousand—much higher than the risk of a fibroid really being a malignant cancer.

Standard teaching also says that if you have no uterus you don't need your ovaries. Wrong! Ovaries are needed for continued estrogen protection, and this is clearly seen in the higher rates of CAD and osteoporosis in surgically menopausal women. Also, the ovary continues to make testosterone, which is responsible for libido in women; there are frequent complaints of lack of sexual interest among women whose ovaries have been removed. And we are just beginning to learn about other products made by the ovary. The bottom line is, ovaries are important for more than just having babies.

Gynecologists terrorize women about the fear of ovarian cancer, asking, "Why leave in an organ that might become cancerous—the type of cancer that can't easily be screened for until it's too late?" It's true that ovarian cancer is often deadly, since it's asymptomatic until the later stages. But when you consider the realities, the lifetime risk of ovarian cancer in a fifty-year-old woman is only 1.2 percent, endometrial cancer only 2.4 percent, and cervical cancer only 0.6 percent. Surely these statistics must affect decisions about

---

POSSIBLE COMPLICATIONS OF HYSTERECTOMY

Postoperative:
    Fever
    Bleeding
    Need for a blood transfusion
    Cardiopulmonary event (such as a blood clot to the lung)

Long term:
    Early ovarian failure (early menopause)
    Decreased libido
    Painful intercourse caused by shortened vagina or vaginal scarring
    Vaginal atrophy or granulation
    Urinary problems
    Constipation
    Depression

hysterectomies. In addition, newer diagnostic techniques like high-resolution transvaginal ultrasound for evaluating ovaries, and MRI for distinguishing fibroids from cancers, are now available to help make diagnoses without resorting to premature surgery.

So the question is: How does a woman make an informed decision about hysterectomy?

If your problem is heavy bleeding and pain caused by fibroids, you have to determine whether it is interfering with your quality of life. Most often, fibroids are not risk factors for either cancer or infertility, so the real issue has to be whether or not you can live with them. If you decide you can't, there are other treatments that are less dramatic than hysterectomy.

A myomectomy is a procedure to excise fibroids from the uterus without removing the uterus. Hysteroscopic myomectomy, a new technique using a scope to locate the problem causing bleeding by submucus fibroids and remove them, has lower morbidity and less blood loss. Newer drugs, called GNRH agonists, can shrink fibroids temporarily, although menopause will be induced during their use, and are not a long-term solution.

Fibroids are benign growths of uterine muscle. In and of themselves, they are not problematic. When they put pressure on or obstruct neighboring organs or cause excessive bleeding, treatment is required. Fibroids are far more common in African-American women, as well as in obese women. Oral contraceptive use can decrease their development.

Occasionally, fibroids on the outside of the uterus can twist or degenerate and become an acute surgical emergency, or protrude through the cervix to simulate a delivery. Mostly they are asymptomatic, but they can cause a dull backache, painful menstruation, or painful intercourse.

Fibroids were once thought to be associated with infertility, but newer studies show this is seldom the case unless fibroids are blocking a fallopian tube. However, fibroids can complicate the course of a pregnancy, especially if they are near the placenta. This is a bigger problem for women today since they are delaying pregnancy into their thirties, which is the time of greatest fibroid growth.

Dysfunctional uterine bleeding due to hormone imbalance is another reason given for hysterectomy. But a high percentage of dysfunctional uterine bleeding can be treated medically. Sometimes over-the-counter aids like ibuprofen will stem the abnormal flow. Other times, progesterone can be effective. Endometrial ablation is a relatively new procedure that may be helpful in treating abnormal bleeding caused by fibroids or hormone imbalance. A hysteroscope is used to look into the uterus, then with a laser, the entire uterine lining is destroyed. This usually controls the bleeding, although sometimes the procedure needs to be repeated. Long-term effects are not yet known. If a surgically aggressive approach is necessary, a D&C should certainly precede any consideration of a hysterectomy.

Uterine prolapse can often be approached nonsurgically with a pessary, a device much like a diaphragm that holds organs in place. Pelvic floor muscles can be strengthened with exercises. Hysterectomy is a highly questionable solution, since one of the common outcomes of removing the uterus is prolapse of the other organs if the remaining ligaments weren't reconstructed properly. However, when the uterus actually hangs out of the body, hysterectomy may be the only solution. It is, in fact, the condition that plagued Victorian women prior to the invention of safe hysterectomies. This surgical advance was clearly a medical benefit; it only became a problem when it was used unnecessarily rather than when it was genuinely needed.

Ten percent of hysterectomies are performed to treat chronic pelvic pain, although its source might well be gastrointestinal, urinary, musculoskeletal, or hormonal. We now know that between 40 and 60 percent of women who report chronic pelvic pain were sexually abused as children, and their pain might be a repressed memory response to the abuse. Clearly, hysterectomy won't help them. In fact almost a quarter of the women who receive hysterectomies for chronic pelvic pain continue to have pain.

Adenomyosis is another cause of chronic pelvic pain leading to hysterectomy. It is similar to endometriosis except that the uterine tissue migrates into the wall of the uterus instead of growing outside the uterus. The uterus is enlarged and menstrual periods are heavy and painful. It is most common in women during their forties and early fifties. Until recently, the only way to diagnose the problem was to examine the uterus after a hysterectomy. Recently, however, MRI has been found to accurately identify adenomyosis before surgery. Hormonal therapy that is sometimes effective in treating endometriosis, is ineffective for treating adenomyosis.

Although a hysterectomy might be indicated for severe endometriosis, massive postpartum hemorrhaging, some ectopic pregnancies, and cancer, it should never be casually prescribed. It's important that you and your doctor work as partners, and that you not just accept the dictate, "It must come out," without discussing nonsurgical options. This is also a good time to get more than one opinion. Talk to both a nonsurgeon and a surgeon practicing with a different group.

Some gynecologists are rigid about removing the ovaries when they remove the uterus, especially for women over forty-five. Don't just accept that. Ask why other organs must be removed because of a problem in one organ. Demand a specific compelling reason, not the usual, "It might become cancerous." You now know that the risk of that is slim, and the benefits of keeping your ovaries are great. Even when the uterus is the only organ removed, premature menopause is more likely, probably because of a compromised blood flow to the ovaries during surgery.

CHALLENGING THE SOCIAL ORDER

During the past hundred years, we have witnessed a change in the pattern of women's cycles. Industrialization has played a major role in health. With better nutrition, women are getting their periods much earlier. One hundred years ago, a girl would begin menstruating when she was seventeen and get married shortly after. Because she had many pregnancies and long periods of breast-feeding, she would have relatively few periods in her life. Compared with today's woman, she had few ovulatory cycles. She was also more likely to suffer sexually transmitted infections and childbirth consequences.

Our overall health picture has certainly improved since then, but modern women also experience the consequences of the change. Since girls get their periods earlier, they also become sexual earlier—with all the complex decisions that accompany that transition, especially since we have come to separate sex from childbearing.

More dramatically, women today are in a position unique in all of human history. More women may decide to delay childbirth into their forties or choose to have no children at all. As a consequence, many women will have forty years of periods—some 480 menstrual cycles and 480 ovulatory cycles. What are the implications? The answer is, we don't know for sure since it's a relatively new phenomenon.

Some experts say that if you are a young woman with a family history of breast cancer, your best protection might be to have your first child before age thirty, breast-feed for an extended period, then have many children. This sounds like a startling prescription! But it goes to the heart of our interconnectedness with culture. How do women make socially responsible choices that will also be in their own best health interests? And more important, how does society change to reflect the needs of women?

It's no secret that the reason many women are waiting to start families is because of the pressure they feel to fit themselves into a male-oriented career track. Especially in highly competitive professions, women who take time off to start families in their twenties and thirties are severely penalized in their prospects. We've defined career success according to what's normal for men and have convinced ourselves that it's the "natural" order of things to barrel through—go to college right away, jump into a partnership track, climb the ladder as fast as you can. That may be the natural order of things for men, but it doesn't always work in the best interests of women.

A social order that is truly inclusive of women would be responsive to their unique timelines and would consider birthing and childraising to be important, rewarding parts of life—something to be shared by all.

COMMON QUESTIONS ABOUT PERIODS

Is it okay to have sex during my period?

Some women have found that sex is the best prescription for relieving menstrual cramps. Studies confirm that vaginal and uterine contractions that accompany orgasm might reduce pelvic cramps and backaches.

However, your concern might be one of hygiene, aesthetics, or cultural values. Or you might not feel very sexy during your period. The decision is a personal one between you and your partner. Some studies indicate that men seem to have less of a problem than women do with the idea. But the guiding principle should be whether you feel emotionally and physically comfortable.

How can I prepare my daughter for the start of her period?

Many women of our generation have horror stories to tell about starting to menstruate. Thirty or forty years ago, it was not uncommon for young girls to receive no preparation at all. I have heard women talk about how they were convinced they were bleeding to death, or how their mothers were so embarrassed they simply shoved a box of sanitary napkins at them and let them fend for themselves. I imagine that there isn't a woman alive who doesn't remember an embarrassing incident or a moment of panic about her period. We were ill-prepared to handle a monthly blood flow, and our mothers were poorly equipped to help us.

Today, most parents are determined that their own daughters will know in advance what to expect and find a level of comfort with this normal life event. Some have adopted rituals to celebrate the transition into womanhood. I think this is a lovely idea. But in the process, it's helpful to balance the celebration with some good practical information about what it's like to have a period.

Tell stories from your own experience; let your daughter know that it's natural to feel uncomfortable, to occasionally have an accident, to have trouble coping with the mess. Also talk to her about some of the physiological symptoms she might experience—a little bloating, cramps—and suggest ways to alleviate them. Try to avoid using terms or descriptions that imply menstruation is a sickness or an abnormality, so your daughter can come to view it as an ordinary event in her life, not a pathological condition.

I've heard that tampons can cause toxic shock syndrome. Are they safe to use?

Toxic shock syndrome (TSS) is a serious condition that has been linked with the use of tampons. The syndrome was discovered when otherwise healthy women began suffering severe symptoms—high fever, rash, low blood pressure, vomiting, diarrhea, and kidney and liver failure. After several women died of TSS, the Institute of Medicine formed a committee to study the matter. It found that 92 percent of women who suffered TSS during menstruation were tampon users. In particular, high-absorbency tampons made of polyester foam and carboxymethylcellulose were considered culprits, and these are no longer on the market. However, tampons are a relatively recent invention, and we still don't know all we should about their effects on our vaginas.

TSS is relatively rare, but experts recommend that all tampon users protect themselves by using the lowest absorbency tampon possible, preferably cotton, and avoid deodorized or perfumed brands. Tampons should be changed at least every four hours during the day and be discontinued at night, since the bacteria that cause TSS thrive in the absence of oxygen.

Are vaginal infections more likely during my period?

Yes. Yeast that can colonize the vagina may increase in the alkaline pH environment that occurs premenstrually. Urinary tract infections can occur during menstruation if a tampon remains in place too long and bacteria spread.

What effect does hormone replacement therapy have on the growth of fibroids?

Fibroids rarely grow under the influence of hormone replacement therapy. If you already have fibroids, that should not deter you from starting HRT. Studies are needed to assess the problems, if any, with HRT for women with fibroids.

Sometimes there are thick blood clots in my menstrual flow. Does that mean that something is wrong?

Clotting can occur during normal menstruation. However, if your periods are unusually heavy and include many clots, it may indicate the presence of fibroids or other growths. Clots can also be caused by an IUD. I suggest that if you experience anything that is abnormal to your usual menstrual experience, have it checked out.

I have terrible bleeding, bloating, and back pain from my fibroids. My lower abdomen protrudes, and I must constantly wear a pad. Yet I am very concerned about getting a hysterectomy. What should I do?

Sometimes a hysterectomy offers a major improvement in a woman's quality of life, so we shouldn't be rigid in our thinking. If all methods short of hysterectomy have failed, you should probably go ahead. As long as it's your choice, the benefits can sometimes outweigh the disadvantages of hysterectomy.

My mother had a hysterectomy. Does that mean I'll need one, too?

Chances are, your mother had a hysterectomy because it was the procedure of choice for menstrual abnormalities. I'm seeing a rash of women in my office these days who don't know when to expect menopause because their mothers had early hysterectomies. There's no reason to believe that you'll need one. If you do develop fibroids, try to find a woman's health specialist who doesn't consider hysterectomy the first treatment of choice.

I had a complete hysterectomy, with my uterus and ovaries removed. Do I still need an annual Pap smear?

After the loss of your uterus and cervix for noncancerous reasons, the Pap test offers little information. It can be used to evaluate estrogen replacement therapy or help diagnose infections. Cancer of the vagina is rare, except for women whose mothers took DES. However, you should still be screened for cancer of the vulva, and even if a Pap is not done, the external genitalia should be examined, as even melanomas can appear there. Women who have had hysterectomies for cervical cancer should continue having Pap tests to rule out recurrence or vaginal cancer, which may be associated with HPV.

If your ovaries are not removed along with the uterus, you should have them palpated by your doctor at least yearly. If a doctor feels something abnormal, a sonogram and CA125 should be done to collect evidence of malignancy.

How do I know I'm menopausal if I've had a hysterectomy?

Menopause can be suspected when your monthly rhythm changes. Don't forget that even though you have lost the external manifestation of your ovarian cycle, the cycle still goes on and gives its usual cyclic symptoms. If you aren't aware of any cyclical signs and aren't experiencing menopausal symptoms like hot flashes, a routine blood test to check FSH levels should be conducted at your annual physical.

RESOURCES

ORGANIZATIONS
American Fertility Society
2131 Magnolia Avenue, Suite 201
Birmingham, AL 35256
205-978-5000

Endometriosis Treatment Program
St. Charles Medical Center
2500 N.E. Neff Road
Bend, OR 97701
800-446-2177, x7563

The Resource Center
American College of Obstetricians and Gynecologists
600 Maryland Avenue SW
Washington, DC 20024
202-863-2518

PUBLICATIONS
Body Talk pamphlets—*For Girls Growing Up* and *For Parents of Girls*— can be ordered from the Publications Department, Center for Research on Women, Wellesley College, Wellesley, MA 02181.

The Journal of Reproductive Medicine
P.O. Drawer 12425
8324 Olive Street
St. Louis, MO 63132

12
PREGNANCY AND BEYOND
A Lifelong Effect

~~~

The myth of pregnancy is that it is strictly a gynecological event. In this century, the medical specialty of OB/GYN has controlled reproduction, and a rigid barrier has developed between it and other health issues. Based on the way our health care system is structured, one would think that pregnancy confined itself to the uterus. But the opposite is true. Pregnancy (and the potential for pregnancy) has a systemic influence throughout a woman's life.

For the past thirty years, the women's health movement has been focused on reproductive issues—from contraception to childbirth. While these efforts have benefited women in many ways, by supplying information and encouraging self-determination, in the long run this limited focus has served to reinforce the bias, socially and within the medical profession, that women's health is centered in the reproductive organs. It's not that far removed from the era when women were defined as uteri surrounded by other body parts. I have a great deal of respect for the women and clinicians who fought on the forefront of women's health and achieved reproductive rights. But now it is time that we broaden the focus. We must begin a discussion of pregnancy from the perspective of the whole woman.

I want to introduce you to a new way of looking at pregnancy and health. This chapter is not the usual guide to having a baby. I am interested here in describing the connection between your reproductive life and your total health. You cannot fully take charge of your lifetime health unless you understand this connection, yet it is rarely if ever described in standard books about women's health or pregnancy. My interest here is not so much on the event of having a baby as it is on the lifetime health implications of pregnancy as well as the effects of not having children at all. Don't skip this chapter if you are childless and plan to remain so. Your life is affected by the potential for pregnancy even if you never become pregnant. That knowledge and understanding is part of a woman-centered rather than an infant-centered approach.

THE MEDICALIZATION OF PREGNANCY

Pregnancy and birth have traditionally been social and cultural events for women, but in this century we have seen them become medicalized. Childbirth has been moved from the home to the hospital; it carries a diagnostic code that makes it reimbursible by insurers. While there's no question that modern medical technology has made childbirth less dangerous to women and infants, somewhere along the way we have gutted the core of what was once a woman-centered process.

In previous eras, when midwives assisted most women in labor, they were more than technicians. They were friends who kept a woman company and supported her through a painful and frightening crisis—which childbearing was, since many women died in this process. Midwives organized the rest of the family to support the needs of the laboring woman, and spent time with her after the birth, teaching her about nursing and child care. Compare that to the sterile process of obstetrician-assisted birthing we have today. A pregnant woman is examined every month in a clinical environment, with ultrasound technology on hand to monitor the development of the fetus. She might be sent to a hospital where probes are put onto the fetus's scalp while it is still in the womb to monitor fetal heartbeats and look for signs of distress. During this procedure, the woman is placed in a position that is most comfortable for the doctor. She is given an enema to make it more aesthetic for the doctor. Until recently, she was even put to sleep and excluded from the process altogether. All of this can occur—and often does—with very little communication between the woman and her doctor. The doctor is performing the task as a technician for whom this is a common procedure, while the woman struggles with the emotional impact of an event that may have major consequences for her and her child.

This is not to say that women don't benefit from scientific advances that allow us to survive childbirth and stay healthy well into our eighties. But technology alone has limited benefit in a medical environment that is not woman-centered.

An excellent example of the medicalization of childbirth has been the rise in the number of Caesarians performed. It is now the most common surgical procedure for women. Although research shows that only about twelve to fifteen percent of all deliveries actually require such drastic intervention, doctors continue to perform Caesarians whenever there are complications during labor. Given that the Caesarian rate in the U.S. in 1992 was 22.6 percent, one could calculate that $1.3 billion dollars was spent on unnecessary surgeries.

Given the number of Caesarians performed every year versus the estimated need for them, we have to assume that in many cases surgery is not necessary. So why do so many doctors perform Caesarians? Studies on this question have documented that the main difference between an obstetrician who performs many Caesarians and one who performs them rarely is professional bias. Some doctors find them easier, less traumatic for the fetus, and more convenient. Some are concerned about malpractice litigation, if there is a problem with the baby.

A number of years ago, two doctors created controversy when they speculated in the British journal, *Clinical Obstetrics and Gynaecology,* "It may well be that during the next 40 years the allowance of a vaginal delivery or attempted vaginal delivery may need to be justified in each particular instance." Their contention was shocking, but you can see how such a scenario might evolve, given the popularity of the procedure.

Doctors who perform Caesarians often tell women how much better the procedure is for their babies. They talk about unbruised heads and smooth torsoes, infants unmarked by forceps and untraumatized by the rugged journey down the birth canal. Although absolutely no studies have ever shown that Caesarian-delivered babies are in any way healthier or less traumatized than their naturally delivered counterparts, this has been a favorite argument. It is an example of the devaluation of the woman and the glorification of the fetus—a trend that is similarly seen in the antiabortion and anti-birth-control movements. Sometimes women who refuse Caesarians are accused of willfully endangering their babies.

Those who argue that Caesarians might ultimately become the option of the future ignore the massive insult to the body that any major surgery implies. We should not be misled into believing that this is a "simple" surgery. It is major and invasive. Women who undergo Caesarians are vulnerable to the dangers of surgery, as well as to the complications that are common in the aftermath. One report estimates that half the women who undergo Caesarians have serious complications, including hemorrhaging and infections. Another study showed a more than 20 percent increase in uterine infections following Caesarians, compared to only 1.45 percent in vaginal deliveries. Most women report pain, gas, and weakness for weeks and even months after delivery. That's not to mention the disfigurement, permanent injury to abdominal muscles, and the risks associated with blood transfusions.

On the other hand, natural labor isn't benign. It can be associated with severe tears of the vagina, leading to a false connection between the rectum and vagina. Tears around the anus can damage the anal sphincter and cause

CHOOSE A WOMAN-CENTERED OBSTETRICIAN

Don't wait until you're ready to deliver to find out what your obstetrician's attitudes are about Caesarians, the use of drugs to induce labor, or other procedures. Before you select an obstetrician, find out the following:

1. What percentage of the doctor's deliveries are Caesarian? (Above 15 percent is a concern.)
2. What are the doctor's attitudes about when Caesarian delivery is appropriate? Get specifics.
3. Does your doctor believe that a first Caesarian requires subsequent Caesarian deliveries? This belief has been discredited, but many doctors still go along with the old assumption.
4. Under what conditions does your doctor think it is appropriate to use drugs to induce labor?
5. Can your doctor provide maximum medical care while keeping "medicalization" to a minimum?
6. Does your doctor educate you about the changes occurring in your body, prepare you for the ordeal of labor, and work with you as a partner in the process?

fecal incontinence. Tissues can be stretched to the point of uterine prolapse (where the uterus literally hangs outside of the body). Trauma to the bladder can lead to urinary retention and other bladder conditions.

By being well educated and decisive before your pregnancy, or in its early days, you can avoid finding yourself in the delivery room having procedures performed that you might have objected to when you were feeling less anxious and vulnerable.

WHAT HAPPENS TO YOUR BODY AT PREGNANCY?

The vast physiologic changes that accompany pregnancy tell us something about the female organism. Only women's bodies are so constructed that they can adapt to a radically different state. Consider what occurs at pregnancy:

▶ Blood volume expands by as much as 50 percent, and the heart chambers enlarge to accommodate this extra volume. Blood is pumped more efficiently, allowing the chambers to return to a normal size after each contraction.

▶ The heart muscle grows thicker; the changes are similar to those that occur with endurance training.

▶ The heart beats more rapidly.

▶ Cardiac output increases by 30 to 50 percent—a measure of the amount of blood that is pumped through the circulatory system. Between 10 and 20 percent of the blood goes to the uterus alone, while enhanced blood flow also reaches the kidneys, skin, and breasts.

▶ Collagen within the blood vessels softens; changes in vascular tone (including dilation of the veins and arteries) occur to accommodate the increased blood volume.

▶ The respiratory rate increases and the amount of air moved increases by 40 percent.

▶ Blood pressure drops.

▶ The kidneys and ureters dilate, allowing the bladder to hold double the capacity of urine.

▶ The amount of fluid filtered by the kidneys increases, and there is a change in the filtering and absorption process.

▶ The hormone relaxin, which is involved in the softening of the cervix, also causes a softening in the ligaments and changes the shape of the pelvis.

▶ Motility along the gastrointestinal tract is slowed, and there is less production of gastric acid.

▶ The immune system is suppressed to allow for the presence of a fetus (which carries the foreign antigens from the father).

▶ Alterations in the thickness of the eye lens and the composition of tears can lead to vision changes.

▶ During the first half of pregnancy, estrogen stimulates the release of insulin and enhances the regulation of glucose. In the second half, hormones made by the placenta counter the effects of insulin.

These normal physiologic occurrences can change you in ways that are both positive and negative. If you have a medical condition or are at risk for one, it might be affected by pregnancy. I'll describe a number of the most common pregnancy-sensitive conditions. You might find the details a bit grim; pregnancy and childbirth are, after all, usually happy events. But rather than seeing this as a pessimistic portrayal of the things that could go wrong, use it to arm yourself with knowledge that will help you prepare realistically and fully for your pregnancy.

As you read these details, you'll see that every system and bodily function is involved. Consider your own personal profile and risk factors in light of these factors, and discuss these issues with your doctor.

Cardiovascular Function

Owing to your body's need for enhanced blood flow, your heart works much harder in pregnancy. Its chambers dilate and contract harder in the first twenty weeks to force out more blood with each beat. It also beats faster in the first twenty weeks. Palpitations and shortness of breath are common. For a normal, healthy woman, these changes are not harmful. However, for those with congenital heart disease or rheumatic heart disease, the normal changes can be too stressful and cause heart failure.

Blood Vessel Changes

When the normal physiologic increase in blood volume occurs, sometimes the blood vessels can't contain all the extra fluids. Your hands, feet, and face might swell. If you have high blood pressure, the condition can worsen. Pregnant women have a thirteen times greater risk of stroke and five times the risk of a burst blood vessel in the brain as nonpregnant women. Pressure from the uterus can backflow in the veins, increasing the risk of phlebitis or blood clot. Pulmonary embolism, where a piece of clot in a vein breaks off and travels to the lung, accounts for 15 percent of all obstetrical deaths. Swelling of tissues can also put pressure on the nerves, causing carpal tunnel syndrome (compression of a nerve to the hand) and Bell's palsy (weakening of a facial muscle).

Renal and Urologic Disorders

Urinary tract infections are common during pregnancy, but they are often asymptomatic and can trigger premature labor. In particular, pregnancy imposes a real renal stress on women with lupus or diabetes. The enlarged uterus can block urine flow and cause kidney swelling and failure. Birth trauma can also tear bladders and cause incontinence due to prolapse.

Mineral Absorption

The stages of women's lives might directly affect their susceptibility to environmental toxins. Pregnancy, lactation, and menopause are all times of intense activity in women's bones, which serve as storage compartments for minerals, and in fat tissues which concentrate levels of PCBs, DDT, and dioxin. During these physiologically active times in a woman's life, toxins (such as pesticides, PCBs, and dioxin) that have accumulated over her lifetime in these storage compartments may be mobilized into the bloodstream and affect other organs. In particular, lead might cause damage to brain tissue and DDT to breast tissue.

Dermatologic Changes

Pregnancy increases the production of melanin, causing darkening of the skin. You might see a brownish discoloration of your cheeks, known as the mask of pregnancy. Freckles, moles, and discoloration might also occur around the areola of your nipples.

Hormones also affect hair growth, and you may experience some shedding of hair in the third month after delivery. Stretch marks and vascular spider veins occur in 90 percent of pregnant women. Some women experience itching of the skin, which then resolves after delivery—although it may occur again in subsequent pregnancies or with use of oral contraceptives. Flare-ups of venereal warts can also occur in the genital skin.

Orthopedic Disorders

Softening of the connective tissue (collagen) is necessary to widen the pelvis and create the birth canal. But other tissues soften, too. Be aware that back sprains and herniated disks are common, as are problems in the ligaments of the knees and the pelvis.

Gastrointestinal Problems

High estrogen levels can encourage gallstone formation. It's not so unusual for new mothers to return to the hospital to have their gallbladders removed. High progesterone levels cause slowing of the intestines leading to constipation; reflux of acid stomach contents into the esophagus causes heartburn.

In the last months of pregnancy, pressure in the uterus can crowd the stomach and intestines and make it difficult to eat and eliminate. Protrusion of hemorrhoids is common.

Nutritional Changes

When you are pregnant, you have an enormous need for iron to make more blood and calcium to form fetal bones. Anemia is common in pregnancy, and osteoporosis causes some pregnant women to fracture their hips and vertebrae due to calcium mobilization from the mother's bones to use for fetal bone growth.

Endocrine Disorders

Gestational diabetes affects 4 to 6 percent of pregnant women. (See Chapter 7.) It causes many risks to both mother and fetus, while placing the mother at risk for diabetes later in life.

Thyroid diseases are common, especially after pregnancy. (See Chapter 10.) A condition can also develop in which the pituitary gland swells and outstrips its blood supply, leading to pituitary failure after delivery.

Another relatively common, though very serious, condition is ectopic pregnancy, a condition caused by the embryo growing in the fallopian tube. Ectopic pregnancy can be detected by a pelvic exam and ultrasound. There is no way a fetus can survive in the fallopian tube, so this doesn't constitute a viable pregnancy. Rupture of the tube is an emergency because it causes massive internal hemorrhaging. It is the leading cause of maternal death during the first three months of pregnancy. Rupture occurs most often to nonwhite women, and the incidence increases in all women as they age. Over the last ten years, the rate of ectopic pregnancy has quadrupled owing to the rise of pelvic inflammatory disease (PID). One episode of PID may increase your risk of ectopic pregnancy tenfold.

In addition to the "normal" changes that occur with pregnancy, it can also put you at risk for other conditions, including heart or renal failure of unknown cause; amniotic fluid embolism—a fatal passing of amniotic fluid through the blood during delivery; and failure of the blood vessels to dilate to accommodate increased blood volume, leading to life-threatening conditions. In roughly one in 2,000 pregnancies in the United States, tumors arise from the trophoblast, the layer of cells that line the placenta. The result is failure of the fetus to thrive. On rare occasions, malignancies can develop in the placental tissue even after a normal pregnancy. Make sure your doctor has all the information necessary to help decrease your risk of any pregnancy-related complications. It is remarkable to me that although much is made of the potential complications of aborting a pregnancy (which are relatively rare), women are not fully informed about the potential complications of *continuing* a pregnancy.

Pregnancy Changes You Forever

It never occurred to me until my first son was born that his birthday was also an important marker in my own life. Most of us are so used to seeing pregnancy as a fetus-centered event concluding in the birth of a child that we've failed to appreciate its importance to the woman.

There are both positive and negative consequences to pregnancy. As an individual woman, you must evaluate your risks and benefits in light of other risk factors. If you are childless, you have a different set of risks and benefits. But let's keep the issue of risks in perspective. You can make yourself crazy—and many women do—worrying about whether to have children, when to have children, if late childbearing is hazardous to your health, or whether remaining childless is good or bad from a personal health standpoint. Remember, risks must always be considered in a total context. No single factor is sufficient to make a determination. Use the following information in that spirit and avoid making rigid assumptions.

Let's also appreciate that the decision to have a child is a serious one. It's something that you have a choice about. You should not feel pressured by a false idea of biological imperative. Indeed, control over our reproductive life is arguably the most important advance women have made in this century. We mustn't carelessly toss this freedom away or give up the personal power we have fought so hard to gain. Rather, we should let our knowledge of risks give us even more control as we plan for healthy lives.

Be aware of the ways in which your reproductive history affects you for life—whether you choose to have children or not.

Parity (meaning the condition of having borne a child) has been associated with both protection from and risk for certain medical conditions.

Parity offers protection against breast, endometrial, and colon cancers. Several studies also note significant decreases in ovarian cancer among women who have given birth more than once.

Parity is known to increase the risk for diabetes, cervical cancer, hypertension, and CAD. Multiparity (giving birth more than once) is associated with lower HDL cholesterol levels, even after factoring in age, menopausal status, smoking, obesity, and other contributors. Women who have more children are at higher risk for Type II diabetes and impaired glucose tolerance; the risk is double if there is a family history of diabetes. Parity is closely related to obesity, regardless of other social or demographic factors. Although maternal mortality has been dramatically reduced in the last one hundred years, nonwhite women are still three times as likely as Caucasian women to die of pregnancy related causes. The risk to African-American women is the highest of all racial groups.

Carolyn, thirty-four, had an uneventful pregnancy until her eighth month when she was diagnosed with gestational diabetes—although she was of normal weight and had gained only twenty pounds during her pregnancy. Carol's diabetes was controlled with diet, and her OB/GYN doctor and I followed her very carefully for the remainder of her pregnancy. She had a normal delivery and a beautiful baby.

After her baby was born, Carol moved to another state, and I lost touch with her for about ten years. When she moved back to New York, two kids and fifty pounds later, she was busy, exhausted, and beside herself—a full-time mom who rarely exercised, couldn't get control of her weight, and couldn't shake her fatigue.

Then, suddenly, Carol began to experience strange symptoms. She was losing weight and urinating so frequently that she couldn't sleep. Her vision was so blurred she couldn't read. Alarmed, she found my phone number and called me.

I was glad to see Carol again, but I was saddened by what had occurred in the ten years since her first son's birth. I wasn't surprised to find that Carol now had full-blown diabetes. As a woman with gestational diabetes, she was at higher risk for developing diabetes later—and indeed, she had. What I found most frustrating was that no doctor had counseled her in the past ten years to eat a healthy diet and to get regular exercise so that she could avoid weight gain and thereby decrease her risk for adult onset diabetes. She had been poorly served by physicians who weren't making a connection between her short-lived gestational diabetes and her long-term risks.

Carol's visit to me was a wake-up call to self-care. I urged her to start taking care of herself and to stop putting herself last on the list. I spoke with Carol's husband about her need for support—including a nutritional change for the whole family and support for time away to exercise. With good lifestyle counseling, I hoped to avoid having to treat Carol with medication. So far, the plan has worked. Carol has been able to control her diabetes with

---

HOW PREGNANCY AFFECTS YOUR RISKS

Long-term risks for certain conditions are influenced by pregnancy. Studies have shown different mortality patterns among women who have had children versus those who have not.

The Risk Goes Down for . . .
  Breast cancer
  Ovarian cancer
  Uterine cancer
  Uterine fibroids

The Risk Goes Up for . . .
  Diabetes
  Heart disease
  Hypertension
  Gallbladder disease

diet and exercise. But the point is, had she been better informed and motivated to take charge, she might have avoided diabetes altogether.

THE POST-PREGNANCY MOOD EFFECT

Most women think of pregnancy as an event that lasts approximately nine months, after which their bodies return to "normal." But the tangible effects of pregnancy linger. Plummeting hormone levels after delivery are a high-risk time for postpartum depression. Estrogen, progesterone, endorphins, cortisol, and thyroid hormones are all involved.

"Baby Blues," a mild postpartum mood alteration, occurs on the third or fourth day after childbirth and can last for up to two weeks. This depression is often not taken seriously, but it is a legitimate phenomenon that afflicts up to 80 percent of all women. Postpartum depression is a more serious state beginning at six weeks to four months after delivery. It can last as long as two years. Prenatal depression is a good predictor of risk. So is prior postpartum depression. Postpartum depression should be treated aggressively for the sake of the woman and her relationship with her child.

This is a hard condition to accept because it seems to contradict everything we think a new mother should be feeling. The birth of a child is supposed to be a joyful, life-affirming event, so where does the depression come from? Women who suffer from postpartum depression usually feel terribly guilty and confused. It might help to know that postpartum depression is almost certainly hormonal, and can sometimes be related to an immune system disorder like thyroiditis. It also responds to antidepressants.

The incidence of postpartum depression is far lower following abortions than term pregnancies. There is no scientific evidence to support a diagnosis of post-abortion depression. When it does occur, it is usually in the context of pre-abortion depression. Transient sadness, guilt, and regret are normal feelings following abortion, but studies have shown that the predominant feeling is one of relief.

Miscarriage is more complex. The trauma of miscarriage is heightened by the conspiracy of silence surrounding the event. There is no established ritual for mourning a fetal death; women are expected to go on with their lives without suffering anything more than a sense of disappointment. But even early in the pregnancy, the emotional commitment and expectations are there, along with the psychological reactions triggered by hormonal changes. A miscarriage has an impact.

In spite of the hormonal and medical bases for postpartum depression, clinicians have found that the best predictor of outcome is a woman's relationship with her partner. For this reason, both men and women should be educated about what to expect after a baby is born. Physical side effects as well as hormonally-induced depression should be fully understood and anticipated—just as couples prepare for the childbirth itself.

HEALTHY PREGNANCY . . . AND BEYOND

Early and regular prenatal care has been identified as the single most important factor in a healthy pregnancy. Yet, 35 percent of African-American women and 20 percent of white women do not receive early prenatal care because they have no access or cannot afford it. Four in ten pregnant women have incomes below fifteen thousand dollars a year, and nearly 40 percent have no medical insurance to cover pregnancy. There is a huge coverage gap between the very poor, who are covered by Medicaid, and those above the strictly defined poverty level, who are not eligible for benefits. But even women who are eligible for Medicaid aren't guaranteed state-of-the-art care. Often, there is no coverage for complications or for special screening procedures like amniocentesis. The health of women and their children will continue to be at risk if the system itself fails to address these issues. It is a terrible breakdown in ethics and responsibility that in an affluent society, where access to the best medical care in the world exists for those who can afford it, large segments of the population receive care on a par with that of Third World nations.

While it's not possible to transform the problem of access to prenatal care overnight, we can begin individually to do our part through self-education and empowerment. That is what we hope to accomplish with this book and with other efforts on women's behalf. The woman-centered society we anticipate and strive for would affirm the choice of motherhood as well as the choice to remain childless. Mothers and their children would not sink to the bottom of the social and economic ladder, but be supported and allowed to flourish. Pregnancy would be viewed as a natural life event rather than a troublesome interruption of a woman's career. Reproductive freedom would be a core factor of every woman's life, and the choice to have children or remain childless would be equally respected.

Common Questions about Pregnancy

I have chosen to remain childless. Does this place me at greater risk for diseases later in life?

There are some data showing that having children offers women protection against breast, endometrial, and colon cancers, as well as a possible decrease in the risk of ovarian cancer. However, these risk factors must be considered in the context of your other risks. Also remember that many women who develop breast cancer have no known risk factors. I would discourage any woman from making a decision about childbearing based solely on these data. We did not fight so hard for reproductive freedom only to conclude that childless women are less healthy! In today's society, the decision to remain childless should be considered every bit as valid as the decision to bear children. Women contemplating childlessness may want to use oral contraceptives to decrease their risk of ovarian and endometrial cancers.

My first child was delivered by Caesarian. Must I have my next child by Caesarian, too?

It used to be the rule of thumb: Once a C-section, always a C-section. Doctors were afraid that the pressure of a vaginal delivery might rupture the site of the incision. Today, the wisdom is reversed, and unless complications are present, you can expect a vaginal delivery even if your previous child was a C-section.

Is it safe to have my baby at home?

The groundswell of interest in home birthing is a direct outcome of the invisibility women feel by being powerless within the medical system. I believe women and their families should be encouraged to make the childbirth process as natural and personally comfortable as possible. However, you have to keep medical considerations at the forefront. Although childbirth is natural, it is not necessarily benign.

Some hospitals have established birthing rooms in an effort to make the process feel more intimate. The goal is to offer the intimacy of home with the protection of a hospital. Needless to say, the effort often falls short, but it is a step in the right direction. There are also more than one hundred birthing centers in the United States, some utilizing nurse midwives. These centers are connected to hospitals in case rapid emergency care is needed.

How soon after childbirth should I resume birth control?

As soon as you begin sexual activity, which can be about six weeks after delivery, you should use contraceptives. It's possible to get pregnant right away, even if you are breast-feeding.

I am having my first child at forty. Am I at greater risk for complications?

The pregnancy rate of women ages forty to forty-five is 30 percent that of women in their twenties. As women age, the rate of miscarriages increases. There is more likelihood of chromosomal abnormalities. Fibroids are more common in this age group and can complicate conception and pregnancy. Older women are also more vulnerable to hypertension, toxemia, and diabetes. In general, older women have a sevenfold increase in incidences of maternal death and a much higher rate of obstetrical complications. (Consult your doctor for a preconception evaluation to understand your risks.)

Are fertility drugs safe?

In addition to the burden of infertility caused by pelvic inflammatory disease, fertility declines with advancing age—the burden of delaying pregnancy. In 1988 2 million women had already been exposed to fertility drugs used in the burgeoning business of advanced reproductive technologies. Drug sales for clomiphene doubled from 1973 to 1991. To date, two studies have been published indicating increased risk of ovarian cancer in women exposed to these medications, especially clomiphene when used in many cycles. In women with no family history of ovarian cancer, risk is increased to two to three times that of the general population (1.8 percent lifetime risk). As with all medical treatments, risk must be weighed against the benefits, both biologically and socially, of childbearing.

RESOURCES

ORGANIZATIONS
American Adoption Congress
P.O. Box 23641
Washington, DC 20024

COPE (Coping with the Overall Pregnancy Experience)
37 Clarendon Street
Boston, MA 02116

Midwives Alliance of North America
30 South Main Street
Concord, NH 03301

National Association of Childbearing Centers
Box 1, Route 1
Perkiomenville, PA 18074
215-234-8068

PUBLICATIONS
Caesarian Prevention Clarion
Caesarian Prevention Movement
P.O. Box 152
Syracuse, NY 13210

Journal of Nurse-Midwifery
52 Vanderbilt Avenue
New York, NY 10017

Mothering
P.O. Box 2208
Albuquerque, NM 87103

13

THE MENOPAUSE YEARS
Time to Take Stock

~~~

In 1991, a Seattle woman was denied permission by the State Department of Licensing for a customized license plate reading MENOPOZ. In a letter explaining its decision, the Department wrote, "It has come to our attention that the phrase used on your personalized license plate, MENOPOZ, is offensive to good taste and dignity."

What a perfect commentary on our cultural squeamishness about women and their natural functions! As I mentioned earlier, women's physiologic processes have always been in the closet. They are an embarrassment to both sexes and usually dealt with covertly. When the physiologic process at hand is menopause, it is treated with delicacy and distance, regarded as an inevitable yet humiliating event that is best left unnoted. Our attitudes are based on a lengthy history of misinformation and cultural bias.

Prior to the twentieth century, menopause was seen as a physiological crisis—a disease. It was also the grim portent of a life that had outworn its purpose—as Columbat de l'Isere noted in his *Treatise of the Disease of Females,* "Compelled to yield to the power of time, women now cease to exist for the species, and hence forward live only for themselves. Their features are stamped with the impress of age and their genital organs are sealed with the signet of sterility . . . [The menopausal woman] now resembles a de-throned queen, or rather a goddess whose adorers no longer frequent her shrine."

Even as recently as thirty years ago, some medical experts were defining menopause as a pathological state. In 1963, Dr. Robert A. Wilson (the man who popularized HRT) wrote in *Feminine Forever* that "a large percentage of women . . . acquire a vapid cow-like feeling . . . the world appears as though through a grey veil and they live as docile, harmless creatures, missing most of life's values."

In 1987, a medical textbook prepared doctors to treat menopausal women by saying, "Emotional instability is another outstanding feature of this phase of life. Nervousness and anxiety are extremely frequent. The patient may feel that the end of her useful life has come, that now she is old, that she has lost her appeal as a woman, and that nothing is left to her. She cries easily; she flares up at her family and friends; she is irritable and may have difficulty in composing her thoughts or her reactions."

To judge by our literature, menopause is the end of the road for women; if not a real death, then certainly a "death" of all that is worthwhile about being female. The bias is so pervasive that we must work hard to find replacement images of power and self-worth. Sometimes those images come from other cultures.

The characterization of menopause as the end of a woman's worth in society has been a decidedly Western view. In many nonWestern cultures, menopause is considered a positive point in a woman's life, signalling the beginning not the end of her power. This view is most common in societies where women of childbearing age have little or no access to power because they are valued only for their potential as breeders and sexual beings. Menopause releases them from subordination. Their cultures allow them access to political power once they relinquish their reproductive power, and menopause becomes a welcome time in their lives. We might argue with the fundamental philosophies of these cultures, which consider young childbearing women as dangerously sexual. Nevertheless, the empowerment of older women is fascinating to observe.

The Yoruba of West Africa, for example, allow only older women to travel freely and participate in trade. Among the Mandurucu of South America, the oldest woman holds authority over the household. In Plains Cree and Winnebago Indian cultures, postmenopausal women can become shamans. The Navajo elevate postmenopausal women to the positions of spiritual leaders and healers.

Although menopause is a biological event, it takes place in a cultural milieu. The way it is perceived in wider society naturally affects the way we experience it. In America, we often find menopause to be a double whammy: A blow to self-esteem that is the result of both agism and sexism. Some of the most pained women I have met are those who have depended on physical beauty and youth for their identities. We are a culture that prizes youth and sexuality. And even though older women do not lose their sexuality, there is a prevalent perception that they are not sexual. We strip them of that quality, even as we accept and admire sexual virility in older men. We see older women as neutered, even though all that has happened is that they have stopped ovulating.

Rather than reinforce the stigma of "menopausal" when referring to women at this point in their lives, I prefer to think about the midlife woman.

WHO IS THE MIDLIFE WOMAN?

The midlife woman is hardly over the hill! Indeed, she is right at the center of the action. She is most likely to be a mother; nine out of ten midlife women have at least one child, and many others want a child. She is sexually active—more so if she's divorced—and still needs birth control and regular screening for sexually transmitted diseases. She is unlikely to be one of two parents, staying at home to care for a family—a traditional model now represented by only 10 percent of American women. Chances are, she's a divorced single parent; one-third of all first marriages and one-half of all second marriages end in divorce, resulting in a decreased standard of living for 70 percent of divorced women, even as it represents an increased standard of living for 40 percent of divorced men.

The midlife woman is part of a group that begins to have health problems, something which increases with age. Half of the women in this group have high blood pressure, one-third are overweight, and one-third smoke.

The midlife woman is more than just someone "suffering menopause." Decline of ovarian functions is merely a background against which the script of social circumstances, health, and illness unfolds. Let's remember this as we look more closely at one of women's most misunderstood natural events.

At last, we have started to redefine menopause. In 1991, the Massachusetts Women's Health Study reported that "menopause, as a natural event, appears to have no major impact on health or human behavior. Any increase in symptomatology appears to be relatively small and transitory . . . The majority of women barely notice the menopause and health care utilization does not increase during menopause."

Most of my patients actually feel freed up and energized. For these women, menopause marks a time of life when the sense of self is stronger than ever, accomplishments are many, and personal power is at its peak. They enjoy being mature women, with all the respect that status brings. They are invigorated by their release from the fear of pregnancy and the new thrill of experiencing sexuality without a link to reproduction.

A fifty-year-old woman told me, "I would love my face and body to look younger. But there is no way I'd want to return to a younger age because I am so much more put together now than I have ever been in my life."

Menopause is not a disease. It is a normal life event. I don't like to talk about "treating menopause." Rather, I treat the symptoms that sometimes accompany menopause and the physiological changes that result from estrogen deficiency. Unfortunately, many gynecologists today are actively pursuing the menopausal patient. Looking to extend their reach into this "booming" population, gynecologists have called for the creation of a specialty in "climacteric medicine," defining this period as ranging from thirty-five to sixty-five years of age. Women are being described as premenopausal, perimenopausal, or postmenopausal, as if the end of ovulation were a life-defining medical event. Although this may be one way gynecologists evolve into primary care of older women, the approach is still reproductively centered. Essentially, doctors are creating patients, diseases, and dollars; in business terms, it's "carving out the market."

In 1900, fewer than five million American women were older than fifty-two, the average age menopause occurs. By the year 2000, more than twenty-one million women will reach age fifty, at a rate of about 1.3 million a year. Today, the average woman's life expectancy is approaching eighty—meaning that we will spend more than one-third of our lives in this "menopausal" state. Women need to resist medicine's reach into the medicalized market of menopause. We must understand that menopause itself is not the problem. We need to shift our thinking to a "woman as norm" model in which we appreciate the relationship between our ovarian hormones and the rest of our body. If all of our organs are accustomed to an estrogen-rich millieu, it makes sense that an estrogen-depleted state will facilitate degeneration and enhance vulnerability to disease—a different process from what occurs in aging men.

Today, we can expect to live more than one-third of our life span after menopause. Older women, often outliving their male partners, are prematurely asked to retire from the mainstream of life at age sixty-five, as men do; they crowd hospitals and nursing homes. I believe we must reclaim this period in our lives and advocate for health and social vitality. We must demand that medicine define the postmenopausal woman in a way that maintains her femininity and her uniqueness, despite waning estrogen levels. Medicine contributes to the "neutering" of older women by comparing postmenopausal women to men. But even though they stop ovulating and their estrogen levels decline, older women are still women, not men!

WHAT HAPPENS AT MENOPAUSE?

Although life spans have increased by several decades, the timing of menopause has remained consistent, occurring for most women between the ages of forty-eight and fifty-five. The greatest differences are seen among smokers, who seem to enter menopause two or more years earlier than nonsmokers. Women who haven't had children also tend to have earlier menopause. And, of course, many women experience early "man-made" menopause when they are given hysterectomies and oophorectomies in their thirties and forties.

We have a tendency to think of menopause as a single event—the dividing line between youth and age. In reality, it is a process that happens gradually, the culmination of changes that have been occurring in your body for a number of years.

Simply put, menopause is a biological milestone signaling the completion of reproductive years, just as adolescence is a period that marks the onset of reproductive ability. When you are born, your ovaries contain a lifetime supply of eggs, which diminishes over time. By the time you reach menopause, the ovarian follicles—the multicellular structure that contains the eggs and produces female hormones—are depleted. This process does not happen overnight. Rather, the gradual decline of ovarian function and in the production of estrogen and progesterone usually begins a few years before the cessation of menses.

We are now sophisticated enough to know that the nonovulating (or postmenopausal) ovary is not an inert organ. Hormones and other substances continue to be produced in altered amounts. What's more, each woman's ovaries can follow a different course. Highly sensitive ultrasound tells us that the postmenopausal ovary is alive; we are seeing cysts grow in women who, according to traditional medical teaching, shouldn't have growths.

Unfortunately, also as a result of "tradition," these women are brought into operating rooms to have their ovaries removed.

Furthermore, the ovary doesn't just act on its own. Newly sophisticated studies reveal the brain's role in menopause. Changes in the timekeeping functions of the brain (called circadian rhythms) affect neurohormones that may then contribute to the age-related slowing of ovarian function.

Cross-cultural studies also tell us that menopause is not experienced the same way by all women. Expectations play a major role in symptom reporting, and those who perceive menopause to be an adverse event report more symptoms. Diet may also play a role; women in Asia who consume diets low in fat and high in herbs and soy products that contain plant forms of estrogen, rarely report hot flashes. It is also clear that in societies where women acquire social, religious, or political power in the postmenopausal years, symptoms are minimal.

THE MYTH OF MENOPAUSAL DEPRESSION

My women patients have sometimes shrugged off their feelings of depression by saying, "I guess it's just menopause." One woman reported how her husband angrily called her "a menopausal witch." Of this insult she said calmly, "You know, he's right. I think menopause is turning me into a shrew."

There are many reasons why women suffer depression, but in the sense of cause and effect, it looks as if menopause is not one of them. Experts now believe that the increased irritability or lack of energy many women report might simply be the result of sleep disturbances caused by overt or subclinical flushes. In fact, when men were awakened and prohibited from entering deep sleep, researchers found them irritable and depressed.

It is understandable that we'd assume a link between menopause and depression, since it fits so well with our prejudices against aging in women. But the evidence is to the contrary. Of 7,500 women who participated in the Massachusetts Women's Health Study, 70 percent reported relief or neutral feelings about the end of their menses. Although rates of depression were slightly higher in the group, it did not appear to be a menopause-related clinical state; depression was transitory and seemed to be linked to discomfort with menopausal symptoms like hot flashes. The strongest risk factor for menopausal depression is premenopausal depression, and preexisting depression is associated with more menopausal symptoms.

Not surprisingly, some studies have shown that women who experience the most intense feelings of depression around menopause are those who have relied on childbearing for their identities. Other factors correlating with depression are stress in interpersonal relationships, changes in marital status, and a decline in physical health.

There have been reports that some women experience depression as a result of estrogen replacement. Sometimes trying a different hormonal replacement can eliminate this side effect. With progesterone use, switching to the "natural" form (micronized progesterone) can help. Obviously, more research is needed.

CHECKING IT OUT

I view midlife, as I prefer to call this period around the menopause, as a time to take stock. It is when we prepare for the third trimester of life by moving beyond being reproductively focused to total women's health. In this broader context, we take stock of health risks that might predict problems in older age. It's a good time to change lifestyle habits or begin preventive therapy. As pediatrics focuses on nutrition and behavior in adolescents, preparing them for healthy young adulthood, we need to do the same for midlife women.

As you approach menopause, your menstrual function might undergo subtle changes. Clinical studies show that only about 10 percent of women will experience a sudden stoppage of menstruation. The norm is less clearly recognized. Seventy percent report a time of abnormal periods—either unusual length between periods or lighter bleeding. Another 18 percent report heavier bleeding or irregular bleeding between cycles.

If you are experiencing any symptoms—be they irregular periods, the cessation of menses, or flashes—I suggest that it is time for you to get a full physical, to make sure that some other condition is not causing the symptoms.

Don't assume that your bleeding irregularities are menopausal. For one thing, until your periods stop completely, you may still be fertile. The first thing to rule out if you are missing a period is pregnancy, since 80 percent of midlife women are sexually active. A Portland, Oregon, woman holds the record for the oldest pregnancy, conceiving at the age of fifty-seven years and one hundred twenty days. Don't assume it can't happen! Demographics among midlife women are very different now and are often not appreciated by physicians. Only one out of four is married and living with a husband; many midlife divorced, widowed, or single women are sexually active; they are twice as likely as married women to have more than one sexual partner. The statistics about midlife reproductive events are dramatic: half of all births to women over forty are unintended, and one-third of all conceptions are aborted. Midlife women are quite sexual, and health practitioners cannot assume a midlife woman is not at risk for pregnancy or sexually transmitted diseases.

Cora, a forty-four-year-old woman, came in for a checkup, and she mentioned that she was somewhat concerned because she hadn't had a period in six weeks—a very unusual occurence for her. She thought something was wrong. Remember, even though we experience our periods as annoyances, there is something very reassuring about their regularity. You expect them to be there, and equate them with a sense of normalcy. When suddenly you don't get a period, it's a matter of great concern.

So I asked Cora, "Could you be pregnant?"

She was momentarily taken aback. "Oh, no," she said. "I've never been able to get pregnant, and besides, I'm forty-four now. I don't think I could be pregnant."

I reminded Cora that forty-four-year-old women could indeed get pregnant.

She was suddenly fascinated. "Well," she said, shaking her head and laughing a little. "I hadn't thought of that. It would be an interesting thing in my life if I was pregnant."

Cora turned out not to be pregnant, but I've seen it happen. Change of life pregnancies are relatively common, especially now when women are deliberately delaying parenthood. The point is, a midlife woman needs to continue using birth control. Don't make assumptions about your fertility based on your age.

FLASHES: THE MARK OF MENOPAUSE

In Western cultures, one of the most common signs of menopause is the "hot flash," described as "recurrent, transient periods of flushing, sweating, and a sensation of heat, often accompanied by palpitations, feelings of anxiety, and sometimes followed by chills." Most women experience minor or no discomfort, but for others this can be a severe condition that robs a woman of sleep, makes her uncomfortable, and embarrasses her when she sweats in public.

When a woman in her forties or early fifties begins to experience flashing or night sweats, she is likely to automatically assume, "It's menopause." But here again, it's important to check it out. Night sweats can accompany tumors, infections, hyperthyroidism, or diabetes. And if you're already on hormone replacement therapy, a hot flash means you are not fully absorbing estrogen.

What exactly is a hot flash? The hallmark of a hot flash is a sudden feeling of warmth throughout the upper part of the body with a reddening of the neck and face. Sweating occurs, followed by a cold, clammy sensation, chills, or shivers. Flashes vary in intensity, frequency, and duration within any one woman and also among different women. They can be as often as hourly or never occur at all. Sometimes an aura precedes a hot flash by several seconds. During this period the heart rate increases and is experienced as palpitations. There may be a wave of nausea and a sensation of dizziness, which might be accompanied by anxiety or dread—a sensation easily confused with a panic attack.

Flashes can begin before the time of menstrual irregularity and they can last forever, although the average time is about six months. They have a diurnal rhythm with a peak intensity at night and lesser intensity when the temperature is low. They can be precipitated by stress, caffeine, alcohol, spicy foods, and skin-to-skin contact.

Aside from flashes, women may experience a general state of "unwellness": fatigue, dizziness, irritability, apprehension, insomnia, altered libido, poor concentration and memory, headache, neck stiffness, and mood fluctuations. The important thing to remember is that most women have no symptoms, so don't write off any of the above symptoms to menopause. Check them out.

UNDERSTANDING HORMONE REPLACEMENT

Phyllis was a new patient whom I saw for the first time when she was a few years past menopause. Her husband had recently died after a long illness, and now Phyllis was paying more attention to her health. She came in for a routine checkup. I asked her whether or not she had given any thought to hormone replacement therapy.

Her immediate reaction was very negative. "No, I don't want it," she said firmly. "I'm very healthy, my mother is still going strong at eighty, and I've never had a single hot flash. I'm perfectly fine without hormones. Besides, I don't like to take things that aren't natural if I don't have to."

Like Phyllis, many women relate the need to take hormones to the severity of menopausal symptoms. If they feel fine, why bother? As I began to educate Phyllis about some of the benefits of estrogen replacement beyond specific menopausal symptoms, her eyes were opened. She was unaware that estrogen could decrease her risk of heart disease and keep her bones strong. I also attacked the theory that taking hormones wasn't natural. "Living for many years beyond menopause isn't natural," I told her. "Humans are the only species that have a significant life span beyond our fertile period, and that has only been true for us in this century."

When you consider all of the ways that modern medicine has given us a new lease on life—less death in childbirth, antibiotics for treating infections, and so on—it's clear that these are not "natural" in the strictest sense of the word. But few people would support turning back the clock to a time when technology and knowledge were not available to treat disease. I strongly believe that we should embrace the knowledge that we have and continue exploring the remarkable protective influences of estrogen on women's health.

As I explained my beliefs about the role of modern medicine and the positive influences of estrogen, Phyllis began nodding her head. She admitted that she had never considered how recent a phenomenon long life spans were. It gave her something to think about. "But," she asked, "won't estrogen replacement put me at risk for breast cancer?"

It happened that Phyllis didn't have risk factors associated with breast cancer, so I explained that in her case, the risks of being low in estrogen were probably much greater.

I could empathize with Phyllis's concerns—not only those she voiced but also the unspoken feelings. A lot of women look at being on medication as a signal that they've crossed a line and can now be called "old." They avoid hormone replacement therapy because they're not informed about it and see it as just another "medication." They are wary of doctors' prescriptions for hormones, especially when they're not studied fully before finding their way into common practice.

Although the data about the benefits of hormone replacement therapy are voluminous, the prospective randomized clinical trials necessary to conclusively show efficacy are only now being done. So there is reason for healthy skepticism. That being said, I still believe we can make reasonably informed decisions while awaiting confirmation if we do it together in a mutually understood way. Hormone replacement therapy is not just a matter of going to a doctor and getting a prescription for medication. It's an opportunity to be an active participant in your health care. You have to help the doctor monitor your progress. You have to know what you're taking, when you're taking it, how to take it, what side effects to look for, what routine screening tests you should be getting, and what kind of follow-up is indicated. HRT is part of a lifestyle program, not just a pill.

Education begins with the realization that a low estrogen level affects more than just fertility. It has an important effect on other tissues in your body as well—both short and long term. There are estrogen receptors in nearly every tissue in the body. So, instead of considering ovaries as a separate entity, consider how they are related to every other organ system—the cardiovascular system, the skeletal system, the urogenital tissue, the brain, the colon, and the immune system.

There's no sure way to predict what the transition called menopause will be like for you. I've seen women whose long-term migraine problems ended at menopause. Others first started getting migraines at menopause. Some are completely energized, feeling at the peak of life, while others are fatigued and feeling vulnerable. Some will tolerate estrogen well, others will need to try several formulations before they find one that works, and others may not feel well on any.

This isn't just a pill. There is a wide range of treatments within this category. HRT is not yet a science; it's more like an applied craft. A replacement program must be carefully formulated according to each woman's needs and preferences. Needs are defined by symptoms, current medical problems, and risks for future illness. Preferences take into account feelings about taking pills, fear of complications, distaste for continuing menstruation, and the ability to afford treatment. I can think of no other area where education and collaboration are more important.

DECISIONS TO MAKE

Let's look at some of the issues that will inform your judgment about hormone replacement therapy.

1. Should You Take Hormone Replacement Therapy?

There are three reasons to consider HRT: Relief of menopausal symptoms, maintenance of urogenital health, and prevention of disease. All midlife women are at risk for shrinkage, weakness, and atrophy of tissues that have estrogen receptors. As we age, most of us are at risk for degenerative processes like cardiovascular disease, cancer, frailty, and mental decline, although 46,000 women die annually of breast cancer, 400,000 die from cardiovascular disease, and 300,000 fracture hips. HRT should be a decision that you and your physician reach after assessing your needs and preferences.

2. Should You Take Estrogen Alone or with Progestins?

When estrogens were first prescribed in the 1960s, their introduction was followed by an eightfold increase in endometrial cancer during the 1970s. That was because doctors failed to appreciate the effect of "unopposed" estrogen on the uterus. We now know that when progesterone is added, the enhanced risk of cancer to the uterus is eliminated and no increase in risk of breast cancer is seen. There has also been a fear that progesterone might blunt the beneficial effects that estrogen has on lipids and therefore on coronary artery disease, but recent studies have shown this not to be so. Women who have had hysterectomies/oophorectomies should receive estrogen alone. All other women require progesterone.

Some women have unpleasant side effects to progesterone, including fluid retention and irritability or depression. This is where craft takes over from science. Doctors are experimenting with decreasing the time women need to spend on progesterone—for example, prescribing it only every three months. Some use a progesterone-filled IUD to target the hormone only to the lining of the uterus and avoid systemic effect; this requires annual changing of the IUD. Still other doctors avoid progesterone altogether and monitor women regularly with endometrial sampling and ultrasound. Progesterone's down side may be minimized when a natural rather than a synthetic substance is used, but micronized progesterone is not easily found in the United States at this time and is considerably more expensive.

3. If You Need Progesterone, Is Cyclic or Continuous Therapy the Best?

When progesterone was first added on to estrogen replacement, doctors tried to mimic a natural cycle—estrogen for three weeks, progesterone added in the third week, and nothing in the fourth week when bleeding occurred. Some women, however, would experience a return of symptoms during the off week. Regimens were then expanded to daily estrogen, with progesterone added for ten to twelve days of the month (best remembered by following the calendar days one through twelve). Bleeding would still occur at the end of the progesterone.

To eliminate bleeding altogether, a continuous combined regimen was developed. Estrogen is taken daily along with a lower dose of progesterone. On this regimen, the uterine lining eventually atrophies and bleeding stops. Unfortunately, there is a good deal of spotting during the first six months of the regimen, especially for newly menopausal women. But after that, the bleeding should stop.

4. How Do You Know if HRT Is Working?

I always insist on yearly physicals so that we can review our assessment of needs and preferences. At one extreme, hormone replacement maximizes its effect with current use; that is, once you stop, your risks for CAD, osteoporosis, and other conditions start again. On the other hand, women often feel more comfortable knowing HRT can always be stopped if problems develop. We are currently expecting a lot of important information on HRT from studies begun now, and we need to continuously update our practices. Stay tuned!

When I monitor my patients who are on HRT, I look for effectiveness of treatment. Are all flashes gone? If not, you may not be fully absorbing the hormones. Each woman has her own pattern of absorption and modification by the liver. That's why blood levels are inaccurate even when taking pure estradiol (Estrace). Premarin, the most commonly used preparation in the United States, contains a mixture of estrogens that have already been modified. So, if you are taking estrogen orally, a good way to assess its effectiveness is by noting the presence of any persistent flashes, and by having a vaginal smear taken when you get a Pap smear to see whether estrogen is successfully thickening the vaginal wall. If a patient of mine doesn't seem to be experiencing the full hormonal effect, I will sometimes increase the dose or add a bit of local estrogen vaginal cream.

Transdermal estrogen ("the patch") is the only way to get accurately measured blood levels of estrogen because it goes directly to your blood. However, while studies of osteoporosis have shown the patch to be effective, none has been done yet on CAD. It is possible that the patch won't have the same effect, since oral estrogen enhances HDL and lowers LDL cholesterol when it is absorbed and passes through the liver. The other down side of the patch is local skin irritation and the need to change it twice a week. Even so, there are certain circumstances when I prefer to use the patch. They are:

1. **Gallstones.** When a woman has known gallstones, I use the patch because oral estrogen enhances gallstone formation.

2. **Smokers.** Smoking increases the metabolism of estrogen, which is why smokers have earlier menopause, greater risk of infertility, increased frequency of hirsutism (hairiness), and more fractures due to osteoporosis. This may be less pronounced for transdermal, as compared to orally ingested, estrogen.

3. **Migraine** sufferers: Menopausal transdermal estrogen has relieved migraines in those women who once had severe premenstrual headaches. The patch can reduce migraines in women who continue to get them using oral estrogen.

4. **High triglycerides:** Oral estrogen can sometimes worsen elevated triglyceride levels—an important risk factor associated with CAD in women.

Bone density tests can also document whether estrogen is effective. If enough estrogen is being absorbed and enough calcium ingested, bone density should remain stable or even improve. Bone density testing is controversial from a cost-effectiveness point of view; if you're going to be on HRT anyway and do all the other preventive therapies, why spend money to document a number? On the other hand, if you have known osteoporosis, it is important to know if your therapy is working. I also tend to do bone density tests for women who are unsure about starting HRT or those who can't take estrogen.

Some practitioners follow all women on HRT with yearly endometrial sampling and ultrasound. Clearly, this is overutilization of reimbursable technology. My practice is more focused. The only time I do more than a physical exam is when unusual vaginal bleeding occurs—a possible sign of endometrial cancer—or when I'm following a woman who is on less than a monthly progesterone regimen. Ultrasound is getting so sensitive in ruling out endometrial cancer that it may replace endometrial sampling as the standard of care in the future.

Be wary about having your body constantly monitored by technology. It reinforces a "woman as disease" feeling, contributes to an overall sense of fear, and generates costs for the health care system.

WEIGHING THE BENEFITS AND RISKS OF TAKING HORMONES

Janet was a fifty-five-year-old woman who had a hysterectomy when she was forty because of endometrial cancer. At that time, she had been told by her gynecologist never to take estrogen. Since that had been fifteen years ago, I told her it was time to reopen the subject. She was vehement. "He said never."

It took me two years to get Janet to agree to a bone density test. She had significant bone loss. I said, "Please, do yourself a favor. Go back to your gynecologist and reopen the subject." So she walked into his office and told him why she was there, and he replied, "What! You mean you're not on estrogen?"

I believe that for most women, the risk of not taking estrogen outweighs the risk of taking it. But ultimately, it boils down to a personal choice related to your own health considerations and individual priorities. Take the issue of breast cancer. If you look at it by the numbers, the potential risk of heart disease absolutely swamps the risk of breast cancer. Yet, I have had women tell me point blank, "I would rather die of a heart attack than lose a breast."

I encourage my patients to carefully weigh all the data before making a decision. For example, it has long been assumed that if you've had breast cancer, you should never take hormones. Now we're beginning to study whether or not this needs to be the case, especially for women who have breast cancer when they're young. We've observed that pregnancy, which is an elevated estrogen state, does not cause a re-emergence of breast cancer in these women. So we have to study whether or not estrogen replacement will do so.

From a purely statistical standpoint, the evidence clearly marks heart disease as the higher risk factor for most women. Among one hundred women fifty-five years and older, 26.6 will die of heart disease compared to 5.9 of breast cancer and only 1.5 of endometrial cancer.

Having said this, it's also important to say that estrogen is not the be-all and end-all. There are other ways to protect yourself against heart disease and osteoporosis. As I pointed out in Chapter 5, even if you take estrogen, smoking, diabetes, and a high-fat diet all contribute to heart disease. We know that for some reason diabetics aren't protected from heart disease by their hormones, so we have to ask, if hormones didn't protect them before menopause, why should they protect them after menopause?

Furthermore, there are many other ways you can protect yourself. There is early research on a drug called tamoxifen, which is given to women who have had breast cancer. This drug not only appears to prolong disease-free survival rates in women with breast cancer (especially in women over fifty), it also is associated with an estrogen-like decrease in total cholesterol, an increase in HDL cholesterol, and protection against bone loss. Tamoxifen may ultimately prove to be the solution for women who can't take estrogen replacement because of breast cancer. Unfortunately, tamoxifen is associated with an increased risk of endometrial cancer—another example of the ways we must juggle risks.

Calcium and exercise are essential even when taking HRT, but they are especially crucial for preventing osteoporosis in women who choose not to take HRT.

Taking Control

The first thing you can do to take control is to find a women's health specialist who will manage your total care now and in the future. As we discussed earlier, this is not always easy to do, since a gynecologist might not be looking at your heart or bones, while an internist will not necessarily know how to evaluate abnormal bleeding or how to prescribe HRT.

Traditionally, gynecologists focused on the reproductive years and weren't trained to deliver medical care to older women. Now, they're attempting to make menopause a subspecialty in order to extend their patient care base. While this is one way to broaden services to women, the multifaceted needs of a menopausal woman cry out for a women's health specialty!

The next thing you need is a commitment to your own health. HRT is not a magic pill. It requires active involvement. Studies have found that there is a very high discontinuation rate among women on hormone replacement. Some women don't want to bleed. Some don't want to take pills. Some get bloated or feel depressed. But I believe that the high rate of discontinuation of hormone therapy is the result of ignorance among doctors, not patients. If doctors fail to adequately educate women about the importance of hormones and how to use them, women will find the idea of hormones too burdensome.

One survey of women who did not continue taking their prescription during the first year found that most of them stopped because they didn't really understand why they were taking hormones in the first place. The compliance rate is much higher among women who are well educated about the treatment. Know why you're taking them and feel comfortable about it. If you don't feel comfortable, HRT is not for you, no matter how much your doctor may encourage its use.

It's possible that your doctor might not even suggest hormone replacement, and you have to be alert to that, too. Since the evidence is so strong that it has important benefits, why are more doctors not informing their patients about its use? One study of physician prescribing practices found that many doctors based their recommendation on whether or not women had menopause-related symptoms and low cancer risk. These women were given estrogen. If there were no symptoms and even the slightest cancer risk, estrogen wasn't mentioned. Another study showed that younger doctors and female doctors were more inclined to recommend estrogen. There are no "shoulds" about HRT other than enabling all women to make informed decisions in collaboration with their health care providers.

ALTERNATIVE WAYS TO MINIMIZE MENOPAUSAL SYMPTOMS

If you cannot take hormones, or choose not to, there are still things you can do to minimize the discomfort and inconvenience of menopausal symptoms. Some of these suggestions are common sense. Others are compiled from anecdotal reports of women.

1. Wear layered clothing, so you can remove items if you feel overheated during the day.
2. Avoid caffeine and alcohol; they can trigger flashes in some women.
3. Certain medications, such as those prescribed to lower blood pressure, can bring on flashes. If this is a problem, ask your doctor to prescribe a different formula.
4. A tepid shower can help bring down body temperature.
5. Use a lubricating cream like K-Y jelly, Replens, or Astroglyde for vaginal dryness or itching.
6. Nonabsorbable or minimally absorbable estrogen cream can add lubrication to the vagina without systemic effect.
7. Vitamin E is sometimes used to improve mood, reduce hot flashes, and promote vaginal lubrication, although the reports are only anecdotal.
8. Ginseng, a root that contains plant estrogen, and Dong Xai and alfalfa are sometimes taken to limit symptoms.
9. Yam extracts that contain a plant form of progesterone may control sweats and flushes.

When you're making a decision about what is right for you, always keep in mind that science is influenced by cultural biases. We see this bias repeatedly in the failure of doctors to talk to their menopausal patients about hormone replacement. As one expert in the field quipped, "If we had a male hormone replacement that was as effective as ERT in women, men would be buying it in the supermarket."

COMMON QUESTIONS ABOUT MENOPAUSE

When should estrogen replacement begin?

The sooner the better. Rapid bone loss occurs in the first five years after menopause. However, it is never too late to start HRT.

Will a seventy-year-old woman who has never taken estrogen benefit by starting it that late?

Absolutely. I began a seventy-year-old hypertensive woman on estrogen to keep her heart healthy and prevent stroke. Even at seventy, estrogen still has protective effects. In fact, it is important for secondary prevention in women with known CAD. I include estrogen as part of my treatment for women who have suffered heart attacks. In a study conducted by Leisure World, women with previous heart attacks, strokes, or high blood pressure had a 50 percent reduction in death from subsequent strokes or heart attacks. In women with severe CAD, estrogen users had a 97 percent survival rate at five years compared with 81 percent for nonusers.

What happens if I smoke while I'm on HRT?

Smoking counters the protective action of estrogen. A woman who undergoes HRT and smokes has essentially the same risk profile as a nonsmoker who doesn't take estrogen.

My doctor recommended clonidine patches for my hot flashes. Is that the same as HRT?

Clonidine is a drug designed to lower blood pressure. It has sometimes been used in the form of transdermal patches to treat hot flashes in menopausal women. However, there are potential side effects including dizziness, dry mouth, fatigue, and nausea. Furthermore, clonidine won't diminish other menopausal symptoms. Nor will it offer the other benefits of hormones— including protection against coronary artery disease and osteoporosis.

I have a normal cholesterol count. Would I still benefit from HRT?

Yes. Estrogen also acts directly on blood vessels and inhibits the growth of atherosclerotic plaque in their walls. Enhancing HDL cholesterol levels accounts for only 30 percent of estrogen's beneficial effect.

Does menopause cause an altered libido?

Libido is determined by psychological as well as biological factors. Biologically, testosterone is responsible for libido in both men and women. Since the ovaries and adrenal glands continue to make testosterone after menopause, this is not an issue for women who have not had their ovaries removed. Even then, not all women suffer a loss of libido. For those who do, a combination replacement pill called Estratest is used. We do not prescribe testosterone casually for women who want to enhance their sexual interest, because of testosterone's unfavorable effect on lipids and its tendency to cause hirsutism (hairiness).

Will estrogen make me gain weight?

Women naturally gain weight with age and especially after menopause or when their ovaries are surgically removed. After menopause, muscle mass decreases and body fat increases even if weight remains unchanged. We see this in both African-American and Caucasian women. This weight appears predominantly on the trunk and around the abdomen—weight associated with increased risk for CAD. Estrogen replacement seems to prevent this redistribution of fat.

My mother had early onset of Alzheimer's disease. Is that a risk factor to consider in taking HRT?

Estrogen receptors are clearly found in adult brains. In research settings, estrogen has been found to improve the ability to learn new material and to enhance short-term memory. There is also evidence that estrogen given to women with early Alzheimer's may retard the deterioration of memory that is the hallmark of this disease.

RESOURCES

ORGANIZATIONS
National Women's Health Network
514 Tenth Street, NW
Washington, DC 20004
Publishes newsletter on women's health issues.

Older Women's League
666 Eleventh Street, NW
Suite 700
Washington, DC 20001
Publishes newsletter on women's issues.

Women's Association for Research in Menopause
(W.A.R.M.)
128 East 56th Street
New York, NY 10022

Women's International Pharmacy
(for micronized progesterone)
5708 Manona Drive
Madison, WI 53716
800-279-5708
608-221-7800

PUBLICATIONS
The Complete Book of Menopause: Every Woman's Guide to Good Health
by Landau, Cyr, Moulton
Grossett/Putnam, 1994

A Friend Indeed (newsletter)
Box 515
Place du Parc Station
Montreal, Canada H2W2PI
514-843-5730

Hot Flash
The National Action Forum for Midlife and Older Women
Box 816
Stony Brook, NY 11790-0609

Menopause News
2074 Union Street
Suite 10
San Francisco, CA 94123

Menopause Today
Planned Parenthood Federation of America
810 Seventh Avenue
New York, NY 10019

The Silent Passage (revised expanded edition)
by Gail Sheehy
Pocket Books, 1993

TAPES
Menopause: A Time of Transition
Produced by Planned Parenthood Education Department
1660 Bush Street
San Francisco, CA 94109

FOUR

MIND
AND BODY
TOGETHER

14
THE EMOTIONALLY HEALTHY WOMAN
Staying Well in Mind and Body

~~~~

There is a common misunderstanding that woman-centered health is merely an expanded focus from reproductive organs to hearts, bones, lungs, colons, and bladders. But to merely add more body parts and organs to the focus only further fragments women's care. To be woman-centered, health care must include the psychological, behavioral, social, and cultural arenas in which women exist, and she must be looked at as a total person. Only in this comprehensive environment of care are health and healing possible.

Anna, a young Latina patient, was a case in point. Anna was hurting. She once confided in me, "My health problem is that I'm a woman." She said it in a joking manner, but I could see that she really meant it. After years of seeking help for chronic pelvic pain that seemed to have no origin, and unsuccessful psychotherapy that never lifted her depression, she had learned to accept that it was her lot in life to have "female pain" and to be unhappy.

As Anna grew comfortable with me, she talked about her experiences growing up in an explosive household. She remembers frequently cowering in a corner when her father became enraged and beat her mother. He drank heavily, and he was also angry because Anna's mother had been unable to have more than one child—a less desirable girl. Once Anna saw her father rape her mother, and she was herself raped by an uncle when she was eleven. She never told anyone, because he threatened he would harm her if she did.

Now Anna was thirty and she had three children. Each birth had been difficult and had intensified her pelvic pain. But as she looked ahead, she saw many more children in her future. She had pleaded with her husband and her priest to allow birth control, but both had insisted that birth control was out of the question. If she became pregnant, it was God's will. Anna was a good Catholic and she believed this was true. Her husband also accused her of inventing the excuse of pelvic pain to avoid having sex with him. Sometimes she wondered if he was right; certainly, no doctor could find a medical cause.

Anna was an intelligent, articulate woman, but that did not rescue her from her pain and depression. A lifetime of hearing the powerful messages from her culture and religion convinced her that she could expect no more than what she had.

I listened to Anna's story of suffering, and I heard in her words the belittling verdict of our history: That women's pain is not real, that our depression should be overcome by will, that we are victims of our circumstances.

Anna's experience was indicative of a women's health crisis rarely mentioned in doctors' offices or medical literature. And in a sense she was right when she said her medical problems were a result of her gender. Being female in the final years of the twentieth century is still a health risk to both mind and body.

THE MIND/BODY CONNECTION

How can a woman like Anna take preventive health measures when she is paralyzed by her circumstances? How can she find help when her pain is so easily dismissed? And how can she take control of her circumstances when she is told that physical and emotional pain are an expected by-product of being a woman?

Many so-called experts truly believe that women are by nature more inclined to experience psychological and behavioral problems. I vehemently challenge that view. Since psychological standards for mental health have been based on a male model, they have traditionally failed to take into account the ways in which women develop differently, make decisions differently, communicate differently, and adapt to experiences differently from men.

Psychological norms describe a well-adjusted person as being one who is independent, autonomous, and assertive. However, this mental health standard fails to acknowledge the way women achieve mental balance differently from men. Modern theories of female development emphasize a self-in-relation model whereby women create a sense of themselves through their relationships with others. Mental health is achieved in an environment of mutual support, not rugged independence.

Both autonomy and support are important, and a healthy human being should develop both. But our culture has historically overemphasized the characteristics valued in men and underemphasized those operative in women. It is in this foreign environment that women must struggle to be themselves and maintain their fragile self-esteem.

We cannot talk about mental health in women without acknowledging the impact of living in a male-dominated society with its accompanying power relations manifested in all aspects of women's lives—intimate relationships, family, educational institutions, places of worship, the workplace, professional life, the legal system, government bureaucracies, and the health care system. None of the institutions in our society reflect female patterns and lifestyles. And the very relationships women need for good health are burdened by the expectation that women remain agreeable and passive and do not ask for what they really need.

Both sexes manifest mental illness. But the cultural domination of male values often allows our institutions to ignore women's real pain while they are quick to diagnose as pathologic behavior in women who step outside gender and sex-role stereotypes. Medicine has also failed to appreciate the role of violence and gender-based abuse as significant etiologic factors in women's mental illness. Rather than pursue the study and treatment of male aggression, male fear of intimacy, and male unrelatedness, medicine has focused on "pathologies" within women. Multiple personality disorders, borderline personality, self-defeating personality disorder, false memory syndrome—all psychiatric labels suggesting that disorder originates inside women themselves, instead of being secondary to abuse, gender-related stress, or the long-term effects of living with male aggression and lack of intimacy.

THE FIGHT FOR SELF-ESTEEM

Fran was a shy young woman who married when she was only eighteen. Her two children were born within a few years, and family life settled in. Fran's husband was an assertive and self-centered man who did well financially and liked to boast about his self-made success. Fran was treated to nice clothes, expensive furnishings, and fancy jewelry, but she was always made to feel that these were her rewards rather than the fruit of her own labors. In addition to caring for the children and household, Fran worked part-time in her husband's store. I say her husband's store because he owned everything in his own name—the home, business, and all bank accounts. Fran was given everything she needed, but it was at his discretion. Furthermore, he verbally abused her, demeaning her ideas, thoughts, and opinions. Fran's two sons, taking the lead from their father, made her feel stupid, insecure, and isolated in her own home.

In her forties, Fran had some plastic surgery that went awry. Instead of being transformed into the beauty she had dreamed about, she hated her looks. This was the insult that put her over the edge. Her precariously balanced integrity and her poor self-esteem eroded into full-blown depression. No medication worked. Her husband and sons derided Fran for being so weak and unable to pull herself together. Fran couldn't cope and didn't know how to deal with the pain in her life. She became a patient, going from one doctor to another with illness upon illness. She found that the sick role allowed her to demand care and attention; it gave her a way to extricate herself from the degradation of her life.

Fran went on to suffer a number of sicknesses related to her frail immune system—lupus, chronic pain, and a perforated ucler. She gained sixty pounds and felt very fat. She developed an addiction to sedatives to quiet her nerves.

Fran's husband and children refused to throw her a lifeline when she was clearly drowning. Instead, they blamed her even more, and her husband threatened divorce. Fran finally gave in, unable to bear the pain of her life any longer, and committed suicide. Her story is tragic and all too familiar. Who is to say how much of her problem was genetic predisposition, how much the result of an unsupportive environment, and how much a neurochemical imbalance? And does it really matter? Fran's story shows that good health is intimately linked with self-esteem.

Self-esteem, a learned and dynamic sense of who we are and how we value ourselves, underlies all of our health behavior. On some level, you probably know that quite well. When you are feeling strong and full of self-worth, life's ups and downs don't send you reeling. You are not afraid to develop a variety of quality relationships or to explore a diversity of skills and activities. Your equilibrium is more easily reestablished when you've been upset. You're more realistic in knowing that you can't please everyone all of the time. You have a sense of balance and perspective.

A woman with low self-esteem finds herself living in an unfriendly world. She sees herself as a helpless victim of fate whose life is outside of her control. She is unable to hold a sense of self-worth without the constant reinforcement of others, and when they don't provide that reinforcement, she is lost. A minor slight, failure, or rejection can trigger a prolonged despondency. She lacks the skills to cope with these assaults to her dignity since she needs the reassurance of others to maintain her emotional equilibrium. Friendships often fail because she is overly needy.

The road to self-esteem is paved in childhood and it is nurtured (or not) by adult caretakers. A child's core relationships are formed within the family circle, and later the wider community. These relationships become the building blocks of self-esteem. Children depend on adults for positive reinforcement because they are incapable of developing self-esteem on their own. If a child has emotionally remote parents, she will struggle to learn and feel bonding. If she is made to feel inadequate or unworthy, if she is made to feel ashamed of the way she looks, if she is demeaned for stating her opinions, if she is told she won't amount to anything, if she is blamed when things go wrong, she will grow into adulthood with an absence of self-esteem.

When a woman is conditioned to feel negatively about herself, and when that view is reinforced by lack of support and intimacy in adult relationships, she becomes vulnerable to many psychological and medical problems either directly or as a consequence of poor health behavior.

Being able to care for oneself is a basic factor in having good health behavior—like following a special diet if you are diabetic, or exercising to reduce your risk of CAD. Self-esteem is necessary for avoiding high-risk behavior like unprotected intercourse, substance abuse, or smoking. Being able to give to oneself is a necessary precondition to following a good cancer screening program or complying with a therapeutic regimen.

Few women come to a sense of self-esteem easily, even when they are raised in loving homes. Most of us wage a lifelong battle for self-esteem because it is not our cultural birthright. Indeed, we are socialized to be compliant, self-blaming, ashamed of the way we look or what we say, and overly responsible for the well-being of others, often at our own expense. The daily indignities that chip away at women's self-esteem start very early in life, and by the time they reach adulthood, many women believe that it is normal and even okay to feel dissatisfied with their faces and bodies, to be unable to express their opinions with authority, to be demeaned about their sexuality, and to be chronically unable to form fulfilling relationships.

Even professionals who should know better often think nothing of insulting women or making casual statements that leave them shaking with humiliation. These doctors don't realize how naturally their male biases have entered into the doctor-patient encounter.

A patient of mine who was very overweight complained of persistent headaches. At her insistence, I referred her to a neurologist, although I believed her headaches were probably stress related.

Later, she returned to me, subdued by the experience. After some coaxing, I learned that in the process of taking her history, the neurologist asked if she was sexually active. She told him no. When he asked why not, she shyly said that she guessed it was because she was overweight and didn't feel too good about herself. The doctor laughed off her embarrassment. He said, "Even hippopotamuses have sex!"

She was absolutely mortified, and she had cried bitter tears after leaving his office. Rather than offer a healing hand or a listening ear, this doctor had joined the ranks of those who contributed to her demeaned state and sense of helplessness.

WHO'S AT RISK FOR DEPRESSION?

Although depression in women is too often shrugged off as being a volatile mix of hormones and overemotionalism, the roots of depression run much deeper. It is a sad commentary on our lack of understanding that depression in women is misdiagnosed in as many as 50 percent of all cases. It is also telling that 70 percent of prescriptions for antidepressant medications go to women. Drugs are a favorite method for treating social ills.

Although women are often treated from the standpoint of "It's all in your head," science has advanced far beyond that stereotypical explanation. We now appreciate more fully that so-called mental disorders have a biochemical basis—that the body produces a physical response to life experiences.

I believe that there are four pathways to depression in women:

1. **Genetic predisposition**
2. **External events and status in the community**
3. **Neurochemical changes in response to external events**
4. **The internal interpretation of what occurred**

These four pathways are not separate and distinct like parallel highways. Often they merge so that it takes a special effort to distinguish one from the other. Within the broad category of depression, there are many gray areas. We must become more rigorous in determining the root causes of depression—for example, not assuming a hormonal link when an environmental or social issue is driving the depression; or recognizing that external trauma can leave a neurochemical imprint.

Symptoms of depression and psychiatric illness should be examined for both biochemical and psychosocial causes. We should be sensitive to the fact that the presentation of depressive symptoms can be clues to the existence of previous trauma. For example, consider anxiety, which is characterized by a wide range of symptoms including palpitations, tremulousness, sweating, diarrhea, worry, insomnia, abdominal pain, and persistent headaches. There might be a biological source, such as hyperthyroidism or mitral valve prolapse. But anxiety may also be a sign of extreme stress, a warning that abusive conditions exist, or a symptom of posttraumatic stress disorder.

Likewise, panic attacks, which are intense feelings of fear and discomfort characterized by shortness of breath, agoraphobia (the fear of going out) or claustrophobia (the fear of being confined), might be biochemical, caused by a neurotransmitter imbalance or an overly sensitive "suffocation alarm"—a primitive reflex. They might be an inherited trait, or they may be the long-term result of trauma or abuse.

Recently, Sylvia, a new patient, came for a checkup, and in the course of our conversation, she began to tell me how worried she was that "out of the blue" she was having panic attacks. Sylvia said that every time she or her son left the house, she was convinced they would never see each other again. She would be overwhelmed with a pounding heart, trouble breathing, sometimes crying. "At first," Sylvia said, "my husband tried to reason with me. He would say, 'Now, you know, you're going to see Todd again.' Eventually, when reason didn't work, he just got mad. Now, he yells, 'Will you please snap out of it!' "

The problem is, Sylvia could neither reason away her panic, nor snap out of it. The transmissions to her brain were signaling danger, and it was quite real. I recommended a good therapist whose task would be to determine the pathway to Sylvia's panic attacks, and possibly treat her with medication and psychotherapy.

Mental health is an area where the patient must be her own advocate, since doctors commonly misdiagnose or fail to recognize symptoms of psychological disorders. The World Health Organization claims that 40 percent of problems seen in primary care settings are psychological. Yet, our physicians are untrained to deal with common psychological disorders in women: depression, violence, substance abuse, and eating disorders.

Depression can also be caused by external circumstances, and a woman's relationship to them. A woman with low self-esteem will have a difficult time coping with small traumas, and everyday experiences will lead to a loss of self-confirmation. And any woman will struggle to maintain equilibrium in the face of these dilemmas:

▶ Emotional loss, even when there is no single event, like the loss of a parent, occurs in the everyday life of women, leading to a confirmation of loss of self (or self in relation).

▶ Being a witness to traumatic or violent events.

▶ Being a victim of gender-based discrimination or exclusion, which leads to a sense of powerlessness, isolation, and low self-esteem.

▶ The double whammy of also being a minority, elderly, lesbian, or other woman whose status is defined as unconventional, inappropriate, or less worthy.

▶ Poverty. In the United States, up to 75 percent of people living in poverty are women and children.

▶ The experience of being in an unsatisfying or abusive relationship. It is interesting to note that while marriage typically confers a protection against depression in men, married women are three times more likely to be depressed than either men or single women. Unhappily married women report being isolated and lonely with relationships of inequality and emotional distance, and many women in unhappy marriages are depressed.

▶ Being a lifelong caretaker—first of children, then of aging parents, then of an infirm spouse. For many women, the stress and restrictions of being caretakers lasts most of their lives. Dual caretaking increases the risk of depression, since caring for others may entail not caring for self.

▶ Being a working mother places tremendous strain on women, especially when they have no access to viable day care, little or no help in child care from spouses, or still bear the primary responsibility for running the household.

We know that there is a direct correlation between chronic stress and health; it is a major risk factor in gastrointestinal disorders, heart attacks, diabetes, autoimmunity, and cancer. Stress is a universal condition, but it is also highly individual, since women respond differently to external circumstances. For example, a woman with high self-esteem and strong, supportive relationships might better adapt to the stress of losing a loved one or being a working mother than another woman. For those with poor internal and external resources, stress can wear on the system until it creates an overload that both damages organs and leads to depression.

Stress is a tricky thing to define because for so long we have used it as a catchall to describe every unpleasant or difficult event. The current structure of the health care system, perpetuates the belief that there is a medical response to every misfortune or feeling of discontent. We all live with stress, but some of us are more prone than others to respond to stress in a destructive way. Chronic stress (which may be psychosocial or biological) such as pain, isolation, confinement, and lack of control can lead to structural changes in the brain that kindle progressively more autonomous acute symptoms. These stressors can literally alter the hormonal balance, and cause multiple organ damage through depletion and wear and tear. It can diminish immune response and cause vulnerability to infection, the growth of viruses, and the inability to ward off cancer cells.

Some of the most effective research on stress has been done with animals, since we don't accuse them, as we do humans, of being neurotic or having imagined symptoms when they respond to stimuli. In one study on the effects of stress, monkeys that were isolated from the others demonstrated traits of depression, anxiety, compulsive disorders, and panic. They also consumed more alcohol. Researchers concluded that the stress of isolation sent their neurotransmitter pathways out of kilter. And they recognized very similar responses in humans who were subjected to stress.

Women are often accused of being hypochondriacs or overreacting to common, everyday circumstances. But when a woman shows up in my office who seems overly distressed by a minor symptom, my ears perk up because I recognize a sign of chronic stress. You see, most of us have the ability to screen out most of the irritating bodily sensations we experience. But during times of stress, the rheostat gets turned up and everything is experienced much more dramatically. An astute physician will stop and ask about stress and the underlying psychic state of the patient. If the doctor says, "Oh, don't worry, nothing is wrong with you," the stressed patient will experience only transient relief. Soon she'll find another focus.

SIGNS OF BIOLOGICAL DEPRESSION

▶ You feel down, sad, depressed.
▶ You've lost the ability to feel pleasure, even from the things that you used to love.
▶ You've lost your appetite or eat compulsively.
▶ You have trouble sleeping even though you feel exhausted. Or you sleep to excess.
▶ Your movements and speech feel sluggish—as if you were in slow motion.
▶ You have little energy or interest in activities.
▶ Your libido has changed.
▶ You feel inadequate and unworthy.
▶ You can't concentrate, and you may feel agitated.
▶ You feel gloomy all the time and sometimes have thoughts about death or suicide.

Although 80 percent of suicide completers are men, the majority of suicide attempts are made by women. The most common method for women, accounting for 90 percent of attempts, is drug overdose. Most completed suicides for both men and women involve firearms, and the presence of such weapons in the home is a major factor in suicide deaths. Perhaps the higher rate of completed suicides in men is due to their choice of more lethal methods.

One reason for gender differences in suicide is the different prevalence of depression and alcoholism. Depression is twice as common in women and is highly correlated with suicide attempts. However, women may be less likely to complete suicide attempts because they seek treatment. Suicides are highest among white women, compared to women of color.

A disturbing recent trend has been the aggressive marketing of firearms to the female population, allegedly for the purpose of self-defense. Yet statistics show that firearms in the house are 43 times more likely to be used for suicide or homicide or to cause accidental death than to be used for protection.

Depressive symptoms can sometimes be a clue that some form of physical, sexual, or verbal abuse is occurring in a woman's life, or has occurred in the past. That is why we cannot adequately address depression in women unless we also address the epidemics of violence and abuse that place millions of women in physical and emotional danger every year.

AN EPIDEMIC OF VIOLENCE

When I mentioned to a colleague that my book on women-centered health included a discussion of violence, he didn't immediately see the connection. "Doesn't that topic go in a different kind of book?" he asked. "Something more sociological?"

"That is precisely the problem," I told him. "Even aware, caring professionals like you think that a woman's heatlh can exist independently of her environment. If a plague were infecting two to four million people every year, we would be frantically trying to stop it. But that's how many women are affected by domestic violence, and we don't think it's relevant to health."

Violence against women is a major health issue whose medical cost is so enormous that it's hard to calculate. One study done at Rush Medical Center in Chicago found that the average cost for medical services to abused women, children, and the elderly was $1,633 per person per year, amounting to an estimated average national cost of 857.3 million dollars per year.

Yet it has remained largely in the closet. Both the medical establishment and law enforcement agencies have basically looked the other way and refused to tackle this massive indignity and serious health problem directly. As recently as the end of the last century, the courts refused to outlaw spousal violence, instead limiting the beating of one's wife to a stick no bigger than a husband's thumb—thus the phrase "rule of thumb." Furthermore, views of violence against women are often cast in terms of how it affects others—the police officers who intervene, the children who witness it, or the fetuses that are aborted because of it. Less concern seems to be directed toward the women who suffer it. Because of fear and prior experience with unresponsive medical and legal authorities, it is estimated that over half of all domestic violence incidents go unreported. And over 90 percent of abused women never discuss it with their physicians. Only one in thirty-five battered women gets appropriately diagnosed by medical personnel. Yet estimates show that battered women account for 35 percent of emergency room visits, 23 percent of prenatal visits, and 58 percent of rape victims over age thirty.

When I talk about violence, I am, of course, referring to the prevalence of overt battering, murder, and rape that are daily occurrences in our society.

But I am also referring to the more insidious culture of violence that permits sexual harrassment, intimidation, and degradation.

I daresay if men were the victims of recurrent violence to the extent that women are, it would become a national priority. As it is, even in the most devastating cases of rape, women are often revictimized by a justice system that tries to blame them, and battered wives are suspected of provoking the violence by their behavior. Remarkably, even in medicine, all of the studies are done on "the victim," with barely any mention of "the perpetrator."

For some men, violence is a primary means of problem solving. Violence to men by men usually occurs in the street between strangers. Violence against women most often occurs in the home and is perpetrated by a male intimate. Women are 2.5 times as likely to be killed by a husband as by a stranger.

According to the Commonwealth Fund, 3.9 million cases of physical domestic violence occur every year, and 20.7 million women are verbally or emotionally abused by their partners. Furthermore, 53 percent of men who abuse their partners also abuse their children, while another one-third threaten to. And 28 percent of battered wives who stay also abuse their children, while an additional 6 percent threaten abuse. The cycle continues from one generation to another. Studies show that children raised in violent homes identify along gender lines. Boys become abusive and girls become victims. It is a madness that will continue unless we decide to end it.

Statistics indicate that abuse may be the single most common reason for injury in women—more than automobile accidents, mugging, and rape combined. In fact, physical and sexual abuse of women is so prevalent that it has been characterized as a normal aspect of female development. Homicide is the fourth leading cause of injury death among females, and the leading cause of occupational injury death for women. Forty-six percent of maternal deaths surveyed in Cook County, Illinois, were due to injuries. Pregnancy is a risk factor for battering.

Abused women who look for support from the health care system find little help. Physicians and emergency room personnel are poorly trained and often uncomfortable raising questions about abuse. One survey conducted among physicians affiliated with a large urban health maintenance organization found them repeatedly using the image of a Pandora's box when describing their reluctance to address domestic violence. As one said, ". . . you just don't ask a question that you know is going to open a Pandora's box. Even if it crosses your mind, you don't ask."

THE CRISIS OF VIOLENCE

For those who believe that violence against women is someone else's problem, the statistics prove otherwise. These statistics provide sobering evidence of the real cost to everyone:

▶ Nearly 25 percent of all women in the United States will be abused by a current or former partner at some time in their lives.
▶ Forty-seven percent of husbands who beat their wives do so three or more times a year.
▶ Approximately 52 percent of female murder victims are killed by a current or former partner.
▶ Fourteen percent of ever-married women have reported being raped by a current or former husband.
▶ Rape is a significant form of abuse in 54 percent of abuse cases.
▶ 10 percent of mothers' rape or murder is witnessed by their children.

Furthermore, battered women account for:

▶ 22 to 35 percent of women seeking care for any reason in emergency rooms;
▶ 19 to 30 percent of all injuries seen in emergency rooms;
▶ 14 percent of all cases seen in internal medicine clinics;
▶ 25 percent of attempted suicides;
▶ 25 percent of cases seen by emergency psychiatric services;
▶ 23 percent of pregnant women seeking prenatal care;
▶ 45 to 59 percent of mothers of abused children;
▶ 58 percent of women over thirty who have been raped.
   Men as perpetrators account for 92 percent of sexual abuse of girls and 84 percent of abuse of boys.

Strikingly, fear of offending the patient was one of the strongest concerns physicians expressed. One doctor said, "I'm not wanting to touch on something that they are uncomfortable with. . . . It has to do with both of us, our levels of comfort. And also I don't want to be nosing around into somebody else's business."

In spite of published statistics to the contrary, the majority of the physicians felt that domestic violence was uncommon in the general population, so they didn't pursue it. "You know, it's not the major medical issue you see in your practice," said one. "You don't have time to deal with all this," said another.

A clear example of the reluctance of medical personnel to confront abuse is seen in the following case study published by the New York City Family Violence Task Force:

"A hospital employee who did not work in the emergency room, but who often passed through the area, frequently saw the same woman waiting to see a doctor. After several weeks, the hospital worker approached the woman and said, 'I'm beginning to feel like I know you. Why are you here so often?' The patient began to cry and her story spilled out. She said that no one had ever asked her why she was there so often or how she got so many injuries. She said that she was being increasingly battered by her husband, and that she had been to the hospital on many separate occasions for stitches, a broken arm, X rays for broken ribs, and several other injuries."

Obviously, this woman was a victim of violence. Surely no doctor, nurse, or technician who treated her during her many visits to the hospital could have concluded otherwise. No one believed she was accident prone. The signs were all there. So, why was she never asked?

One problem is that the subject of domestic violence is rife with myths. Among them:

VIOLENCE ONLY OCCURS IN LOWER SOCIOECONOMIC GROUPS. While certain groups of women seem to be at somewhat higher risk, there is no single cultural profile. Domestic violence is primarily reported in lower socioeconomic groups because people in those groups tend to use public emergency facilities, while wealthier patients use private doctors who are less prone to make reports. All groups, regardless of race, religion, or socioeconomic conditions, are subject to domestic violence.

WOMEN MUST LIKE IT, OTHERWISE, THEY'D LEAVE. Studies have shown that battered women are not masochistic. They stay in abusive relationships for many reasons, including intimidation, low self-esteem, and economics. Leaving is often the trigger that leads to a woman's violent death. Forty percent of all female homicide victims are killed by their husbands. Leaving can be deadly!

WOMEN BRING ABUSE UPON THEMSELVES. The source of violence resides with the abuser, not the abused. Unfortunately, even victims of abuse often believe this myth. Women will say, "I should have known better than to say that." Or, "I know I make him angry." They think they can stop the abuse by changing their behavior—perhaps becoming more compliant, or giving in to the abuser on important issues. Victims of abuse can lose their sense of reality, and because their self-esteem is low, they often accept the abuser's explanation that they did something to provoke the violence. Some women do deliberately provoke the violence, but this is actually a way of minimizing its force—for example, provoking a fight before he gets more drunk, or before the kids get home from school.

VIOLENCE IS ALWAYS VISIBLE AND UNQUESTIONABLE. Many doctors surveyed about domestic violence were untrained to look for signs beyond those of physical battering. A startling number of them were reluctant to believe women even when they said they were being battered. As one doctor said, "Some people will say things that I may tend not to believe. I may not have a reason to believe them . . . because for some people there may be a secondary gain in trying to say something." These doctors said that in order to believe domestic violence occurred, they must have full evidence—including physical marks and often the confirmation of other family members.

This attitude is not only insulting but also ignorant. Domestic violence is not always provable in a clinical sense. Sadly, women are getting the message that unless they have already been severely beaten, no one will listen. But the development of an abuse situation is often more subtle, including many forms of emotional abuse before the first physically violent act occurs.

Even when there is violence, that's not always enough. I hear people say, "Why didn't she have him arrested? Look at what he did to her?" As it stands now, a woman who has been beaten by a spouse or partner has little to gain and much to lose if she presses charges against him. The legal process is lengthy and inconclusive, and chances are, the man will serve little or no time in jail. He is still available to abuse her again. A restraining order is a piece of paper that provides little protection against a violent man. Sometimes a battered woman feels safer saying nothing.

ARE YOU BEING ABUSED?

Michele, a patient in her early forties, the mother of two children, complained of depression and fatigue. "I just drag around the house. I don't know what's causing this," she said. She felt embarrassed to be complaining. "My life is good compared to most people," she told me. "But I can't seem to shake this feeling."

Michele was married to a very successful man who made excellent money as a film producer. They lived in a beautiful house and were able to send their children to the best schools. In many ways, Michele said, she was living the life she had dreamed about while growing up in a poor, working class family. So, why was she depressed?

Further exploration revealed that during the past two years, Michele had been drinking heavily in the evenings, and she sometimes took amphetamines to keep her weight down. Her husband often worked very late, and she felt lonely. Sometimes, when he arrived home hours later than expected, they would have bitter fights.

I asked Michele if during those fights her husband had ever struck her. "Oh, no," she said. "He would never do that. His way is to ignore me—to leave the room and refuse to speak."

Several weeks earlier, Michele's twelve-year-old daughter had asked her point-blank, "Is dad having an affair?"

"I was shocked," Michele said. "I had suspected it myself, but I didn't think my children would have thought about it. Then came the final blow when my ten-year-old son started crying and said, 'Don't yell at daddy all the time. He might leave!' "

Michele was tortured with guilt. "I want my children to feel safe and happy," she said. "I realize my behavior has made them insecure."

Her behavior!

I was struck by how easily Michele accepted the idea that her husband's behavior was her fault. Her children blamed her, too. Already, I imagined the message was being passed along to her young daughter: Don't make waves if you want to keep a man. I felt very sad for Michele.

Although she would never define her relationship as an abusive one, I believed Michele was being emotionally abused. She did not feel valued or loved in her relationship. Her husband was unresponsive to her needs. And there was a threat hanging over her head—the one suggested by her son: Unless she toed the line, her husband would punish her and her children by leaving. It was a heavy burden for her to carry.

Michele's story was a reminder that violence against women doesn't usually begin with physical battering—and it may not even end there. It's abuse when you feel threatened or intimidated, too.

Domestic violence, when it comes, rarely happens without warning.

Experts who have studied the experiences of battered women have identified a three-stage Battered Woman Syndrome.

Stage One is the tension-building stage. This involves name calling, intimidation, withdrawal, or general meanness.

Stage Two escalates to physical injury—pushing, kicking, slapping, and beating.

ARE YOU ABUSED?

Physical Abuse:
▶ Being pushed, shoved, slapped, punched, kicked, choked
▶ Being assaulted with a weapon
▶ Being held down, tied down, restrained
▶ Being left in a dangerous place
▶ Being refused help when you're hurt or sick

Emotional Abuse and Coercive Control:
▶ Being threatened with harm
▶ Being isolated physically and socially
▶ Being subjected to extreme jealousy and possessiveness
▶ Being subjected to deprivation
▶ Being intimidated
▶ Being degraded and humiliated
▶ Being called names, constantly criticized, insulted, and belittled
▶ Being falsely accused and blamed for everything
▶ Being ignored, dismissed, or ridiculed
▶ Being lied to
▶ Being frightened or intimidated

Sexual Abuse:
▶ Being made to perform sexual acts against your will
▶ Being hurt physically during sex
▶ Being coerced to have sex without protection against pregnancy or sexually transmitted diseases
▶ Being criticized and called sexually degrading names

Stage Three is retreat. Often abusive men become extremely apologetic, beg for forgiveness, and swear it will never happen again.

But as time goes by, the first and second stages increase in intensity and the third stage becomes less frequent.

Domestic violence is an escalating cycle. It's about establishing power and control, not love. I have heard women protest that a husband or boyfriend only hit them once; it was out of character and certainly wouldn't happen again. But if a man believes that physical force is the only way to make a woman do what he wants—and hitting a woman even once demonstrates that he does—the behavioral basis already exists for future violence. There's little to stop it from happening again. Recent research does show that mandatory arrest can decrease the likelihood of subsequent violence against women. However, no police officer or judge has the absolute authority to stop your partner from abusing you.

Lesbian couples are not immune from domestic violence. In fact, it is reported to occur among as many as one third of lesbian couples. Until recently, this problem has gone virtually unnoted in organizations and shelters working with battered women.

Because abuse takes many forms, you may not be sure if you're being abused—and you may feel so bad that you can't make an objective judgment. Although my patient Doris's husband never hit her, his violence against her was clear. He didn't say a word when he took her beloved cat and threw it against a wall, smashing its skull. Messages of coercive control come in other forms than direct physical attack. If you think you might be a victim, ask yourself these questions:

► Are you in a relationship in which you have been physically hurt or threatened by your partner?
► Are you in a relationship in which you feel you are treated badly?
► Has your partner ever destroyed objects or pets you cared about?
► Has your partner ever threatened or abused your children?
► Has your partner ever forced you to have sex when you didn't want to, or forced you to engage in sex acts that made you uncomfortable?
► Do you ever feel afraid of your partner?
► Has your partner ever prevented you from leaving the house, seeing friends, getting a job, or continuing your education?
► Does your partner become physically or verbally abusive when he uses alcohol?

▶ Do you have guns or other weapons in your home? Has your partner ever threatened to use them when he was angry?

WHEN VIOLENCE IS MISINTERPRETED AS SEXUAL

Many people still blame women for rape. In a random sampling of 598 Minnesota adults, more than 50 percent agreed with statements like, "a woman who goes to the home . . . of a man on the first date implies she is willing to have sex," and "in the majority of rapes, the victim was promiscuous or had a bad reputation."

Women who pursue the arrest and conviction of their rapists learn all too well that society is waiting to find an excuse for the rape by blaming the victim. Rape victims who submit without a fight are often accused of not trying hard enough to prevent the rape—never mind that they may have had a knife to their throat or a gun to their head. It's almost as if society expects women threatened with rape to take the path of those early Christian virgin martyrs who chose death rather than submit.

Even if a woman fights hard against the would-be rapist, she still must submit to a microscopic review of her own moral fiber: What was she wearing? What was she doing? Why was she walking down that street? Was she being provocative? Was she often provocative? Had she ever been sexually active before? Did she encourage her rapist? Did she want to be raped? Did she enjoy being raped?—and so on. Ultimately, it is the woman who is on trial. She is raped again by the process of justice at a time when she is struggling with physical and emotional scars from the trauma. It's not surprising that so many women do not report rape or pursue the conviction of their rapists.

We are a morally rigid society, comfortable when troubling questions are settled in definitive ways. We are conditioned to believe that behavior has consequences and that there is a cause-and-effect relationship between what a woman does and what happened to her.

It is very hard for us to grasp that victims of violence do not bring on that violence—especially if we judge their behavior to have been provocative. There is clearly something missing in our culture that protects women against uncontrolled male violence. We can learn something about the implications of this missing element by observing Native American history. Native Americans had many ways to protect women until their culture was destroyed. But since being overtaken by American culture, Native American women have extraordinarily high rates of physical and sexual abuse.

A close look at the Navajos will show how violence against their women is mirrored by the violence done to their culture. Traditional Navajo society honored women; indeed, its major holy people were women. Female puberty was noted with elaborate celebrations, with no similar ritual for boys. Navajos were matriarchal, and husbands moved into the wife's village, rather than the opposite. There were strong taboos against men making sexual advances toward women other than their wives, and divorce laws were simple. If a husband misbehaved, he would come home to find his saddle in front of the family dwelling—a clear sign that he was to leave. However, the culture was destroyed when Navajo children were forced to attend U.S. federal boarding schools. Family structure, respect for women, and moral values were lost. Since that time, physical and sexual abuse of Navajo women have become commonplace, leading to high rates of depression and alcoholism.

Society has a particularly hard time accepting the idea of acquaintance or date rape, even though rape is more likely to be committed by someone you know. Face it. It's much more comforting to imagine a rapist as the scary monster of our nightmares than as the good neighbor, loving father, or attractive classmate. Women themselves find it difficult to believe they are in danger when they're in a social situation. This is a denial of the fact that the men we know and like are capable of violence. It also dismisses the effects of our socialization. Women (especially Caucasian women) are socialized to view men as rescuers and protectors, not threats. For this reason, we are not taught to protect ourselves either physically or verbally.

In acquaintance or date rapes, women are often made to bear the burden of blame, while the men are considered less responsible for their behavior. A classroom study conducted on one college campus demonstrated this vividly. Students were told the story of a woman who was raped after a party. Some of the students were told that the man was drunk at the time; others were told that the rape victim was drunk. Those students who were told that the man was drunk held him less responsible for his behavior. Those told that the woman was drunk held her more responsible for being raped. Furthermore, one-third to one-half of college men indicate that they would rape a woman if assured they would not be caught; one-fifth report that they have forced a woman to have sex against her will.

Recently, there has been an effort on college campuses to address the problem of date rape by instituting guidelines and regulations informing sexual behavior. This is an urgent matter. In more than 80 percent of rapes on college campuses, the victim is acquainted with the rapist; in 50 percent of the cases, the rape happens on a date. Although many young men have criticized sex codes as unnecessary, confusing, and intrusive, most women have reacted with relief. Sex codes have given them a vocabulary with which to react to unwanted sexual advances.

DEFINING SEXUAL CONSENT

1. **If your date consults with you about your feeling about whether to have sex, be honest.**
2. **When in doubt, trust your instincts. If you feel wary about going to his apartment, don't go. Err on the side of caution.**
3. **You can't identify a rapist by physical appearance.**
4. **You have the right to decline sex without feeling that you will hurt the man's feelings by insinuating rejection. You always have the right to say "no."**
5. **Try to be consistent and only say "no" when you mean "no." It is not necessary for you to play hard to get by saying "no" when you mean "yes."**
6. **You need not feel that you must always be submissive, waiting for the appropriate moment to consent. You can make the first move.**
   —adapted from Project SAFETEAM

Rape is a violent act that is not about lust but about power and control. But a man does not have to violate a woman physically in order to abuse her sexually. Sexual harassment is a different variation of the same theme. Thanks to Anita Hill and the subsequent tightening of legal definitions of sexual harassment, there has been more focus on the topic in recent years. But many men are still scratching their heads and refusing to hear the seriousness of the issue. They think women are making mountains out of mole hills and depriving men of their normal "harmless" fun. A large percentage of men still believe that sexual harassment only exists when there is a direct link between a sexual act and job protection—a variation of the old casting couch.

An interesting new study shows that "objectification" experiences (being made to feel like a sex object) can lead to depression in women. The minor insults we all feel when male coworkers stare at our breasts while talking to us, when men make catcalls or lewd remarks as we pass them on the street, or when we are referred to as a "piece of ass" are objectification experiences.

In fact, we have grown far more sophisticated in our ability to recognize that women rightfully feel harassed, humiliated, and unable to perform when they are demeaned because of their gender. Behavior that might be considered sexual harassment includes:

- ▶ Unwelcome sexual remarks or questions
- ▶ Sexually explicit jokes, teasing, or name calling
- ▶ Suggestive looks or gestures
- ▶ Unwelcome pressuring for dates
- ▶ Unwelcome touching or nearness
- ▶ Pressure for sex
- ▶ Letters, phone calls, pictures, written material
- ▶ Attempted or actual sexual assault

I think it's a specious argument for men to complain that the rules have changed and they're confused about the guidelines. Most people, men and women alike, can recognize harassing behavior. For one thing, it's usually unwelcome. For another, it's usually inappropriate to the work environment. Finally, it's usually demeaning to women.

Women are beginning to fight back through the courts, and by drafting legislation. Two women on the Supreme Court, Sandra Day O'Connor and Ruth Bader Ginsburg, were responsible for sending a clear warning that sexual harassment in the workplace would not be tolerated by the courts. But it's also important that we address the source of antiwomen behavior. It's not enough to offer legal protection to victims. We must also strive to cure the pathology—sexism.

We must also educate women about how to take care of themselves following sexual assault. According to the National Women's Study, fewer than 20 percent of survivors had medical examinations following their assault, and of those examined, nearly three-fourths did not request information about HIV infection. Ideally, all survivors should be medically evaluated and counseled, and follow-up should be provided. All rape survivors should be screened and prophylactically treated for STDs and injuries. HIV testing should be done with informed consent, first at six weeks, then at six months after the assault. Unfortunately, mandatory HIV testing of perpetrators only exists in thirty-two states, and fifteen of those authorize post-conviction testing only.

PHYSICAL AND PSYCHOLOGICAL BURDENS OF SEXUAL ASSAULT

▶ Fear
▶ Loss of self-esteem
▶ Relationship problems
▶ Poor social adjustment
▶ Sexual dysfunction
▶ Depression
▶ Obsessive-compulsive behavior
▶ Anxiety
▶ Posttraumatic stress disorder
▶ Sexually transmitted diseases
▶ Unplanned pregnancy
▶ Suicide

THE SECRET SHAME OF CHILDHOOD SEXUAL ABUSE

Whenever a woman comes to me who seems depressed or anxious or who has multiple unspecified complaints, my antennae go up. Since there is no real distinction between mind and body, I always consider the possibility that physical complaints are more than physically based.

Kathy was a woman in her late fifties that I had been following for high blood pressure. She showed up at my office one day, several weeks before her scheduled physical, saying she just wanted to check on her blood pressure. My antennae went up right away. I suspected there was more.

I invited Kathy to sit down and talk. "Something doesn't seem quite right to me," I told her. "Let's talk about your concern. What else is going on in your life?"

She began to tell me about a woman friend whose husband had recently died. Kathy and her husband had been close to the other couple for many years, and Kathy said she felt very sad about his death. As she spoke, tears were rolling down her cheeks, and she had a very hard time maintaining her composure.

I asked her how long ago her friend's husband had died, and she said about eight months ago. That alerted me. It had been eight months and she was still sobbing in my office. I thought her reaction was a little bit intense. So we talked about it some more, and I asked if she was able to tell anyone about her feelings.

Kathy nodded. "Yes, I talk to my friend, his wife, all the time." Then she paused as if struck by a sudden thought. "Doctor," she asked, "is it possible that something from your childhood can affect you later on in life?"

"Yes," I said. "Of course."

She went on talking about her friend, indicating that she had told Kathy painful secrets from her past. "I don't know, my friend is able to say these things to me, but I can't tell her how I feel . . ." her voice trailed off.

I was beginning to put the pieces together. I could see she was struggling, and I knew I would have to help her put her experience into words.

"From what you've told me, I'm getting the idea that your friend was abused sexually as a child."

"Yes," she said quietly. "That's right." She stared at her hands.

I took a chance. "And did that happen to you?"

She continued to stare at her hands and the tears began to flow again. "Yes."

And then she told me what was really troubling her. When she was a child, her father had sexually abused her. Recently her own daughter had given birth to a child and she was terrified about her son-in-law being left alone with the baby. All of the feelings that had been locked inside for so long were flooding back. She told me that she had never spoken about this to anyone. For most of her adult life she had blocked it out. But suddenly it was on her mind all of the time and she couldn't cope with her feelings and fears.

When I first began studying the issue of childhood sexual abuse, I was stunned by its prevalence. According to statistics, more than 20 percent of women will be sexually abused by the time they reach adulthood. How was it possible that such an evil was being perpetrated against so many of our children and we have been so blind to it? As I began to share my discovery with other women, I quickly learned that it wasn't a subject one could talk about randomly. Too many women had personal experiences of their own. And, by the way, I did not learn about childhood sexual abuse in medical school. Even today, medical students are lucky to have one lecture on the subject—hardly enough to be fully informed about treating women.

Indeed, experts now tell us that 50 percent of all psychiatric patients have childhood histories of severe chronic physical and/or sexual abuse.

There are many reasons why childhood sexual abuse has remained so firmly in the closet. But I believe the primary reason is that people simply can't face it. We believe the family is a safe haven, especially for children. Our attitudes about the virtues of family are so strong that we literally choose not to see what is too painful to accept.

Perhaps the best example is the way in which the psychiatric profession itself has historically denied the existence of childhood sexual abuse. In 1896, Sigmund Freud made the startling declaration that the hysteria so prevalent among women had its roots in childhood sexual abuse. When he tried to present this view, the Vienna Psychoanalytical Society refused to publish his paper. Freud eventually gave up his position and reemerged with the Oedipal theory. Thus the claim of sexual abuse was relegated to the world of imaginary complaints.

Even today, we are loathe to believe claims of sexual abuse, especially since children are believed to be such unreliable reporters.

When adults come forth to claim that they were subjected to sexual abuse as children, their families often take the side of the accused brother, uncle, father, or friend. There is special difficulty believing women who realize they were abused later in life after repressing the memory for decades. People wonder how, if something so traumatic really happened, you could possibly repress it for so many years?

The answer has to do with the dynamics of posttraumatic stress disorder. Although traumatic experiences are stored in memory, they might be expressed in other ways. Essentially, there is no cognitive memory, only repressed memory. Scientists have learned that humans adapt biologically to inescapable stress by literally skipping the cognitive process and responding in a mode of fight or flight.

People with PTSD (Post Traumatic Stress Disorder) may lack a clear perception of the traumatic event, but they show behavioral signs that we can recognize. Often, there is an impaired capacity to modulate emotional responses, so we might see panic, withdrawal, or dissociation (becoming emotionally disconnected).

PTSD reached acceptance in relation to the experiences of men who had served in combat—in particular, Vietnam. Doctors observed a pattern of trauma responses, sometimes occurring many decades after the Vietnam War. By studying veterans and other trauma victims neurobiologists learned that in high-stress situations, an emotional "memory" is established. This memory may be completely unavailable cognitively; a person might have no clear recollection of the event. But at some later point, a new stress might jog the emotional memory and place the individual right back in an emotional state of trauma. My patient, Myra, reclaimed her memories of sexual abuse by her brother, starting at age four, when she was having knee surgery at age forty-three. When Myra was given general anesthesia, a tube was passed down her throat to help her breathe. That it did, but it also stimulated the memories of forced oral sex. Similar experiences are being documented in dentists' offices where stories of childhood sexual abuse are correlated with stress-related dental problems, breaking dental appointments, and experiencing PTSD-like symptoms while at the dentist.

Our greater understanding of PTSD has been a life saver for thousands of veterans. Not surprisingly, however, our profession became fixated on the actual experience of combat as the stress; it has only been in the past year or so that PTSD has been legitimized for women who served as nurses in Vietnam.

There is tremendous evidence that PTSD occurs all the time in women who were sexually abused as children. Many physical problems, risky social behaviors, and mental illnesses can be traced to childhood sexual abuse. We are learning to recognize the signs—even those that appear to be more subtle.

Some women who were abused as children act out their repressed preoccupation with the trauma event by being of assistance to other trauma victims. Others identify directly with the trauma. Veterans go on to become mercenaries. Incest victims become prostitutes or adult self-mutilators. Victims report having a vague sense of apprehension, boredom, or anxiety when they're not involved in activities reminiscent of the trauma.

One of my patients was a case in point.

Angela, a thirty-three-year-old woman, suffered recurring symptoms, including palpitations, chest pains, fatigue, and a number of nonspecific complaints. She was a frequent visitor to my office. Once she even took herself to a cardiologist because she didn't think I was treating her aggressively enough.

Angela had been taking birth control pills for many years, and she spoke very bitterly about never wanting to have children. When her sister was ill and Angela had taken care of her daughter, she said it was a very big trauma to have the child around.

I knew something was going on with Angela beyond her physical complaints, but no matter how I probed, I couldn't get to the issue.

Then one day, Angela came to my office to talk about how she might lose some weight. She was very overweight at the time, and it was really making her unhappy. In the process of talking, I asked her what she did with her time when she wasn't working. She told me she worked in a rape crisis center—and then, out of the blue, she volunteered that she'd been repeatedly abused by an uncle when she was a child. Angela admitted that she'd never dealt with it, and it was a lingering source of pain.

Finally, I knew what was bothering her. And I realized that instead of finding help for her own trauma, Angela, in the way of many trauma victims, was actually reliving it through the experiences of others. Fortunately, I was able to get Angela into counseling.

THE LONG-TERM EFFECTS OF CHILDHOOD SEXUAL ABUSE

In comparison with women not reporting a history of childhood sexual abuse, those who do more commonly:

▶ Show evidence of sexual disturbance or dysfunction
▶ Have anxiety, fear, panic, and phobias
▶ Have depression and depressive symptoms
▶ Have revictimization experiences
▶ Have suicidal attitudes and behavior
▶ Predisposition to somatization (localizing psychic disorders to a body part) and chronic pain syndromes—like chronic pelvic pain, migraines, irritable bowel syndrome
▶ Use the health care system far more often and have surgery more often, as the state of hypervigilance makes them more sensitive to pain perception, more reactive to environmental irritants, and less able to cope with common ailments
▶ Suffer eating disorders
▶ Are often substance abusers or alcoholics
▶ Engage in risky behavior such as unprotected sex (a significant number of HIV-positive women have histories of sexual abuse)
▶ Are overrepresented among women in psychiatric institutions—misdiagnosed as schizophrenic and unresponsive to treatment
▶ Become engaged in criminal behavior, often including becoming abusers themselves
▶ Are promiscuous, often leading to teenage pregnancies and prostitution

STANDING UP FOR YOURSELF

Marilyn was a young woman patient who seemed very overinvested in trivial symptoms. She came to my office frequently, whenever she had an ache or a pain. I noticed that she was unusually worried about minor symptoms for a young woman in generally good health. One day, she came in complaining of a sore throat and after I examined her, I asked, as I am prone to do, what else was going on in her life.

Marilyn opened up to me and poured out her story. It seems her husband of five years was seeing another woman, and he was quite up front about it. He basically told Marilyn that the only reason he was still living with her was because he didn't have enough money to leave. She sadly described to me how he would come home at night, still smelling of his mistress's perfume, and get into bed with her.

I looked at Marilyn, such a young, pretty, bright woman, and I said very bluntly, "You don't have to take this. Your husband is being sadistic. Why are you allowing it to happen?"

She didn't respond one way or another, and I didn't see her again for several months. But one day she arrived in my office and she said, "I have to tell you, you said something to me the last time I was here about how I was allowing myself to be abused. I heard that in a way I'd never heard it before. Within one month of my last visit, I left my husband, found my own apartment near the school where I teach, and started getting involved in the mayoral campaign. I'm learning a lot about myself and the choices I make. I don't want my next relationship to turn out this way." She shook her head, remembering the torment of her married life. "I was frightened to leave. I knew it was wrong, but I didn't think I could live on my own. Well, you know what? I like living on my own!"

I would tell any woman that abuse, whether physical, sexual, or emotional, is unacceptable. It is a health issue as urgent as any other. But leaving an abusive relationship isn't always a simple matter. Many women are afraid for their lives and the lives of their children. They lack independent resources, family, friends, and jobs. They need help in order to leave.

In my opinion, providing the foundation of this help is the responsibility of the health care system. We are the ones who see the battered women return time and again to emergency rooms. We are the ones who see women showing up more often than necessary in the waiting rooms of our offices. We are the ones who hear the cries for help, whether they're voiced openly or not. A health care system that advocated for women would not allow such a large percentage of them to slip through the cracks. We would not, as some doctors admit to doing, turn away and say nothing about the bruises or somatic complaints or other signs that indicate abuse. Nor would we treat depression by dispensing drugs and platitudes instead of digging for the source.

A woman-centered health care system would refocus its research and clinical energies from the study and treatment of victims to the quest for a solution to the problem of male violence. It is the only epidemic I know of where people aren't mobilizing to figure out how to stop it—only to treat the women who are its victims. How different things would be if our profession mobilized around the goal of diagnosing, treating, and eliminating male violence.

COMMON QUESTIONS ABOUT DEPRESSION

I always feel more depressed in the winter and I've heard of something called Seasonal Affective Disorder. What is it and what can be done about it?

Studies have shown that an estimated ten million Americans suffer from Seasonal Affective Disorder, or SAD. These people, often women who live in northern climates, seem to have a special sensitivity to changes in light which leaves them depressed during winter months. This is different from the normal moodiness or cabin fever people experience during the winter. It is a real illness and can be effectively treated with special lights. There's even a national organization, listed at the end of this chapter.

How can I tell if my depression is chemically based or the result of my circumstances?

No tests have been refined to determine the exact cause of an individual's depression. But I would suggest that it is erroneous to state it as an either/or situation. That's like asking, "Is it real or is it in my head?" and I hope you can see the fallacy of that question. The pathways to depression often connect. For example, if you are getting a divorce, you might feel depressed about it. But your ultimate ability to cope with your sadness probably depends on a combination of genetics, past experiences that have encoded a "memory" in your biochemical structure, and the actual details of your current circumstances. On the other hand, some depression is entirely caused by biochemical imbalances. Both can be treated effectively with drugs that boost the activity of certain neurotransmitters. I also believe that we should not wait until depression is very severe before resorting to medication. I have often seen women suffer tremendously, even while in psychotherapy, because of misconceptions about who should take antidepressants and when.

Are there any drugs that help build self-esteem?

Not specifically, although a course of certain antidepressants in combination with psychotherapy might help achieve that result. Prozac, a new antidepressant drug that has been receiving a lot of attention, seems to help some people function with renewed vigor and hope, with a minimum of side effects.

Let me add that some people have the impression that taking antidepressants is not a valid way to feel better. They think that authentic self-realization should occur independently of drugs—that it's "cheating" to take a pill that makes you view your life with more clarity or optimism. But I consider the use of antidepressants in a therapeutic environment as a valuable aid. It's no different from using a blood pressure medication while you lose weight, exercise, and improve your general health habits.

Aren't women responsible for sending the wrong signals about their willingness to have sex on dates?

Saying that date rape occurs is not the same as saying that women should not take responsibility for their words and actions. But that's different from saying that women bring rape on themselves. Remember, women are the victims of rape, not the perpetrators. Acquaintance and date rape are more complex than stranger rape because they occur in an environment where many assumptions have already been formed about the meaning of behavior and "signals." While men have been socialized to be aggressive (some coercive and some violent) to get what they want, women have been conditioned to be compliant and to avoid making waves. If they lack a strong sense of self, they might be afraid to assert themselves. But even when they do, men don't always read a definite no as being a no, since pornography and male myths present a picture of women not really meaning it when they resist. A woman must be very clear and consistent about what is okay and what is not, although she can be very clear and still be raped by a date. Many people laugh at the guidelines imposed on some college campuses that require verbal permission every step of the way during a sexual encounter. But as awkward as this seems to some women, because they are unaccustomed to this shift in power, I think it is a good way to train women to assert themselves positively and to train men to take women seriously. The best protection against date rape is for men to behave decently.

RESOURCES

My colleague Karen Johnson has written a superb book for women about becoming emotionally healthy. It is:

Trusting Ourselves: The Complete Guide to Emotional Well-Being for Women
by Karen Johnson, M.D.
Atlantic Monthly Press, 1991

Adult Children of Alcoholics
P.O. Box 3216
Torrance, CA 90505
310-534-1815

Anxiety Disorder Association of America
600 Executive Boulevard, Suite 200
Rockville, MD 20852-3801
301-231-9350

Center to Prevent Handgun Violence
1225 Eye Street, NW, #1100
Washington, DC 20005
202-289-7319

Families Anonymous
P.O. Box 528
Van Nuys, CA 91408
818-989-7841

Incest Survivors Anonymous
P.O. Box 5613
Long Beach, CA 90805-0613
310-428-5599

National Child Abuse Hotline
800-422-4453

National Clearinghouse for the Defense of Battered Women
125 S. 9th St., Suite 302
Philadelphia, PA 19107
215-351-0010

National Organization for Women
NOW Legal Defense & Education Fund
99 Hudson Street
New York, NY 10013
212-925-6635

The National Organization for SAD
Box 40133
Washington, DC 20016

One Voice (A Project of the National Center for Redress of Incest and
Sexual Abuse)
1858 Park Road, NW
Washington, DC 20010
202-667-1160

Self-Help Clearinghouse
800-367-6274
(If you're not certain about whom to call about your specific problem)

National Organization for Victim Assistance
1757 Park Road NW
Washington, DC 20010
202-232-6682 (for counseling and business)
800-879-6682 (for information and referrals)

National Council on Child Abuse and Family Violence
1155 Connecticut Ave, NW, Suite 300
Washington, DC 20036
202-429-6695

15

HEALTHY SEXUALITY

A Woman's Way

~~~

What does it mean for a woman to be sexual? In our culture, that depends upon whom you ask. The prevailing social attitude (based on male preferences) is that a sexual woman is young, slim but full breasted, compliant yet quietly seductive, and physically beautiful.

This standard is arbitrary, romantic, and not in the least bit valid. All women are sexual beings, regardless of our age, appearance, race, weight, social status, or even sexual activity. Older women are sexual. Celibate women are sexual. Women who have had mastectomies are sexual. Obese women are sexual. Disabled women are sexual. Your sexuality is an essential part of your nature. It doesn't matter who you are or how you look. Every woman deserves to have her sexuality treated with respect.

But the battle for dignity is not easily won, for we live in a sexist world. Throughout history and across virtually every culture, women's sexuality has been devalued. Male-centered sex was a concept successfully reinforced by Freud in the nineteenth century. Freud taught that women were traumatized by not having penises. Many were so envious of the male organ that they acted out their pathology in antisocial ways. In Freud's world, most women's psychosomatic illnesses had their roots in penis envy. In particular, women who expressed sexuality were said to be acting out their desire to be men.

To some extent, this notion remains firmly implanted in our culture today. Overtly sexual women are still viewed as dangerous, predatory, immoral, and even pathological.

In some societies and religious traditions, women are permitted sex only for procreation. To this day, Catholic women are instructed that sex for any other purpose is a sin, as are masturbation and oral sex. In the Muslim faith, women become the property of men, with no legal rights of their own. Men are allowed many wives as well as mistresses, and these women (who are often married as young as age twelve) are held hostage to the sexual whims and brutality of their husbands. A woman who is found having sex with or even kissing a man who is not her husband may, by law, be put to death.

In many Middle Eastern and African societies, clitorectomy is still widely performed on young girls who have reached menarche. The tradition is so pervasive to cultural ideals that there has been little outcry, even though it is intensely painful, demeaning, and subjects women to lifetimes of medical complications and terrible suffering. Sadly, the ceremony itself is conducted by women, not men. Only recently have human rights organizations raised objections to the custom, but I'm certain it will remain prevalent until the women themselves refuse to allow it.

Archaic standards of woman-as-temptress are alive and well today, even in the most contemporary circles. The famous case of the "Preppy Sex Murder" is an example of what occurs daily in the courts of America when women are the victims of sexual violence. In this case, a young man, Robert Chambers, murdered a young woman, Jennifer Levin, in New York's Central Park, following an evening of drinking. It was Chambers's contention that the murder was an accident that occurred when Levin became so sexually aggressive that she caused him pain. During the trial, Levin was reassaulted in death as Chambers's defense team paraded witnesses and used her own diary to prove that she was sexually active. The strategy was to prove her sexual and thereby hold the sexual woman responsible for a man's sexual and violent misconduct. Chambers's sexual behavior was never considered abnormal or discussed in the media. Nor was the credibility of his story that a young woman half his size felled him with sexual violence. He was later allowed to plea bargain for a light prison sentence when it appeared to the prosecution that the jury might acquit him altogether.

So while it may seem in the waning years of the twentieth century as though we've come a long way, women have a tenuous hold on their sexual dignity. Today, too many women develop a sense of their sexuality in the context of violence—childhood sexual abuse, rape, or harassment. Television, films, and pornography reinforce a view of women as sex objects. The attitude is so deeply ingrained that we barely note its existence.

Furthermore, women who behave in a sexually open manner are often held responsible for men's sexual and violent misconduct. Rape remains the only crime where the victim's testimony is not sufficient to convict the abuser.

Disabled women have been rendered invisible and genderless by our society. Physicians make assumptions that disabled women are not sexually active, and they are lax about providing appropriate gynecological exams, STD screening, and contraceptive counseling. Doctors also tend to be less sensitive about rape and abuse in the disabled population—especially disturbing since disabled girls suffer an exceptionally high rate of sexual abuse.

Sadly for women, the sexual revolution of the 1960s was really a male revolution. It succeeded in giving men more access to women's bodies, legitimized multiple partners (which is essentially a male fantasy), and reinforced a male norm of sex as physical, not emotional. Although freer to engage in sex, women still struggle to develop a healthy sexuality.

DEFINING A FEMALE NORM

Every norm that has ever been established for female sexuality has been based on male patterns, perceptions, and distortions. One hundred years ago, it was well known by anatomists that the clitoris was the site of female sexual pleasure, and it was thought that the vagina had no sensation at all. In the mid-twentieth century, physicians believed that the vagina could even be operated on without anesthetic. Yet Freud taught that female sexual maturity was achieved when a woman's focus shifted from her clitoris to her vagina. Generations of women believed they were inadequate and abnormal if they could not achieve a vaginal orgasm—another example of women's way being invalidated.

When Masters and Johnson published their work on the human sexual response cycle, it was applauded as revolutionary. However, it too was another version of the male model. Masters and Johnson succeeded in reducing the essence of sexuality down to a specific sequence of physiological changes, based on the model of the erection— a model that overvalues sexual performance and undervalues personalities, relationships, context, and ethics.

The result of all this distortion has been that most women worry that they're not sexually normal. They deny their actual experience when it does not match what they have been told is normal. It is no wonder that women still struggle with asking for what they want and need, or talking frankly about what would give them pleasure.

Normal sex is still defined as genitally focused, decontextualized, and centered on heterosexual intercourse. Men and women are viewed as different sides of the same coin, with essentially similar physiological responses. The goal of sex is viewed as a genitally-based physical gratification, a perspective that ignores women's drive toward intimacy and emotional communion, as well as their more complex physiological response. The assumption remains that sexuality follows an easy path from interest to orgasm, uninfluenced by everyday problems, anxieties, and fears. The focus is centered on the male erection and the physiology of the erection. There has been a great deal of attention given to finding mechanical and pharmacologic solutions to men's performance problems, while labeling women's sexual dysfunctions according to their inability to comply with men—for example, frigid or anorgasmic or unable to allow penetration, called vaginismus. Where, I wonder, are the diagnostic labels for men, like "intimacy avoidance behavior" or "penis obsession" or "sexual abuser?"

Current descriptions of sexual dysfunction assume that men and women have and want the same kind of sexuality, based on the gender-neutral physiologic profile of Masters and Johnson. But social realities dictate that we are not all the same sexually. Many studies have shown that women rate affection and emotional communication as more important than orgasm in a sexual relationship. This is not to say that women don't care about orgasm as long as they have intimacy. Rather, it says that the intimacy of a sexual act with another person, in which orgasm plays a part, is a full mind-body event for women. Women's sexuality is far more than just having orgasms. It is about a woman's whole life in relationship to herself, her partner, and the world around her. It is about her memories—of pleasure, frustration, abuse—and her fantasies of things yet to come. Sexologist Gina Ogden reported that when women were asked to describe their feelings about sexuality, she often heard them say that their bodily lust related to their emotional feelings of connectedness. In fact, a woman's most potent sexual organ may be her brain! Feminist sexologist Leonore Tiefer adds, "Most women in the world, lacking secure contraception, secure abortion, knowledge about their bodies, or culture or religion-sanctioned rights to pleasure, have a different sexuality from men."

It is possible that women's attitudes about orgasm are based on their relative inexperience with masturbation. Boys masturbate often and talk among themselves about masturbation. Sometimes they even practice masturbation together. Girls, on the other hand, rarely if ever discuss masturbation, and I've never heard of groups of young girls masturbating together. Girls are not taught about their genitals, and they must learn on their own how to achieve orgasm. Many never do, especially if they later find a partner who is not interested in their sexual satisfaction. Only 20 percent of girls have masturbated to orgasm by age fifteen. By age twenty, 65 percent have masturbated to orgasm, but half of these do so in a relationship. For a boy, frequent spontaneous ejaculations, regular handling of his genitals, and his unambiguous experiences with masturbation guarantees an integration of sexual identity into his sense of self.

Medically defined sexual normalcy makes no allowance for the impact of sexual violence, sexual exploitation, denial of reproductive freedom, or socioeconomic conditions on women's sexual behavior. Daily, women are subjected to the threat of job loss, ridicule, rejection, and even rape when they refuse sex. The wide distribution of pornographic materials has contributed to a culture that demeans women and wrongly assumes them to be sexually available. Yet, the medical model assumes that these sociological factors have no bearing on the physiologic responses women have to sex.

WHAT IS SEXUAL IDENTITY?

If heterosexual women have suffered from sexism, lesbian women bear the full weight of cultural disapproval. Between 10 and 20 percent of women choose to have intimate relationships with other women. Homosexuality has always existed; some research appears to show that it is biologically based, rather than simply a preference. But only in recent times have lesbians become an open presence in society, demanding acceptance as they shake the very foundations of male sexual bias. As a population, lesbians have been far more closeted than male homosexuals. There are many reasons. First, any woman who airs her sexuality in public is ridiculed and ostracized. By declaring herself a lesbian, she is performing the taboo act of making a public statement about her sexuality. (How many times have we heard it said of lesbians, "I don't care what they do in private, but why do they have to talk about it?")

Public contempt for lesbians is also based on their assertion that sexual fulfillment is possible (and even preferable) without men. This is a cage-rattling admission in a male-dominated culture. Men tend to take lesbianism personally, as though by preferring women lesbians are commiting an act of hostility toward men. I have often heard men ask lesbians, "What is it that you find unattractive about us?"—as though one choice necessarily invalidates another.

Socially, lesbians have much to fear when they make their sexual identities public, especially if they are mothers. Only recently, there have been two widely publicized cases involving lesbian mothers who were denied custody of their children for no other reason than their sexual identity.

One reason for the bias is that most people tend to think of homosexuality as a rigidly defined deviance. But scientists who have studied sexuality in animals and humans have found that we all have a capacity for bisexuality. Alfred Kinsey was the first to propose the idea of a sexual continuum—that is, people are neither exclusively heterosexual nor homosexual, but fall somewhere along a scale from mostly heterosexual to mostly homosexual. About 10 percent of the American population is predominantly homosexual. Many others consider themselves bisexual. In addition, married "heterosexual" people with children often have homosexual experiences. And a large proportion of teenagers have experimented with same-sex partners.

When we think about sexual desire and identity as being part of a continuum, it helps us transcend the bias against those who are different from us. Indeed, we come to see that we are more similar than different.

"Heterosexism"—the assumption that heterosexuality is the norm—often leaves lesbians feeling invisible within the health care system. When health care providers are not sensitive to lesbian issues or fail to ask about sexual orientation, they cannot address the isolation, stress, and self-esteem problems that come with living "in the closet." They may not be aware that lesbian patients are at higher risk for substance abuse and suicide. Lesbians may be less honest for fear of receiving insensitive care. They may not want to expose themselves by mentioning that birth control is not an issue for them. They may avoid routine gynecological care because of the system's insensitivities. On the other hand, doctors who are poorly informed about lesbian health may deny routine gynecological care, like Pap tests and STD screening, operating from the misconception that lesbians don't get pregnant. Many health care professionals also assume that domestic violence does not occur in lesbian households, a misconception that adds to the health risks for many lesbians.

Physicians are not immune to homophobia—the irrational fear of differing sexual orientations. One California survey reported that 30 percent of physicians said they wouldn't admit a homosexual candidate to medical school; 40 percent would discourage homosexual physicians from becoming psychiatrists or pediatricians; and 40 percent would not refer their patients to homosexual physicians in those specialties.

In a woman-centered health care system, women's varied lifestyles, health issues, and concerns would be an integral part of the training of health providers, delivery of clinical services, and research agendas.

PROBLEMS WITH SEX

A patient in her forties who was newly involved in a sexual relationship with a man, told me shyly, "I have trouble getting aroused." When I asked her to describe what she meant by that, she turned bright red and replied, "You know . . . wet."

It turned out that she was upset because she had trouble lubricating, even though she was sexually attracted to her partner. He took it as a sign that she wasn't interested—not at all the case—and she was desperate for a way to prove to him through greater lubrication that she was sexually interested.

This is a good example of how ignorance and stereotypes pervade our attitudes about what constitutes normal sexual behavior.

When women experience problems with sex, such as pain, arousal difficulties, or poor lubrication, they are often chastised or rejected by their partners. The verdict: "You're frigid."

Once again, women feel that their very core is inadequate when they cannot meet the arbitrary standards for sexual behavior imposed by their partners. Since most people feel strongly that sexual satisfaction is essential to a successful relationship, the pressure to perform is high on both men and women. But neither sex can be considered a machine whose parts are separate from the whole. That's why sexual problems are so hard to discover and treat. They may be related to any number of physical factors, but also to experience, present environment, and attitudes. Rose was a good example.

Rose was a lovely Eastern European woman in her thirties, married with two children, whose in-laws had recently been visiting. She came to me complaining of abdominal pain. I did a complete physical and medical history and found no medical problem. Still, she was not reassured. I sensed there was something else on her mind, but it wasn't until her hand was on the doorknob and she was ready to leave that she hesitated. In that pregnant pause, I asked her, "What's going on at home?" She blushed a deep red and blurted out that it was awful having her in-laws sleeping in the living room and her husband wanting sex. "I hate it," she said miserably.

"Why?" I asked.

She said, "It's no fun for me."

I asked Rose to sit back down and she began to talk about her frustrations. She admitted she had never had an orgasm. (Two children, but no orgasm.) We discussed it, and I gave her a fairly graphic prescription for masturbation and use of a vibrator. She left my office looking a hundred times better.

Sexual uncertainties and problems are not unusual and need not be a source of shame. Sometimes problems have a strictly physical cause; other times, the source is harder to recognize. Just remember, psychosocial reasons for sexual problems are every bit as valid as physical reasons. Also keep in mind that your "problem" might be a perfectly normal experience.

What are the most common problems women experience? Probably the most common is lack of desire. This might be related to depression, boredom, the unacceptability of your partner, or your particular level of sexual appetite. Lack of interest in sex might also be the result of illness, some medications, or alcohol or drug abuse. Most women experience fluctuations of sexual desire consistent with their hormonal cycles, peaking premenstrually and at ovulation. (Oral contraceptives can blunt this normal fluctuation in libido.) Both men and women experience fluctuations in sexual desire during the course of their lives. Sexual appetite exists on a spectrum of intensity, yet our culture overrates the primacy of sexual activity. When partners differ in their degree of sexual appetite, it is often perceived as a problem when it may only be a mismatch in temperament.

Furthermore, women with histories of childhood sexual abuse often have sexual problems as adults. And we too often minimize the many insults and assaults short of sexual abuse or rape that turn women off to sex.

Some women lose interest in sex after surgical removal of the ovary. Ovaries produce testosterone, the hormone responsible for libido in men and women, so estrogen replacement alone may not suffice to restore full sexual potential.

Aversion to sexual activity can sometimes follow abortion, but long-term studies fail to show a permanent loss of libido. However, fear of unwanted pregnancy or lack of access to abortion can have a negative effect on women's libido.

Problems with arousal are hard to measure. There is often a discrepancy between objective arousal (lubrication) and a subjective sense of arousal.

Inability to lubricate might be a strictly physical problem caused by estrogen deficiency, diabetes, or other conditions, but often it is psychological. Fear, stress, and anxiety can stand in the way. For instance, some of the most frustrated women I've seen are those in the throes of infertility evaluation. These women often manifest all types of sexual dysfunction, but the most prevalent is the inability to recapture active, spontaneous, mutually enjoyable sex.

Due to the increases in immigrant populations from Africa, physicians are unfortunately seeing more and more cases of female circumcision. Complications of these procedures, which vary in extent from removal of the clitoris to closure of the vaginal opening, are numerous: anorgasmia and painful intercourse occur, in addition to infection, dysmenorrhea, childbirth complications, and scarring.

Failure to reach orgasm can be a distressing problem for some women, and the hardest to admit to or talk about. I am moved by those women, of all ages, who are so relieved when they finally talk about this topic they thought was unmentionable; they are grateful when I assure them there is nothing shameful about their problem. Indeed, the usual causes of failure to reach orgasm are anxiety, inexperience, and inadequate clitoral stimulation. And sometimes medications can interfere—among them, antidepressants, sedatives, antipsychotics, and blood pressure medication. This fact has received scant attention since most of the pharmacological studies looking at sexual side effects have been done with men—even for drugs used primarily by women!

Sexual problems can also involve difficulties with penetration. Vaginismus is an involuntary contraction of the muscles around the vagina. Its source may be psychological or it may occur in response to pain. Painful intercourse (called dyspareunia) is not uncommon among women. It may be due to inadequate arousal, endometriosis, vaginitis, pelvic inflammatory disease, painful bladder syndrome, or postsurgical complications. Gynecologists, in their belief that vaginas are better "tight" to enhance sexual pleasure for men, may cause pain for women when they redesign the vagina after gynecological surgery. After pelvic irradiation for cancer, vaginas can narrow, and women are given vaginal dilators to make themselves more flexible.

Coital pain is often seen as psychological, and women who report it are referred to psychotherapists. This tendency reminds me of the time before prostaglandins were discovered and a biological explanation for painful periods was found. Researchers have now uncovered a clinical entity, known as vulvar vestibulitis, an inflammation of the tiny glands of the tissue behind the vaginal opening. Typically with this condition, any penetration of the vagina is painful unless touching of the back area is avoided. There is currently no good treatment for this disorder, but ackowledgment and validation can take women a long way out of suffering.

Vaginal atrophy due to estrogen depletion and exacerbated by infrequent intercourse can be very painful for older women, to the extent that they shy away from sex altogether. However, some of the diminished libido older women experience is socially generated. Since the older woman is viewed as neutered and unsexy, she is expected not to be a sexual person. And when older men leave their partners of many years to marry younger women, they are reinforcing the devalued position older women receive in our culture. In truth, postmenopausal women retain their multiorgasmic capacity; if they were multiorgasmic before menopause, they will be the same afterward. Although orgasms may take longer to achieve and be less intense as women age, by and large most women's sexual complaints are about loss of intimacy not decreased frequency of sex. When sex is focused on in a physical way rather than as part of a larger experience, older women are often left feeling ashamed of their own bodies. How, after all, can they compete with the youthful ideals that bombard the media? Yet, viewed from another angle, our older years actually provide a window of opportunity in which to move from genital penis-in-vagina sex to woman-centered sex. There are hidden advantages in older men's diminished capacity for erection. Women can be free to enjoy clitoral stimulation, oral or manual, without the emphasis on intercourse. When men are freed from sexual performance, they may be more motivated toward other forms of intimacy.

TAKING RESPONSIBILITY FOR OUR REPRODUCTIVE POWER

"Voluntary motherhood" was the first organized attempt by American women to assert their reproductive powers and take responsibility for their reproductive lives. It was a critical effort, launched some one hundred years ago, when pregnancy was a hazardous condition women faced throughout their adult lives. Women went into labor not knowing if they would survive. Even so, the movement for reproductive freedom did not spring to life overnight. For many, if not most women, the connection between sex and reproduction guaranteed that men would marry and support them. Lacking economic independence, women needed to be married, and children were the cement of that marital stability.

Contraception and abortion were readily available in the late nineteenth century. It was not until the American Medical Association began its battle to outlaw "irregular practitioners" and midwives that state regulations prohibiting both contraception and abortion came about—regulations that remained in place until the 1960s.

Margaret Sanger, a nurse in New York City's ghettos during the early part of the twentieth century, led the fight for reproductive freedom. Sanger saw the link between contraceptive control and the alleviation of poverty. She believed that all the other rights women were fighting for, such as the right to vote and own property, would be meaningless unless they also had the right to control their own bodies. But it was not until 1965 that contraception became legal to all married couples in the United States. And it was not until 1972, one year before the legalization of abortion, that contraception was legal for unmarried couples.

In the swirl of heated rhetoric that surrounds abortion, misinformation is rampant. From a medical perspective, there is no evidence that abortion is harmful to the health of the mother. It does not endanger future childbearing, and research by the Centers for Disease Control shows there is no increase in ectopic pregnancies, stillbirths, miscarriages, or infertility as a result of abortion. Although many women are sad and weepy after they have had abortions, studies document no lingering psychological aftereffects. The feeling of loss should not be confused with regret. Most women are relieved. Only one in two hundred thousand who have legal first trimester abortions are at risk for dying from the procedure—one-seventh the number of women who die from childbirth. The chance of complications from abortion is mostly affected by how far along the pregnancy is. Ninety-seven percent of women having first trimester abortions experience no complications, and only .05 percent requires further surgery or hospitalization. Complications for second trimester abortions are somewhat higher. Women giving birth are one hundred times more likely to need major surgery for complications. However, the leading reason for delaying abortion is the unavailability of local abortion providers. Astonishingly, 83 percent of U.S. counties have no abortion services at all. Nearly one-third of all OB/GYN residency programs offer no abortion training. Only 12 percent of all programs actually require it.

The mortality rate for abortion is 0.6/1,000; that for childbirth is 6.6/1,000. Carrying a pregnancy to term has eleven times more risk for death than that from abortion. Furthermore, women giving birth are one hundred times more likely than women having abortions to need major abdominal surgery to manage complications.

Four tax dollars are spent for every dollar saved by refusing to fund abortions for Medicaid-eligible women. This translates into a savings of up to $540 million that would be needed for medical and welfare expenses if no public funding for abortion were available in the United States.

Emergency contraceptive measures are easily available in Europe where the "morning after pill" and RU 486 (the "abortion pill") are used. Although the morning after pill has been available in the United States since 1982, no drug company has been willing to market it, few physicians use it, and women are generally unaware of it. Estimates suggest that the number of unintended pregnancies could be reduced by 1.7 million and the number of abortions decreased by eight hundred thousand each year if more women were aware of the morning after pill, and it was made easily available.

All women are entitled to full use of their reproductive power, whether they are teens or midlife women, heterosexual or lesbian, coupled or single, white or of color, financially secure or living in poverty. By reframing sex as reproductive power that women can use proudly and by choice, we can train women to use that power responsibly and prevent men from abusing or sabotaging that power.

CONTRACEPTION AND HEALTH

Abortion is not an isolated issue. It's clear that if 3 million women are getting pregnant by accident every year (1 million of them teenage girls), the fundamental problem of contraception is not being addressed.

The United States has the dubious distinction of leading the industrialized world in the rate of teen pregnancy, teen childbirth, and teen abortion. Today, the rate of pregnancy among teenagers of color is double that of Caucasian teenagers. One of every four African-American children is born to a teenage mother. Teen mothers face lives of inadequate education and poor employment opportunities, as well as unstable marriages or single parenthood. They are at greater risk for living in poverty with its consequential risks to health and development for both mother and child. What's worse is that teen pregnancy is passed on, so that children of teenage mothers become teenage mothers themselves.

Are American teenagers more sexually active than those in other nations? No. Do teens elsewhere use abortion as much as ours do? No. The problem is partially due to the fundamental discomfort Americans have with issues involving sexuality. Our children are often confused and frightened by the conflicting sexual messages bombarding them. They are hungry for love and tenderness, but sexually illiterate.

Only seventeen states and the District of Columbia mandate comprehensive sex education in the schools. As a result, many teenagers remain ignorant about their reproductive functions. The media exacerbate the problem, delivering approximately twenty thousand sexual messages a year—messages that

CONTRACEPTIVES: MAKING A HEALTHY CHOICE

METHOD	PREGNANCY PREVENTION	ASSOCIATED HEALTH BENEFITS	ASSOCIATED HEALTH RISKS
Rhythm or Withdrawal	Poor	No direct benefits	▶ Increased risk of sexually transmitted disease ▶ Increased risk of unwanted pregnancy ▶ Increased risk of cervical cancer
Barrier/ Spermicide (condom, sponge, cervical cap diaphragm)	Moderate to Good (depending on proper use)	▶ Prevention of sexually transmitted diseases (condom) ▶ Decreased risk of cervical cancer ▶ Decreased risk of pelvic infection	▶ Some incidence of irritation from spermicide ▶ Increased risk of urinary tract infection ▶ Increased risk of Toxic Shock Syndrome (especially if barriers are left in place for twenty-four hours)
Intrauterine Device (IUD)	Excellent	▶ Progestin IUD may decrease risk of endometriosis	▶ Potential fertility problems ▶ Potential for excessive menstrual bleeding and pelvic pain ▶ Risk of uterine perforation ▶ Risk of ectopic pregnancy if pregnancy occurs while IUD is in place ▶ Increased risk of iron deficiency ▶ Increased risk of PID

METHOD	PREGNANCY PREVENTION	ASSOCIATED HEALTH BENEFITS	ASSOCIATED HEALTH RISKS
Oral Contraceptive	Excellent	▶ Decreased incidence of PMS ▶ Decreased risk of tubal infertility and PID ▶ Decreased risk of osteoporosis ▶ Decreased risk of ovarian cancer ▶ Decreased risk of endometrial cancer ▶ Decreased risk of ovarian cysts ▶ Decreased risk of benign breast disease ▶ Decreased risk of fibroids	▶ Temporary increased risk of breast cancer in young women ▶ Increased risk of CAD, stroke in smokers of all ages, but especially after thirty-five ▶ Can elevate cholesterol and triglycerides
Tubal Sterilization	Excellent	▶ Decreased risk of ovarian cancer	▶ Permanent infertility ▶ Potential complications of surgery
Injectibles/ Implant (Norplant)	Excellent	▶ Decreased risk of ovarian cancer ▶ Decreased risk of endometrial cancer	▶ Potential for irregular bleeding and spotting ▶ Potential for side effects of chronic progesterone exposure, such as depression
Partner Vasectomy	Excellent (if monogamous)	▶ Indirectly benefits woman because the risk is lower with complications than with female sterilization	▶ Infertility
Emergency Contraceptive ("Morning-after pill")	Excellent	▶ Prevents pregnancy	

encourage casual sexual behavior, often in the context of violence. While our government encourages a "Just say no" policy about teenage sex, it sabotages efforts to inform teens about sexual responsibility and contraception. "Just say no" prevents teen pregnancy the way "Look on the bright side" cures depression. We must talk to our kids about sex, and we must teach them sexual responsibility.

Medicine has played an important role in the evolution of women's sexuality through advances in preventing pregnancy. But we have not done a very good job in educating girls and women (or, for that matter, boys and men) about contraceptive use; nor have we made contraceptives easily available to the poor and underage populations.

Contraception does more than just reduce your risk for unintended pregnancy. It can affect your future fertility, prevent or enhance your risk for cancer and other diseases, and decrease your risk of illness and mortality from pregnancy and childbirth.

An informed decision about birth control must be made in the context of several factors—including its effectiveness, its potential medical risks, and the long-term complications or benefits of use.

SEX AND DISEASE

Sexually transmitted diseases (STDs) are another legacy of the sexual revolution. Until recently, the three classic STDs—gonorrhea, syphilis, and chancroid—had virtually disappeared in industrial nations. However, in the United States, these three diseases are increasing at epidemic rates, especially among urban minority populations. Poverty, social disintegration, prostitution, and sex in exchange for drugs like crack-cocaine have contributed to an alarming new trend. Most disturbing is the emergence of strains that are resistant to drugs.

A recent outbreak of penicillin-resistant gonorrhea in Seattle was initiated in Caucasian and Latino groups but later spread to African-American men seeking prostitutes and prostitutes exchanging sex for crack. The patient profile of this strain is different from that of the 1960s and 1970s when gonorrhea in Seattle usually involved Caucasians and was rarely linked to prostitution. This parallels the national pattern of other STDs such as syphilis.

Syphilis peaked after World War II and was lowest in the 1950s, only to steadily rise again—first among homosexuals and then among the population trading sex for drugs. Chancroid, once a rare infection in the United States that causes genital ulcers, is now appearing in inner city and migrant labor populations. Its appearance has profound health implications, since it may facilitate HIV transmission.

Women are deeply affected by sexually transmitted disease by virtue of its impact on their reproductive life. Among the ravages of STDs are pelvic inflammatory disease, infertility, ectopic pregnancies, and spontaneous abortion. Offspring are affected by premature birth, low birth weight, mental retardation, and infections. During the last decade, the number of cases of involuntary infertility and ectopic pregnancies have quadrupled because of STDs. Today, ectopic pregnancies are the leading cause of pregnancy-related death in African-American women.

Pelvic inflammatory disease (PID) occurs in about 1 percent of all American women, usually resulting from a sexually transmitted disease. Incidences can be three to five times more common than the number of clinically diagnosed cases, since many are asymptomatic. In its worst form, PID causes severe pain and fever, but sometimes the symptoms are mild. Mild or severe, PID works its damage on the reproductive organs, scarring the fallopian tubes and often leading to ectopic pregnancies or infertility. The economic costs of PID and its associated conditions of infertility and ectopic pregnancy in the U.S. were 4.24 billion dollars in 1991 and could rise to 10 billion dollars a year by the turn of the century.

In a woman-centered health care system, men (the primary transporters of STDs) would be the focus of screening and treatment to prevent women from getting infected in the first place. Currently, our health care system expects all sexually active women to see their gynecologists yearly for screening. What about the same guidelines for sexually active men? All women bear a disproportionate impact from STDs on their reproductive lives: pelvic inflammatory disease, infertility, ectopic pregnancies, spontaneous abortions, chronic pelvic pain, painful intercourse, and pelvic scarring. Prematurity, low birth weight, fetal loss, newborn infections, and mental retardation can be caused by STDs during pregnancy. This risk is seven times higher for minority women, because of the epidemic of drug abuse, differences in health-seeking behavior, and the inadequacy of the health care system. During the last decade, the rate of infertility and ectopic pregnancies has quadrupled because of STDs. Clearly, the number-one risk for STDs is multiple partners—a risk somewhat modified by contraceptive use. Other risk factors are: invasive procedures, including abortion; douching; and obstetric instruments used during childbirth. Until we can get our health care system more focused on primary prevention, especially prevention from a woman-centered perspective, let's educate ourselves.

Let's also be aware that STDs can be an outcome of sexual assault. Trichomonas, chlamydia, gonorrhea, and hepatitis B are the most commonly diagnosed STDs after assault. Follow-up exams should be done at two weeks to pick up organisms too few to notice initially. At twelve weeks, blood testing should be done for syphilis and HIV.

Prostitutes are at very high risk for STDs and associated problems. Let's be clear that prostitution is not a career choice. It is the result of women's poverty, homelessness, and addiction. Street prostitutes live in "stables" where they experience extremes of power, control, and violence. Pimps often traffic in women from state to state and country to country. I wonder how we can say that prostitution is a victimless crime when these women have such high rates of battering, drug abuse, STD and HIV positivity, childhood sexual abuse, and suicide? Prostitutes need more than condoms. They need safe shelters, housing, specialized detox and drug treatment programs, education, job training, and long-term psychological and medical care.

ONE ACT OF UNPROTECTED SEX IS ALL IT TAKES

One act of unprotected sex with an infected partner can lead to transmission of a disease. The statistics are sobering. These are the estimated percentages of women who have been infected after only one sexual encounter:

Chlamydia	40%
Gonorrhea	50%
Genital warts	10%
Genital herpes	30%
Hepatitis B	10%
Syphilis	30%
Chancroid	15%
HIV	1%

STD SCREENING

While some STDs are asymptomatic and work their damage silently, others are loud and clear. One of the most common is genital ulcers. Many different types of infection can cause ulcers. Be aware that not all doctors and clinics have the full spectrum of tests available. A full workup includes a blood test for syphilis and a culture for chancroid. Also, since genital ulcers facilitate the transmission of HIV, you should also be tested for it. It's also important to be tested for genital herpes, since 60 percent of infected persons are unaware that they have it. Herpes is more prevalent in women than in men and in African-Americans than in Caucasians. It can manifest itself with blisters or ulcers and flulike symptoms, and tends to recur during menstruation. Not surprisingly, herpes can cause psychological problems, especially for women who do not have steady partners.

Other common forms of STDs manifest with discharge—in particular, gonorrhea and chlamydia. Be aware that chlamydia is often asymptomatic in men and is transmitted to women without their being aware of its presence. The outcome can be devastating—pelvic inflammatory disease, ectopic pregnancy, and infertility. Screening is best done with a simple swab of the cervix, using a DNA probe that quickly and efficiently detects the presence of chlamydia organisms. Sometimes women may have a mild discharge or abnormal vaginal bleeding, especially after sexual intercourse. Treatment of cervical infection is believed to reduce the likelihood of complications, but few studies have shown that the treatment reduces the risk of subsequent PID or decreases the incidence of tubal infertility and ectopic pregnancy.

In Chapter 6 we talked about HPV, the virus associated with cervical cancer. HPV causes warts that can appear anywhere in the external genital region or be internal and found on a Pap test. Male partners of women with HPV are at risk for penile cancer. Not all HPV lesions progress to cervical cancer; some go away in a few months, some stay the same for years, and still others progress very slowly to eventual cancer. The goal of treatment is to remove warts for cosmetic reasons and to alleviate the symptoms. Unfortunately, no therapy has been shown to cure HPV. Annual Pap smears are recommended for women with or without warts.

The hepatitis B virus is commonly acquired as an STD, and those infected have a 6 to 10 percent chance of becoming chronic carriers—meaning they can continue to infect others and be at risk for cirrhosis of the liver or cancer of the liver. Prevention of hepatitis B can now be achieved with a vaccination. In fact, it is becoming a part of the standard immunization program for children. Adults at risk are also advised to get vaccinated.

AIDS—A WOMEN'S HEALTH CRISIS

In 1981, when the first 189 cases of AIDS were reported to the Centers for Disease Control, 75 percent of them were located in New York and California, and 97 percent were men of whom 79 percent were homosexual. It didn't seem as though the frightening new disease posed any risk for women, much less children. Unfortunately, that perception remains common today, even as the statistics change. In 1991, the CDC reported that of the 45 thousand cases found, two-thirds were outside New York and California, more than 11 percent were in women and adolescent girls, and there were 683 new cases in children.

AIDS has become a women's health issue, especially for minority women. In 1991, 76 percent of women testing positive for the HIV virus were nonwhite; African-American women had twelve times the incidence and Latina women six times the incidence when compared with Caucasian women. By 1992, heterosexual transmission surpassed IV drug use as a cause of AIDS in North American women. With the spread of heterosexually transmitted AIDS, all women are at risk.

Like other sexually transmitted diseases, women usually contract the HIV virus from men—either through sexual contact or through infected needles. Transmission accompanies other risk behavior, such as drug use, prostitution, or unprotected sex. HIV-positive women also have a higher incidence of childhood sexual abuse, which may predispose them to promiscuity, drug abuse, failure to practice safe sex, and multiple casual sexual encounters.

Transmission is higher from male to female than female to male. (Female-to-female transmission is rare except among IV drug users.)

Lenny and Carol were both patients of mine until they had a child and moved out of the city. Lenny continued to see me as he commuted to work in the city. Unfortunately, I became the unhappy listener to Lenny's tales of infidelity, which began when Carol was pregnant. I regularly screened him for sexually transmitted infections; Lenny was so full of guilt that he rushed to my office every time he urinated funny or had an irritation. On several occasions, I urged Lenny to seek counseling, but he was in denial about his problem with sexual impulsivity, and he was too frightened to get tested for HIV because of concerns about confidentiality. This went on until Lenny developed a severe case of venereal warts. After diagnosing them, I referred him to a specialist for treatment. I also pressured him to tell his wife and to use a condom with her. I warned him, "You not only risk giving Carol warts, you also place her at risk for cervical cancer." Although Lenny was undisturbed by his infidelity, he couldn't bear the thought of giving Carol cancer. He agreed to abstain from sex or use a condom while he was being treated. But soon after, Carol saw his warts and the truth came out. She felt sickened and betrayed. Lenny's guilt and fear were heightened by his wife's knowledge and by the worsening of his condition. He developed severe recurrent warts that extended to his rectum and required laser surgery. The surgeon insisted on an HIV test and to no one's surprise except Lenny's, he tested HIV positive. Lenny lost his family and destroyed his and their lives in the process. Carol became HIV positive and spent her days living in fear of AIDS and the possibility that her children would also test positive for the virus.

Carol was not someone who fit the profile of the high-risk heterosexual woman. She didn't have multiple partners or use intravenous drugs. Her behavior was no different from that of her HIV-negative peers. Her risk factor was having ongoing sex in a monogamous relationship with a man who, unbeknownst to her, was HIV infected—an important emerging route to HIV transmission in women.

WOMEN'S RISK FACTORS FOR AIDS

1. **Multiple sex partners**
2. **Unprotected sex**
3. **Blood transfusions**
4. **IV drug use**
5. **Sexual relations with IV drug users**
6. **Sexual relations with men who have sex with prostitutes or have multiple partners**
7. **Unprotected anal sex**

There is a clear gender difference in early manifestations of AIDS. For women, recurrent vulvovaginal candidiasis (yeast infection) is the most common early symptom and may be the primary marker for initiating HIV screening in otherwise asymptomatic women. Esophageal candidiasis is also a common early sign in women.

There are also gender differences in women's AIDS-related infections. Kaposi's sarcoma and severe herpes simplex are rare in women. However, HPV is rampant, and cervical cancer may be considered an opportunistic complication of HIV. Cervical cancer is more aggressive in HIV-positive women, so this group should receive Pap smears every six months.

The social impact of AIDS is heavier on women. They must decide whether to have children, whether to terminate a pregnancy (only 30 percent of fetuses acquire the infection), and how to protect their infants. Breast-feeding is dangerous, for example, because the virus could potentially be transmitted through the mother's milk. AIDS infected women must also suffer the burden of knowing they might not survive long enough to raise their children—a particularly urgent issue if they are single parents and the sole support of their families. AIDS disproportionately affects impoverished minority women who fall outside the established medical and social services systems.

REDUCING RISKS AND TRANSFORMING RELATIONSHIPS

The good news for women is that AIDS prevention can be within your control. Women with abusive or violent partners may find it impossible to avoid unsafe sex, but normally you can reduce your risks by using a female condom or by having your partner use a standard condom. Make sure a condom is used with every act of intercourse. Current data show that

---

PROPER USE OF A CONDOM

1. Carefully remove the condom from its wrapper, making sure not to damage it with your fingernails, teeth, or other sharp objects.
2. Put the condom on after the penis is erect and before there has been any genital contact.
3. Make sure there is no air trapped at the tip of the condom.
4. Make sure there is adequate lubrication during intercourse. Use only water-based lubricants (K-Y jelly or glycerine) with latex condoms. Oil-based lubricants can weaken the latex.
5. Hold the condom firmly against the base of the penis during withdrawal and withdraw while the penis is still erect to prevent spillage.

condoms and behavioral changes are more important and effective than any AIDS treatment now available—and will remain so even if a vaccine is found. Once again, we must do more than tell women, "Just use a condom." Women often lack the self-esteem or negotiating skills necessary to convince their male partners to use condoms. These skills need to be taught according to women's diverse sociocultural contexts.

The need to have safe sex has had a major impact on relationships: The starting of one, the ending of one, and the fidelity and honesty within one. Alice and John, both patients of mine, had been going together for what seemed like forever, in spite of resistance from Alice's family because John was not of her religion. This was a couple who loved each other deeply, but at one point the familial pressure became too great and they broke up. During the year they remained apart, John and Alice each had one other sexual partner. They reunited, and I saw them when they came to me for premarital HIV tests. I was very excited for them and quite cavalier about the testing—until Alice's test came back positive. This occurred in the days before positive tests were automatically confirmed by a second more specific test. I called Alice in to talk. It was the hardest time I ever had talking to a patient. "Yes, it could be an error," I said. "It's very hard to get AIDS from just one exposure, especially a heterosexual, nonbisexual, nonintravenous drug user." I heard myself saying these things to reassure both Alice and myself.

Fortunately, Alice's repeat test came back negative. I was quite relieved but at the same time outraged that my patient had been put through this trauma. After much yelling and screaming, I got the lab to determine that they had made a clerical error in recording tests results. Meanwhile, Alice and John had a lesson in trust, a test that pushed the limits of their love for each other to the furthest boundaries. Happily, they came through it better for the experience. This is the rare case.

The need for safe sex may be giving women a wonderful opportunity to reclaim sex their way, in the context of a total relationship. By providing a supportive environment in which women feel free to say No, an environment that discourages casual sex and tells women they don't have to always be sexually available, we can put more control over sexual encounters into the hands of women.

In a woman-centered world, women would cherish and guard their reproductive powers. They would be in charge of deciding the where, when, what, and whom of sexual activity. Contraception would be a high-priority item in research and develement budgets. Mothers would have honest and meaningful conversations with their daughters about sexual expression and reproductive responsibility. Rapists, sexual abusers, and incestuous relatives would be severely punished, and men would receive clear messages that sexual irresponsibility and violence would not be tolerated. Instead of being the "side effects" of the male pursuit of sexual pleasure, children would enter the world planned and cherished.

COMMON QUESTIONS ABOUT SEXUALITY

I'm afraid if I ask my partner for something during sex he'll take it as a criticism.

That's because you assume that "good lovers" automatically know what to do. The idea that a man can be a good lover without understanding how his partner is unique is a myth that has contributed to the dehumanization of sex for women. You and your partner can't know what pleases each of you unless you communicate. If a male partner chooses to take your request as a criticism, that's an issue that should be discussed openly. You might be surprised to find that he's relieved to have the burden of "knowing" taken away from him. Men experience the stress of having to perform, too. Be aware that lesbian couples are not immune from communication and intimacy problems. All individuals may have sexual interests and preferences that cannot be known unless they are expressed.

Is oral sex normal?

Surveys have shown that most couples practice oral sex. But many women feel uncomfortable about it—especially having oral sex performed on them. They are ashamed of the way their genitals feel and taste, or they may be nervous about such a high level of intimacy. I think your question is really whether or not its acceptable for you to engage in oral sex. I believe any sexual behavior between consenting partners is acceptable as long as it is safe, does no harm, and is desired by both. If you do not want to perform oral sex or have it performed on you, don't let your partner pressure you. You have a right to say no without feeling as though you're abnormal.

Does sexual libido decline with age?

The common assumption that your sexual desire declines with age is based on a combination of cultural mythology and misinformation about women. The mythology links sexuality with youth, romance, and childbearing, leading to the assumption that once fertility is ended, so is desire. Among my women patients, I have often found the reverse to be true. Freed from the ever-present fear of pregnancy, some postmenopausal women often experience new levels of sexual pleasure and intimacy.

Misinformation about female physiology can reinforce the myth. For example, some women and their partners link levels of excitement with the amount of vaginal lubrication, and when women find themselves to have more dryness in the perimenopausal years, they take it as a sign of declining interest. Sometimes women are slower to reach arousal as they age. Again, the wrongful assumption gets made that they're not as interested in sex. We must educate ourselves about our sexuality and resist accepting sterotypes that are demeaning. The fact is, women can maintain sexual vitality their entire lives if they wish to, whether they have partners or not. The most important determinant of sexual interest after menopause is sexual interest before menopause.

Can AIDS be transmitted through kissing?

No AIDS cases have been identifed specifically with kissing, although scientists don't know for certain whether or not "wet" kissing is safe. The current guidelines for safe and unsafe sex are as follows:

Safe: massage, hugging, body-to-body rubbing, dry kissing, masturbation.
Possibly Safe: vaginal or anal intercourse with a condom, fellatio with a condom, cunnilingus with a barrier device, hand/finger to genital contact with latex or rubber glove, wet kissing.
Possibly Unsafe: cunnilingus without a barrier, hand/finger to genital contact without a glove.
Unsafe: vaginal or anal intercourse without a condom, fellatio without a condom, semen or urine in the mouth, blood contact (including menstrual blood or sharing IV needles), oral-anal contact.

Is a vaginal infection a sexually transmitted disease?

Vulvovaginal candidiasis, known as a yeast infection, is the most common of all discharge-producing infections (75 percent of all women have it at least once). It is not considered an STD except that sometimes partners of women with recurrent infections harbor candidiasis in their mouths or get a yeast infection in the glans of their penises. Vaginosis is another syndrome that results from replacement of normal vaginal fluid with bacteria that cause a malodorous discharge. Vaginosis can increase the risk of PID and is often seen after a hysterectomy or a delivery. Although not considered exclusively an STD, vaginosis is rarely seen in sexually inactive women.

RESOURCES

AIDS Hotline
National Public Health Service
Atlanta, GA
800-342-AIDS

American Association of Sex Educators, Counselors and Therapists
11 Dupont Circle NW, Suite 220
Washington, DC 20036

National Gay Health Coalition
206 North 35th Street
Philadelphia, PA 19143
215-386-5327

The National Center for Lesbian Rights
1663 Mission Street, Suite 550
San Francisco, CA 94103
415-621-0674

The Alan Guttmacher Institute
120 Wall Street
New York, NY 10005
212-248-1111

16

THE EATING PROBLEM
Body Image versus Healthy Weight

~~~

How many of us have not heard the whispers of guilt when we eat?
"Oh, I shouldn't."

"This is sinful."

"If I eat this, I'll have to starve for a week."

"Don't tempt me."

"I feel so guilty."

Guilt and food go hand in hand for women, although one rarely hears men expressing remorse or embarrassment over what they have eaten. For women, food has become a powerful symbol, a method for judging whether we are good or bad, loved or unloved, in control or out of control. And this desperation is reinforced daily by a culture that makes women pay for every extra pound of weight they gain. In fact, restrained eating is now normal behavior for American women. No surprise in a nation with a billion-dollar-a-year diet industry!

We are obsessed with being thin. As I write this, more than sixty-five million Americans are starting new diets. For most of them, this isn't the first time. By age forty, the average American woman has dieted more than twenty times. And her daughter is getting an early start on the process: 61 percent of eighth-, ninth-, and tenth-grade girls went on weight-loss diets in 1992. Girls can begin their first diets as early as the fourth grade. In a University of California study, 81 percent of ten-year-old girls reported that they were dissatisfied about their weight and were already dieting. And 31 percent of nine-year-old girls worried that they were too fat or would become too fat.

During the past few decades we have seen that the fashionable body has shrunk in direct proportion to women's gains in the workplace and the political arena. When I was young, we saw this with the model Twiggy, who arrived on the scene at the height of the women's movement. Today, we have Kate Moss, a waif-like, anorexic teenager who has risen to become the top model in the country. It doesn't take a social scientist to read the message: When women are showing their power, the forces of our culture shift the ideal to a frail, powerless image.

Overweight people in our society are discriminated against, both socially and professionally. In 1993, a study from the *New England Journal of Medicine* made headlines when it confirmed the socioeconomic burden of obesity. According to the study, overweight children and adolescents were less likely to marry or achieve economic success in adulthood. The researchers admitted that failure to do well in love and work may be more a result of the social stigma of obesity than any other factors.

Studies have demonstrated downward mobility for fat people, especially women. A disproportionate number of fat women are represented in the lowest socioeconomic groups. Fat women tend to have lower incomes than their parents, while thin women have higher incomes. Thin women are more likely to be accepted into elite colleges than fat women, even when their grades and test scores are identical. Fat people also experience more employment discrimination, with women experiencing discrimination at lower weights than men. Thin women tend to marry wealthier men than fat women, most likely because men derive status from the attractiveness of their female partners. However, despite the documentation of discrimination against fat people, it is still widely believed that poverty causes obesity, rather than obesity causing poverty.

There is no question that obesity is a problem for many American women. But the issue has been clouded by false standards of what constitutes being overweight. A recent study of 37,904 women and 26,733 men, conducted by the Centers for Disease Control, showed that among those trying to lose weight, 62 percent of the women and 44 percent of the men were not overweight by current standards. We can't begin to get a handle on the legitimate problem of obesity until we first address the cultural distortions.

Today, only one in ten people on a weight-loss diet is overweight by health standards. The majority of people who diet are aiming for an invisible cultural ideal—and the diet industry is only too happy to oblige, if not cultivate, the obsession. "Looksism," or prejudice based on appearance, is especially troublesome for women who are not Caucasian, middle class, heterosexual, young, thin, and able-bodied.

If you are a woman who has dieted on and off throughout your adult life, chances are your daughter is following the same pattern—whether she needs to lose weight or not. The 1990 national school-based Youth Risk Behavior Survey found substantial differences among boys and girls in the perception of their weight. Girls said they were "too fat" 34 percent of the time, compared with only 15 percent of the time for boys. Forty-four percent of the girls were "trying to lose weight," compared with 15 percent of the boys.

We know that body image plays a major role in self-concept; feeling that you are attractive is important to your sense of self-worth.

In addition to being targets of the 33-billion-dollar diet industry, women are also the objects of a 20-billion-dollar cosmetics industry and a 300-million-dollar cosmetic surgery industry. These industries are all encouraged by the media, whose portrayal of women establishes standards of attractiveness.

In our country, being attractive is equated with being thin. Since studies show that women and young girls consistently exaggerate their body size, that means most women are walking around with a negative self-concept. Studies in nonwhite women, however, show more acceptance of large body size, and these women are less prone to dieting. Although eating disorders are more common among Caucasian women, women of color who are more acculturated have higher rates.

Not long ago, I convinced a friend of mine to start on the antidepressant drug Prozac for her long-standing depression. After a few weeks, she called me up to thank me. She said the first thing that happened to her on the drug was that her body limits went in; she felt thinner. I was interested in her experience because it confirmed my belief that for women, feeling fat is a parallel to being depressed. When a woman's general sense of self-worth is low, one way it gets manifested is as a feeling of being fat. Fear of fat is a state of mind whose only risk factor is being female in this culture. And it belies the reality: Women gain weight with age, even in the face of constant levels of exercise and food intake. In the Healthy Woman Study, all women gained weight with age, and African-American women gained twice as much as Caucasian women. Women who lived alone gained more than married women. Those who increased their physical activity as they got older gained less—but they still gained some.

Because we are so determined to meet the thin ideal, we are easily persuaded by numerous fallacies about the nature of body fat and how we metabolize food. As a doctor and as a woman I look forward to the time when we can look at food as positive nourishment, take pride in our womanly bodies, and end the futile cycle of yo-yo dieting. We can begin that process by educating ourselves. For example, is overeating leading to obesity a medical condition, a habit, or a secondary response to anxiety or stress? We know that stress elevates brain endorphin levels and this has been found to stimulate eating behavior. High carbohydrate intakes can raise serotonin levels, which are lowered by stress and premenstrually. Is eating an addiction, as has been suggested by some or is it just soothing? There are many questions, but one thing is clear: Eating behavior and weight are not clear-cut issues for women.

NOT ALL FAT IS BAD

Recently, I watched a talk show discussion about "Men Who Want Their Wives to Lose Weight." I found the entire tone of the program painful and demeaning to the women who agreed to sit beside their husbands on the stage and tolerate the verbal bashing of the audience. And I was struck by one couple in particular. The woman was not what I would call obese—merely plump, with extra padding in her lower body. At one point she turned to her husband with tears in her eyes and said, "I just want you to love me for who I am." He leaned back in his chair, his face stony and unresponsive, and said, "I can't help it. I just don't feel attracted to you since you gained weight."

Now, this was an unbearably cruel response—especially in front of a national television audience. But another thing struck me. As he leaned back in his chair, the camera caught the husband full-bodied and I could see his belly hanging out over the belt of his pants. The irony of it floored me: This woman was being raked over the coals by her self-righteous husband for having fat on her hips and thighs, when he was the one whose fat placed him at a health risk. It was a clear case of how the cosmetic bias won out over the health issue.

If the issue of weight and body fat were seen in a woman-centered context, that woman would have been considered just fine, while her husband would be under the gun. From strictly a health perspective, hip, thigh, and buttock fat is not a health risk—and is even necessary to support the childbearing functions of women. Evidence strongly suggests that excess body fat in some locations is dangerous, while in others it's not. The premise, referred to as apple versus pear, is that excess android fat in the abdominal area (more common in men) is a real health risk, while excess fat on the hips, thighs, and buttocks (more common in women) is not. Here's why.

While fat in the hips, thighs, and buttocks tends to be stored fat, excess fat cells in the abdominal area are more metabolically active, releasing free fatty acids into the bloodstream. This android fat is associated with high triglyceride and LDL cholesterol and low HDL cholesterol (risk factors for heart disease and seen in adult diabetes), menstrual irregularities, hairiness, and gallbladder disease. In one study of 41,837 women ages fifty-five to sixty-nine, it was found that a high waist/hip ratio (more fat in the abdominal area than in the lower body) was associated with a 60 percent higher relative risk of death.

On the other hand, lower-body fat, more common to women, easily put on and hard to get off, is not released into the bloodstream but stored for a reason. In late pregnancy, fat stores are made available to nourish the fetus. During breast-feeding, they provide the fat content for breast milk. The female hormone estrogen actually encourages fat in the hips, thighs, and buttocks.

From an evolutionary perspective, women who were best able to store energy and nourish their young survived and passed along their genetic tendencies. In many cultures today, women with lower body fat are revered because they are the mothers of the surviving generation; those who have inadequate lower body fat are less likely to become pregnant, carry a fetus to term, or provide nourishment to an infant. This is particularly clear when we observe populations where famine is common. Ironically, the survival of the human race has depended on the very fat that women in modern America are so desperate to shed! Since we are no longer living from feast to famine, as our ancestors did, and in fact live in a calorie-rich environment, the issue is more complex. Especially since the cultural ideal is a very thin woman.

OBESITY AND ILLNESS

What is obesity? Medically defined, it is an excess of body fat that impairs health—approximately 20 percent or more above the recommended weight. Since we are born with a set number of fat cells, obese people don't have more of them; rather, the more fat a person has, the larger the fat cells. The basic mechanism that leads to overweight is an imbalance between caloric intake and energy expenditure, although it is unclear exactly how this imbalance occurs. What is clear is that it is not a simple matter of will power, but a complex disorder of appetite regulation and energy metabolism.

There has been much discussion in recent years about whether obesity is caused by nature or nurture—that is, are you genetically predisposed to be overweight, or is it a condition determined by environmental factors? Scientists have found that both nature and nurture play a role in obesity. For example, obesity is six times as prevalent in women of lower socioeconomic status. Since the same relationship has not been found in men, it is believed that environmental factors for obesity are more active in women. Researchers have also found that children of lean parents grow up to be lean, while children of obese parents grow up to be obese. This is believed to be partially genetic and partially environmental. Most epidemiologic studies suggest that obese people take in the same number of calories, or even fewer, than nonobese people. There is good evidence, however, that obese individuals are less physically active than nonobese individuals.

The accumulation of research about the causes of obesity points to one fact: Obesity is not a simple issue of eating too much, or being out of control. It is certainly not a moral issue. Rather, obesity, like other health conditions, is based on a complex set of behaviors and genetic proclivities. This information also indicates that even if you're not obese, your basic body shape and metabolic system are probably predetermined in the same way as your height. Trying to match an unrealistic body shape ideal may be as futile as trying to grow three inches taller.

In Western society, it is strongly believed that being fat is unhealthy. However, research studies often fail to account for socioeconomic status—the fact that fat people are generally poorer than thin people. Studies also fail to account for dieting behavior. Fat people diet more than thin people, and dieting itself can result in health risks. People who have dieted and then regained their weight have higher mortality rates than those who have never dieted and stayed at the same high weight. Fat people also suffer stress-related health problems because of discrimination and prejudice. Our society has medicalized obesity and unconditionally equated it with illness. This image is so deeply ingrained that it is hard for us to conceive of fat, healthy women.

Given this background, we have come to associate obesity with several common conditions in our culture.

Young overweight people are 5.6 times more likely to have hypertension and twice as likely to have elevated cholesterol levels. They are three times as likely to have diabetes. Weight loss can modify all three risks, but there seems to be less correlation of weight loss and lowering cholesterol in women. Obesity itself is a risk factor for coronary artery disease, especially with a high waist-hip ratio.

Obesity also increases the risk for many cancers: breast, uterine, ovarian, colon, gallbladder, and bile duct. Breast cancer is six times more prevalent in the United States than in Japan; Americans consume an average of one thousand calories a day more than the Japanese, mostly from fat. It is telling that as Japanese move to the United States, their fat consumption increases, as does their breast cancer.

Obesity is also a risk factor for osteoarthritis of the knees, especially in women.

There is not a single clinical trial among women demonstrating that reducing dietary fat (specifically, fatty acids) or obesity decreases the incidence of CAD or cancer and the subsequent mortality. It is still unclear whether being fat or eating fat is the real risk factor. And overall, those with the shortest life spans are at or below the weight chart figures, while those 20 to 40 percent above the weight charts live the longest.

Despite this uncertainty, doctors spend a lot of energy urging patients to lose weight. In one survey, 90 percent of fat women and 70 percent of fat men were told by their physicians to lose weight, even though they had no medical problems. Often, doctors tell people to lose weight no matter what reason they come to the office. Fat women often neglect regular screening, failing to get gynecological exams and Pap smears because of negative interactions with health care providers. They are also reluctant to ask for birth control or seek abortion services for unwanted pregnancies because of the tendency of health care providers to view them as not sexual.

There are few studies that document a relationship between weight loss and improvement in a medical condition. It is assumed, if not proven, that organs working harder in the face of heavier weight will be less stressed after weight loss. Weight loss might also improve depression and anxiety, but not if the loss is minimal or the weight is regained. In fact, the pattern of overeating and dieting may be associated with depression, and it puts women at risk for eating disorders.

DIETING MAKES YOU FAT

Joanne, a forty-three-year-old patient, was characteristic of those pursuing the futile quest for a slim body. She came to see me for other symptoms that she thought might be indicative of a health problem. She outlined her symptoms: chronic fatigue, dry skin, sleeplessness, depression, and most disturbing to her, the inability to lose weight even though she was eating only 900 calories a day. The World Health Organization defines starvation as 900 calories or fewer a day.

As we talked, I learned that Joanne had tried many diets over the years, losing and regaining weight in a yo-yo pattern. She was typical of women dieters in that her methods usually included eating very little food and skipping meals. But scientific evidence is mounting that very low calorie diets don't work, and they lead to a series of medical problems, such as those experienced by Joanne.

The reason semistarvation diets don't work is because you are biologically conditioned to fight weight loss under those circumstances. Your body is trained to protect you from starvation. When you eat very little, your intricately designed physiology fights against what it perceives to be a famine state. There are several ways that occurs.

In the first few weeks on a low-calorie diet, about two-thirds of the weight loss is water, not fat. Contrary to the often repeated claims of "miracle" diet programs, it is impossible for all but the very obese to lose two to four pounds of fat per week. The mechanism for water loss works like this. Most low-calorie diets are also low in carbohydrates, which are needed to generate blood sugar or glucose. If your body is not producing enough glucose to supply your brain and red blood cells, your liver will begin to break down its stored sugar (glycogen) and send it into your bloodstream. When there is no more glycogen, your liver will begin to convert amino acids from your muscle protein into sugar. Both glycogen and amino acids are surrounded by water; as they break down, this water is released and excreted as urine. The water loss is accompanied by the loss of essential nutrients such as potassium, magnesium, calcium, and phosphorus.

When you begin eating normally after a very low calorie diet, your body retains water and salt. This phenomenon, known as refeeding edema, is not fully understood, but it surely exists—as many women who have seen their weight loss evaporate overnight can attest. In animal studies, refeeding is also associated with cardiac arrhythmias, thickening of the heart muscle, hypertension, and a redistribution of fat to the abdominal area.

Another way your body is programmed to protect you from starvation is that when you cut your calorie intake below a certain level, your metabolic rate gradually slows down to burn fuel more efficiently. It becomes harder and harder to lose weight on the same number of calories. That's why Joanne couldn't lose weight, even though she was only eating 900 calories a day.

Slow metabolism also causes other problems. Accompanying symptoms include fatigue, depression, sleep abnormalities, cold intolerance, dry skin, dry hair, loss of hair, constipation, a fall in blood pressure, and dizziness. Furthermore, research shows that the effects of repeated dieting are cumulative. With each diet, weight loss is slower, since your body learns to adapt more efficiently to starvation conditions. This is especially true for women's bodies. And after each diet is completed, the weight is regained more quickly. When you were twenty, it might have been easy for you to drop 10 pounds in a week or two. But if you diet off and on for twenty years, it gradually becomes harder and harder to lose weight. Ninety-eight percent of people who lose weight gain it back within five years. And 90 percent gain back *more* weight than they lost. Dieting itself could be the single most potent cause of obesity in the United States.

After you've been on a semistarvation diet, you have the urge to binge. This isn't because you lack self-control. There are substantial human and animal studies showing that dieting leads to binging. For a person who eats normally, the act of eating food suppresses further appetite. But for a chronic dieter, eating food has the opposite effect: Eating *stimulates* appetite. This is a biological fact, not a psychological one.

Scientists began to understand this phenomenon when they observed the eating patterns of wolves. In the summer, when food is readily available, wolves eat small amounts of food several times a day. But in the winter, they may go several weeks between kills, so when food is available they stuff themselves, then go to sleep to prolong the stores of food. It is believed that our bodies send similar signals when they are starved. Once food is made available, we're conditioned to binge to help us survive until food is available again.

One of the most famous studies on binging that demonstrates this point was conducted at Northwestern University, using two groups of women students. The first group consisted of chronic dieters and the second group consisted of normal eaters. The two groups were asked to taste ice cream. Before the test, they were given one or two milk shakes or nothing. Following a milk shake, the normal eaters consumed less ice cream than they did on empty stomachs. After two milk shakes, they consumed even less. In contrast, the dieters ate more ice cream after consuming one milk shake and still more after consuming two milk shakes.

Failed dieters who assume they have food addictions because eating makes them hungrier may be experiencing the phenomenon of the urge to binge. The conclusion is as simple as it is shocking: Dieting makes you fat!

THE FIVE FALLACIES OF WEIGHT CONTROL

1. **Body fat is the enemy.** Not all body fat is bad. Women need to store fat in their hips, thighs, and buttocks to support pregnancy and breast-feeding. This fat is resistant to weight loss. The real enemy is fat in the abdominal area. This fat can be more easily modulated by diet.
2. **Dieting makes you thin.** If this were true, how do we account for the fact that chronic dieters gain more weight than women who do not diet? There is scientific evidence that the yo-yo pattern of dieting leads to weight gain, not loss. It upsets the metabolic balance, leads to edema, and triggers binging. Dieting does not make you thin. It makes you fat.
3. **Overweight people lack self-control.** The issue of weight is not about control. On the contrary, a woman who diets frequently surely has more "control" than the person who eats whatever she likes. More often, people are overweight because they have tried too hard to control their weight by starving themselves. It takes a lot of self-control to starve yourself.
4. **The thinner the better.** The cultural ideal that thin is best contradicts the biological imperative. It is arbitrary and can be dangerous. Women's physiology is directed toward storing calories. So, when we are in a calorie-rich environment, especially one that encourages eating as a social activity, we gain weight.
5. **If a diet fails, it's your fault, not the diet's.** This is what the multibillion-dollar weight-loss industry would like you to believe. When diets work, the program gets the credit. When they fail, they blame the victim. I can think of no other treatment that is still deemed acceptable in spite of such a high failure rate.

WHAT IS "NORMAL" EATING?

▶ Normal eating does not require a meal plan. It's eating when you are hungry and stopping when you are satisfied.

▶ Normal eating is choosing a food you like and getting enough of it—not just stopping because you think you should.

▶ Normal eating is using moderate constraint in food selection to get the right food, but not being so restrictive as to miss out on pleasurable foods.

▶ Normal eating is giving yourself permission to eat sometimes because you're happy, sad, or bored, or just because it feels good—as long as you have other ways to satisfy those needs, too.

▶ Normal eating can be three meals a day or munching throughout the day. It is flexible, varying in response to hunger, schedule, emotions, and availability of food.

You might be thinking, "Ha! It's easy for her to say," but I assure you it's not. I struggle with body image, too. I'm unhappy about the twenty pounds I gained while writing this book and am frustrated by the fact that they won't budge even when I'm being "good." Although I am fully engaged in many fulfilling and rewarding activities, I still hear the brain chatter so common to women: "I'm fat." I have learned from my own experience how hard it is to be a "normal" eater when the fear of fat is looming so constantly in the background. But I try to ignore the brain chatter when I can. Instead, I find ways to reduce stress, increase activity, eat healthily, and forget about it.

DIETING CAN BE DANGEROUS

When I was young, gynecologists freely dispensed amphetamines to women so they could lose weight. You went in and said, "I'm feeling a little bloated," and it was no problem. You left with a prescription. There are many case histories that track the use of over-the-counter drugs by teenagers and college students. One study, conducted by Michigan State University, found that 45 percent of female students used or had used appetite suppressants, such as Dexatrim, which contain phenylpropanolamine (PPA). These pills are available in drug stores, and variations of them are advertised through the mail. While many doctors believe that diet pills, when used properly, can aid weight loss, we can't ignore the abuse that often accompanies amphetamine use, or the complications that may come from long-term use. When twelve- and thirteen-year olds are engaged in self-medication to maintain arbitrary weight standards, something is wrong. Furthermore, amphetamines and their derivatives have been associated with insomnia, irritability, and rebound depression. Amphetamines have a high potential for addiction, and in severe cases their use can cause arrythmias, seizures, and psychosis.

It has long been believed that being obese increased the risk of gallbladder disease. But a recent study in the Archives of Internal Medicine suggests that dieting, not obesity, may be the culprit. The study showed that in eight weeks of eating a 500 calorie diet, 25 percent of dieters developed gallstones, as demonstrated by ultrasound examinations of the gallbladder before and after the diet. In contrast, equally overweight individuals who did not diet showed no development of gallstones during that same interval.

Wendy Carter was a case in point. She was only sixteen the day her frantic parents rushed her to the hospital. Wendy was found to be suffering a severe and painful gallstone attack. At first, the doctors were puzzled. Gallstones are almost never seen in teenagers, and Wendy appeared to be otherwise healthy. But then they learned that she was a client of Nutri/System—a low-calorie diet program that included prepackaged foods. The mystery was solved. There was a known (though barely publicized) link between rapid weight loss and gallbladder disease, and it was virtually the only explanation for the appearance of gallstones in a healthy teenager.

Fatal irregularities in heartbeat can also occur from semistarvation, as well as potassium and protein deficiencies, menstrual and fertility problems, metabolic disorders, hair loss, depression, and strokes. Studies show that repeated weight loss and gain might be as prominent a risk for CAD as obesity itself, since the risk of dying from heart disease is 70 percent higher in weight cyclers, regardless of their initial weight, blood pressure, smoking habits, cholesterol levels, or physical activity. Recent studies have also shown a link between dieting and osteoporosis.

Dieting can also lead to the development of serious and even fatal eating disorders. According to the National Association of Anorexia Nervosa and Associated Disorders, eight million people suffer from eating disorders.

Anorexia nervosa, which usually afflicts young girls, often begins as a diet that then goes terribly out of control. The fear of being fat is so intense that the victim literally believes herself to be fat, even when she reaches a level of emaciation. Anorexia nervosa is a life-threatening disease: 5 percent of anorexic girls die from cardiac arrhythmias; 15 percent develop chronic problems, with 2 to 5 percent commiting suicide; 5 percent become obese.

Even the 75 percent who regain weight to normal or near normal levels go on to suffer a lifetime of eating-related disorders. Some go on to become bulimic—a pattern of binge eating followed by vomiting.

Bulimia is more difficult to detect than anorexia nervosa, since a bulimic woman might appear to be of normal weight and health. Episodes of binging and purging usually occur in secret and often include regular use of laxatives and diuretics. However, bulimics often have coexisting problems with alcohol or substance abuse and depression.

Many women with experiences of childhood sexual abuse go on to develop eating disorders. In one study, 50 percent of girls with eating disorders reported childhood sexual abuse, compared with 25 percent in a group without eating disorders.

An emerging area of investigation is the link between eating disorders and infertility. In one study, 58 percent of women attending an infertility clinic had previously undisclosed eating disorders. Another study looking at women who vomited excessively in early pregnancy found that most of them had a prior history of eating disorders, and half of them had attended infertility clinics.

Both anorexia nervosa and bulimia are debilitating, life threatening illnesses, whose only cause is the idea that being thin is the only way to achieve a sense of self-worth. It is tragic that we have passed this legacy along to new generations of young women; that women's magazines continue to encourage the false ideals (on their fashion pages if not in their feature articles); that television and films equate thinness with beauty; that in our own homes we talk about weight-loss diets as though women are obliged to subject themselves to a constant battle for control over every bite of food we eat.

In 1990, Democratic Congressman Ron Wyden held an extensive open hearing about diet practices in America. During one session, Wyden's committee heard evidence of how the obsession to be thin has captivated our young people. Noelle Marie Smith's case history was particularly moving. Noelle was a beautiful, vibrant young girl who had everything to live for. But she spent her youth in self-loathing because she believed that she was fat. After six years of starving herself and overdosing on over-the-counter diet pills, Noelle died at age twenty from anorexia nervosa and bulimia. Her father, Tony Smith, addressed the committee on her behalf, and read the poem that Noelle wrote shortly before she died:

As I sit,
I look down—panicked at the thickness
I've seemed to acquire.

I begin to wonder if I'm hungry,
"Oh, not yet," I say
But who am I to say
for I've lost control

It's hard to say if I'm hungry or full

When my stomach goes its full extent
It's on my way to the porcelain bowl.

I heave and hoe with all my might
Until my guts ache all through the night.

The pain, the agony, the hatred I feel
All comes out to my little porcelain bowl.

In circles around and around
if I don't get help, I think I might go down.

The congressional chamber was hushed while Mr. Smith read Noelle's poem. Even the most hardened politician and medical professional could not fail to be moved by Noelle's silent cry for help—a cry that went unanswered. Everyone in the room knew that this young woman should not have died.

We live in the most affluent and medically advanced nation in the world, and it doesn't make sense when our youth die of starvation. Although it might seem that the standards are slowly changing. Noelle's plight is clear evidence that we have a long way to go. We cannot continue to blame the victim. We need to look instead at the forces in our culture that encourage young women to starve themselves, even to death.

Former FDA Commissioner, Dr. Frank Young, estimates that weight-loss related ailments may cost as much as 140 billion dollars a year in preventable health costs for diet-related illnesses, including metabolic disorders, gallbladder disease, menstrual irregularities, hair loss, depression, heart attacks, strokes, anorexia, bulimia, and even sudden death.

We have long been familiar with the psychological costs of dieting. Statistics show that as many as 90 percent of people who lose twenty-five pounds or more on diets gain it back within two years. This failure rate leads inevitably to poorer body image, a feeling of hopelessness, and depression.

RECOGNIZING THE SIGNS OF ANOREXIA

1. **Refusal to maintain body weight over a minimal normal weight for age and height.**
2. **Intense fear of gaining weight or becoming fat, even though one is underweight.**
3. **Distorted view of self as being "fat," even when underweight or emaciated.**
4. **The absence of three consecutive menstrual cycles when these would otherwise be expected to occur.**

—from the American Psychiatric Association

RECOGNIZING THE SIGNS OF BULIMIA

1. **Recurrent episodes of binge eating—rapid consumption of large amounts of food.**
2. **A feeling that one has no control over binges.**
3. **Regular occurrences of self-induced vomiting, use of laxatives or diuretics, strict dieting, or vigorous exercise between binges.**
4. **A minimum average of two binge eating episodes a week for at least three months.**
5. **Persistent overconcern with body shape and weight.**

—from the American Psychiatric Association

A young woman came to me, the twenty-eight-year-old daughter of a patient. She wanted a checkup because she hadn't had a period in eight months. Her gynecologist had confirmed that she wasn't pregnant, then he told her not to worry about it—this sometimes happened. But she was worried about it. It was a clear warning that something was wrong.

As we talked, she reluctantly admitted that she felt depressed and tired, and then she told me in a small voice that for the past year she had sometimes—maybe once or twice a week—induced vomiting after eating in order to maintain her weight. "My husband and I are very socially visible," she said. "It's important for me to look right."

I couldn't help feeling saddened by the sacrifices this woman was making in her health and personal dignity to meet an approved weight standard.

I didn't tell her it was nothing. Nor did I moralize about the dangers of bulimia. I realized it was important for me to address the real issues that were behind the behavior. I talked with her about the dangers of not having a period for eight months, and quietly urged her to consider her health when she was making decisions about eating and body image. I asked to speak with her therapist so we could work together to treat her depression more aggressively. My intention throughout our conversation was to help her see that she had choices and that I, as her partner, would work with her. But deep down, I was furious to see yet another young woman who was torturing her mind and body to meet a false ideal.

MEDICAL COMPLICATIONS OF EATING DISORDERS

ANOREXIA:

- ▶ Anemia
- ▶ Low white blood cell count
- ▶ Low glucose levels
- ▶ Kidney stones
- ▶ Amenorrhea
- ▶ Frequent urination
- ▶ Slowed intestinal motility
- ▶ Cardiac abnormalities
- ▶ High cholesterol
- ▶ Weakness

BULIMIA:

- ▶ Gastric dilation and rupture
- ▶ Esophageal tears and rupture
- ▶ Dehydration
- ▶ Low potassium levels
- ▶ Erosion of dental enamel
- ▶ Esophagitis and sore throat
- ▶ Toxic cardiomyopathy
- ▶ Rectal bleeding and prolapse
- ▶ Abnormal bowel habits
- ▶ Menstrual irregularities

FIND YOUR HEALTHY WEIGHT

How do you know your correct weight? Chances are, you look in a mirror and think, "I look fat," and determine to take off a few pounds. Or you choose an arbitrary number—like 110 pounds—and try to achieve it. Or you think back to when you were twenty-two and decide that the amount you weighed then was the "perfect" weight for you, and you make it your goal to return to that weight. Let's try a less arbitrary approach. Experts in weight control now recommend a two-part test to determine your healthy weight, which includes both your weight (measured on a contemporary age-adjusted table), and your body fat distribution.

How do you know how much you're supposed to weigh? Since the 1940s, Americans have been judging their weight by the standard of the Metropolitan Life Insurance Company's height and weight tables. They give a range of weights, with the midpoint assumed to be the "ideal." Only in the past few years have Metropolitan Life's guidelines, so faithfully followed by millions, been questioned.

It won't surprise you to learn that the Metropolitan tables were largely conducted using data from Caucasian males and ignoring the physiological differences in women. They also gave no consideration to multicultural differences. Furthermore, although we trusted them completely, the evaluations were never conducted in a scientific way. For one thing, they were only done among purchasers of life insurance—not necessarily a representative segment of the population. Also, the methods were sloppy. Some study subjects answered questions about weight on their insurance forms but were never independently weighed. Others were weighed, but there was no attempt to standardize the tests; for example, some wore clothing and shoes while others did not.

Even if the research had been conducted in a more scientific way, there would still be reasons why the Metropolitan tables are inaccurate. First, they didn't consider the percentage of body fat, meaning that a healthy athletic woman might be overweight by the chart, since muscle weighs more than fat. Nor did the charts consider the distribution of weight. By that standard, a healthy woman with lower body fat might be considered too heavy, while a man with no lower body fat but a pot belly, would still be considered in the healthy weight range.

Particularly relevant for women, the standard tables were not age adjusted. A 5 ft. 6 in., twenty-two-year-old woman was evaluated by the same measure as a 5 ft. 6 in., forty-five-year-old woman. Research has shown that women commonly gain some weight with age, so a healthy weight range must be age-adjusted to accurately reflect a healthy weight.

After a long process of study, the National Institutes of Health recently published a new table of healthy weights that are age-adjusted.

THE NEW HEALTHY WEIGHT CHART
AGE-ADAPTED HEALTHY WEIGHTS

HEIGHT	20–29 YRS	30–39 YRS	40–49 YRS	50–59 YRS	60–69 YRS
4'10"	84–111	92–119	99–127	107–135	115–142
4'11"	87–115	95–123	103–131	111–139	119–147
5'0"	90–119	98–127	106–135	114–143	123–152
5'1"	93–123	101–131	110–140	118–148	127–157
5'2"	96–127	105–136	113–144	122–153	131–163
5'3"	99–131	108–140	117–149	126–158	135–168
5'4"	102–135	112–145	121–154	130–163	140–173
5'5"	106–140	115–149	125–159	134–168	144–179
5'6"	109–144	119–154	129–164	138–174	148–184
5'7"	112–148	122–159	133–169	143–179	153–190
5'8"	116–153	126–163	137–174	147–184	158–196
5'9"	119–157	130–168	141–179	151–190	162–201
5'10"	122–162	134–173	145–184	156–195	167–207
5'11"	126–167	137–178	149–190	160–201	172–213
6'0"	129–171	141–183	153–195	165–207	177–219
6'1"	133–176	145–188	157–200	169–213	182–225
6'2"	137–181	149–194	162–206	174–219	187–232
6'3"	141–186	153–199	166–212	179–225	192–238
6'4"	144–191	157–205	171–218	184–231	197–244

In addition to weight, you need to measure your waist-hip ratio to determine whether your belly fat is too high and therefore presents a health risk. There is a simple test you can perform at home:

▶ Stand straight in front of a full-length mirror. Using a tape measure, note the distance around the smallest part of your waist. Be sure the tape is parallel to the floor.
▶ Now measure the distance around the largest part of your buttocks.
▶ Divide your waist measurement by your hip measurement.
▶ The result is your waist/hip ratio. For women, a healthy range is .70 to .75. Above .80 is considered a risk.

Once you have measured your total weight against the age adapted tables and calculated your waist/hip ratio, you can determine how much weight you need to lose—if any—realizing that it may not be realistic to permanently lose more than ten to twenty pounds.

A woman-centered context for weight control emphasizes fitness as the standard. It links your self-esteem with the realization that being healthy and taking care of your body is an empowering activity. With health as your context, you can be released from a lifetime of pursuing a goal that ultimately is unreachable, and often is destructive. Better still, you can pass along this empowering healthy context to your daughters and break the cycle for good.

How to Eat for Health

Women's relationship to food has been so clouded by concerns about willpower and weight control that we sometimes forget the reason we eat in the first place. We must eat to live, and the nutritional makeup of our diets can make the difference between wellness and illness.

Perhaps no other topic has been buried in misinformation the way nutrition has. I see it every day in my practice. My women patients, in particular, always want to talk about their diets, and I'm eager to listen and help them find a healthy nutritional balance. Often, before we can come to a point of talking about eating for health, we must first work through myths and misinformation about eating.

We can't discuss nutrition without first addressing that reality. Sharon, a forty-three-year-old patient, reminded me of that again. Sharon came to me for an initial checkup, a bright, beautiful woman, who began by telling me about her eating disorder. "I'm an overeater, a binger," she said, "and I've been attending Overeaters Anonymous for almost a year." She gave me a dazzling smile. "I'm proud to say that I've now been abstinent for ten months. I've lost thirty-five pounds and am maintaining my weight."

I didn't ask Sharon what she meant by "abstinent." I recognized the language of an organization that borrows from the AA model to treat overeating as an addiction. Sharon went on to tell me something of her life, including the information that she had started taking Prozac two years earlier because of severe panic attacks. Through it all, Sharon's primary focus was on her eating disorder, which never seemed to be helped, no matter how many diets she tried. Overeaters Anonymous was her last stop.

I listened with fascination and empathy as Sharon described the OA meetings—packed with upward of two hundred women, all very much like herself. She told me stories of women who threw food in the trash and poured Ajax over it so they wouldn't be tempted to eat it, only to wash the Ajax off and eat it anyway; women who squirreled away food in their desks or sneaked it from secret stashes in their homes. The stories were familiar. They might strike a chord with many women.

I asked Sharon what she had done to overcome her problem, and she told me seriously that there was no cure, only control. She proceeded to show me the rigid meal plan that she had adopted as her means of control. I looked it over and quickly determined that the meal plan wasn't very balanced. There was too much protein, not enough fiber, and very little variety. Furthermore, the restrictive nature of the plan, which required weighing and measuring every bite of food, was a method that had been shown to fail almost all of the time. I gently tried to move Sharon away from the restrictive framework of a "diet" to the notion of healthy eating, knowing all along that it would be an uphill battle.

As a doctor, I long for the day when women's relationship with food is released from the snare of guilty indulgence—when we can eat happily and healthily for the good of our bodies. But as a woman, I am aware of how knotty this issue has become for us, since I struggle with similar impulses myself. The best way to approach healthy weight is to begin with a realistic goal and avoid "dieting." As someone who has sworn I would never put the weight back on, I can tell you from firsthand experience that you need a lifelong commitment to healthy eating, coupled with an exercise routine that is woven into the fabric of your life. You may want to consult a nutritionist to help you move to a healthier diet. I urge you to invest in your own ability to learn about healthy eating, rather than contributing to the profits of the diet industry.

NUTRIENT KNOW-HOW

Simply put, the food you eat keeps your body functioning. It gives you energy, enables growth and tissue repair, and delivers nutrients throughout the system.

Each food component has its own role to play in the process. Dietary protein replenishes the protein in your body. When you don't eat enough protein, your body can't grow or repair its tissues. Since dietary protein supplies the essential amino acids your body cannot produce on its own, it is necessary to your daily diet. Protein that comes from animals—including meat and dairy products—is considered "complete" since it contains all the amino acids necessary to meet your body's needs. Vegetable protein is incomplete since it lacks crucial amino acids. However, it is possible to get complete protein from a vegetarian diet if you eat foods in certain combinations. Note that vegetarian doesn't necessarily mean low calorie, or even low fat, so don't assume you will automatically lose weight this way.

VEGETABLE COMBINATIONS THAT MAKE COMPLETE PROTEIN

Certain complementary vegetarian foods, eaten together at the same meal, combine to make a "complete" protein. Here are some examples:

Corn tortillas	+ Pinto beans
Peanut butter	+ Whole wheat bread
Rice	+ Beans
Tofu	+ Rice
Black-eyed peas	+ Corn bread

As a rule, Americans don't need to worry about protein deficiencies. Indeed, the opposite is true. The average American diet contains too much protein—especially meat and dairy foods that are high in saturated fat and cholesterol. Surprisingly little protein is needed to maintain good health. For women, high-protein diets contribute to osteoporosis because of the acids that are generated during protein metabolism; the body buffers the acid load by leaching calcium carbonate from the bones.

An average sized thirty-five-year-old woman requires about 50 grams of protein a day. Since each gram of protein contains four calories, that means only 200 of your daily calories need to be protein—roughly equivalent to a small piece of chicken, a glass of milk, and a container of yogurt. (If you skin the chicken before cooking and choose skim milk and low-fat yogurt, you eliminate much of the saturated fat without sacrificing the quality of the protein.)

WHAT'S THE PROTEIN CONTENT?

FOOD	GRAMS
3 ounces ground beef, broiled	21
3.5 ounces chicken, roasted	27
3.5 ounces turkey, roasted	28
3.5 ounces salmon, baked	27
1 cup milk (whole/low-fat/skim)	8
8 ounces yogurt, low-fat plain	12
1 large boiled egg	6

Source: U.S. Department of Agriculture

Most meat and dairy products are high in fat. Fat has received a bad reputation because it has been associated with a variety of health problems, including coronary artery disease and cancer. But in itself, fat is not bad. Your body needs fat to operate, just as it needs protein and carbohydrates. More accurately, your body needs lipids, which not only become storage fats but are also made into hormones and other substances such as cell membranes.

Here's the problem with dietary fat. While your body needs protein, it does not need the kind of fat that comes with animal foods, since it has the capacity to produce that kind of fat itself. What it does not produce (and therefore must have dietarily) is polyunsaturated fatty acids. These are essential to our diet, but in much tinier amounts than we're used to. In fact, we won't suffer a fatty acid deficiency unless we consume fewer than 3 percent of our daily calories this way.

When you compare this picture with the average American diet, the difference is clear. The high-protein, high-fat American diet is in direct opposition to our nutritional needs.

According to most dietary guidelines, a healthy diet should include between 10 and 15 percent protein, and no more than 30 percent fat (two-thirds of it unsaturated). Newer guidelines even suggest that fat intake should not exceed 20 percent of daily calories. At least 50 to 60 percent of your diet should be composed of carbohydrates. There are two forms of carbohydrates: simple sugars and starches (known as complex carbohydrates). Simple sugars are the basic elements of all carbohydrates; starches are formed by complexes of simple sugars called polysaccharides. When you eat starches, your gastro-intenstinal system breaks them down into the simple sugar glucose, which is used for energy. Good sources of complex carbohydrates include all vegetables, cereal, rice, pasta, bread, nuts, grains, and legumes. Fruit is not a complex carbohydrate since it is composed mostly of the simple sugar fructose and water. But it is important to health by virtue of its vitamin, mineral, and fiber content.

There is substantial evidence that fiber, a substance found in plant foods, has many health benefits. There are two types of fiber. Water-insoluble fiber is made from the structural parts of plants and is found in wheat bran, whole wheat, fruit, and vegetable skins. Water-soluble fiber comes mostly from fruit, vegetables, beans, and oats. Insoluble fiber aids the digestive process and adds bulk to the stool for easy elimination. It is one of the primary preventive measures to guard against colon cancer. Soluble fiber is believed to play a role in decreasing blood lipid levels, offering protection against coronary artery disease. And all kinds of fiber seem to help lower blood sugar.

HEALTHY, FIBER-RICH FOODS

A good, fiber-rich diet includes between 20 and 35 grams a day. Here are easy ways to meet your total:

FOOD	AMOUNT	FIBER GRAMS
Low-fat bran muffin	1	4
Whole wheat bread	2 slices	3.2
Brown rice	⅔ cup	3
All-Bran cereal	1 ounce	8.5
Apple	1 medium	3.2
Pear	1 medium	4
Dried figs	2	7.4
Cooked broccoli	¾ cup	5
Cooked spinach	½ cup	6.5
Cooked kidney beans	½ cup	9.7
Cooked lentils	1 cup	9

WHAT'S THE ROLE OF VITAMINS AND MINERALS?

Vitamins and minerals are so readily available in supplement form that we have come to think of them as magic pills. Just walk into any health food store and your senses will be dazzled by the hundreds of curative concoctions formulated from various vitamin and mineral substances. But scientists are still learning about the true nature and function of many of the substances

---

A DAILY DIET OF CALCIUM

Here are three different daily combinations, each comprising approximately 1000 milligrams recommended for most women, and a large percentage of the 1200 milligrams recommended for others. A daily supplement can make up the difference.

Combination 1:

8 ounces skim, low-fat, or whole milk	325 milligrams
1 cup low-fat or whole milk yogurt	300 milligrams
1 cup cooked collard greens	300 milligrams
¼ pound fresh oysters	210 milligrams
TOTAL	1135 milligrams

Combination 2:

8 ounces skim or low-fat milk	325 milligrams
2 cups low-fat cottage cheese	350 milligrams
1 cup cooked broccoli	130 milligrams
1 cup ice milk	150 milligrams
TOTAL	955 milligrams

Combination 3:

¼ cup nonfat dry milk	377 milligrams
¼ pound canned salmon with bones	225 milligrams
1 cup cooked kale	200 milligrams
4 ounces tofu	145 milligrams
TOTAL	947 milligrams

that are being hyped commercially, so it's best to use caution when you step outside the range of those for which clear daily guidelines exist.

To date, only thirteen vitamins have been identified, and requirements for two of them, biotin and pantothenic acid, have not even been established since there has never been a known deficiency. Of the eleven vitamins for which dietary guidelines are available, there are four fat soluble and seven water soluble.

Fat-soluble vitamins are stored in your body's fat and are transported to your cells by blood. If there is an excess, it is not excreted in the urine but remains in your body. For this reason, fat-soluble vitamins must be used carefully to prevent toxicity.

TIPS FOR GETTING YOUR IRON

The recommended dietary allowance for most adult women who are not pregnant or lactating is about 15 milligrams a day. You might think that's easy to achieve by popping an iron supplement. But iron absorption can be hampered or enhanced according to the food source as well as other foods consumed along with it. Here are some suggestions for getting the most out of your iron consumption.

1. **Red meat, especially liver, is the best source of iron. But you don't have to eat a high-fat, high-cholesterol beef meal in order to get your iron. An ounce or two of well trimmed meat in a stir-fry or a casserole can provide you with substantial absorbable iron.**
2. **Eat foods containing vitamin C along with your vegetarian iron sources: Vitamin C promotes iron absorption.**
3. **Coffee and tea, when consumed at the same meal as iron, inhibit its absorption—coffee by as much as 40 percent and tea by as much as 87 percent. Drink your coffee and tea at other times.**
4. **Don't overdo your fiber intake. Too much dietary fiber can interfere with the absorption of iron.**
5. **Cook some of your meal in cast-iron pans. When acidic foods, such as tomato sauce, are cooked in iron pans, some of the iron is leached into the food, providing extra iron in your diet.**

Water-soluble vitamins include vitamin C and the B vitamins. These need to be replenished regularly and the excess is excreted in the urine.

Minerals are inorganic elements that we need to consume dietarily. Some are required in large amounts and are called macrominerals. Others are needed in smaller amounts and are called trace minerals. Seven minerals have established dietary recommendations: calcium, phosphorus, magnesium, iron, zinc, iodine, and selenium.

DEPARTMENT OF AGRICULTURE GUIDELINES FOR WOMEN

g   = gram
μg = microgram (one millionth of a gram)
mg = milligram (1,000 micrograms)
kg = kilogram   (1,000 grams)

	19–24 YRS	25–50 YRS	51+ YRS	PREGNANT	LACTATING
Vitamin A	800 μg	800 μg	800 μg	800 μg	1.3 mg
Vitamin D	10 μg	5 μg	5 μg	10 μg	10 μg
Vitamin E	8 mg	8 mg	8 mg	10 mg	12 mg
Vitamin K	60 μg	65 μg	65 μg	65 μg	65 μg
Vitamin C	60 mg	60 mg	60 mg	70 mg	95 mg
Thiamin (B$_1$)	1.1 mg	1.1 mg	1.1 mg	1.5 mg	1.6 mg
Riboflavin (B$_2$)	1.3 mg	1.3 mg	1.2 mg	1.6 mg	1.8 mg
Niacin	15 mg	15 mg	13 mg	17 mg	20 mg
B$_6$	1.6 mg	1.6 mg	1.6 mg	2.2 mg	2.1 mg
Folacin	180 μg	180 μg	180 μg	400 μg	280 μg
B$_{12}$	2 μg	2 μg	2 μg	2.2 μg	2.6 μg
Calcium	1200 mg	1000 mg	1000–1500 mg	1200 mg	1200 mg
Phosphorus	1200 mg	800 mg	800 mg	1200 mg	1200 mg
Magnesium	280 mg	280 mg	280 mg	320 mg	355 mg
Iron	15 mg	15 mg	10 mg	30 mg	15 mg
Zinc	12 mg	12 mg	12 mg	15 mg	19 mg
Iodine	150 μg	150 μg	150 μg	175 μg	200 μg
Selenium	55 μg	55 μg	55 μg	65 μg	75 μg

CAN DIET KEEP YOU WELL?

Food has been called "the stuff of life" for good reason. It nourishes our systems, regenerates cells, wards off infections, and enables us to flourish. In this respect, it is a matter of common sense to say that there is a connection between nutrition and wellness. In some cases, that connection is vibrantly clear. Diet is certainly a factor in the development of the arterial plaque that signals coronary artery disease. Dietary factors are essential in the prevention of other diseases like osteoporosis and diabetes. When it comes to health, it's safe to say, you are what you eat.

In other areas, the connection between diet and disease is less clear, but the evidence is mounting, especially regarding some forms of cancer.

Current data suggest that as many as 40 percent of cancer deaths in this country (including cancer of the colon, pancreas, breast, ovary, and endometrium) are associated with nutrition.

THE ACTION OF ANTI-CANCER NUTRIENTS

NUTRIENTS	CANCER-FIGHTING ACTION
Vitamins C, E, phenols, polyphenols, antioxidants, soy protein	**Prevent formation of carcinogens or reactive oxygen**
Tea, flavonoids, alkylindoles, dialkysulfides, organic and inorganic selenium compounds	**Blocking agents, lower activation, increase detoxification of carcinogens**
Carotene, retinoids, antioxidants, selenium, calcium, vitamin D	**Suppress formation of abnormal gene structures, decrease rate of cell duplication**

Specific studies are currently under way that test the role of soy protein in the prevention of breast cancer. There are convincing long-term studies that link high-fat diets to breast cancer. While it is unwise at this point to isolate certain nutrients to the exclusion of others (remember, a well rounded diet is important), these promising early studies show just how powerful nutrition's role is in the prevention of disease.

In addition to research that demonstrates specific nutrient links to cancer prevention, overall dietary guidelines are changing to include not only what we eat but the way we eat. Experts believe that the new healthy diet for the nineties is a form of "grazing" that involves eating not three but six (small) meals a day. According to some studies, the same food divided into six meals will reduce cholesterol levels more than if it is eaten in the standard three meals.

KEEP MOVING

A necessary complement to a healthy diet is exercise. The decision you make about the type of exercise you choose is dependent on your current age, condition, and complicating medical factors. Starting an exercise program can be intimidating if you've never done it before, so the first rule of thumb is to choose an activity that you're comfortable doing, start slow, and keep a steady regimen. Regular exercise at a moderate rate is better for your heart and bones than sporadic high-intensity work. Studies indicate that a moderate-paced walk builds bone density more than running. The old rules about "no pain, no gain" no longer apply. Women who exercise while dieting lose more weight than those who only cut calories. Exercise helps you lose abdominal fat, the kind associated with health risks. It can also raise HDL cholesterol and reduce insulin levels, important for the prevention of hypertension, heart disease, and diabetes. Exercise increases muscle mass, which is more metabolically active. So a person who exercises regularly burns more calories even when she is sitting still than a sedentary person. To get conditioned, all you need is twenty minutes of aerobic exercise three times a week. I often give my patients an exercise prescription just as I would prescribe any other therapy. It includes:

▶ Type: aerobic fitness
  —continuous, rhythmic endurance activities of large muscle groups.
▶ Intensity: monitor by heart rate response.
  —maximum HR = 220 minus your age, or maximum achieved on an Exercise Tolerance Test.
  —target HR = 70–85 percent of maximum.
  —initiate with lower intensity, 40–60 percent of maximum.
▶ Duration:
  —warm-up; 5–15 minutes, stretching.
  —exercise; 20–30 minutes,
  —cool-down; 5–10 minutes at lower intensity
▶ Frequency:
  —minimum three times per week, spread out.
▶ Progression:
  —increase duration of exercise by 5–10 minutes every two weeks, up to 45 minutes.
  —when necessary, lower intensity for longer duration is preferable.

PHYSICAL ACTIVITY BURNS CALORIES

ACTIVITY	LEVEL	CALORIES EXPENDED
Bicycling	5½ mph	210/hour
Bicycling	13 mph	660/hour
Bowling	Average	150–270/hour
Calisthenics	Stretching	150/hour
Calisthenics	Vigorous	300/hour
Dancing	Slow	125/hour
Dancing	Fast	350/hour
Hiking	Easy	120/mile
Hiking	Rough	150/mile
Ice Skating	Average	275/hour
Jumping Rope	Vigorous	850/hour
Roller Skating	Average	275/hour
Rowing Machine	Vigorous	750/hour
Running	Average	100/hour
Skiing	Downhill	600/hour
Skiing	Cross Country	150/mile
Skiing	Water	480/hour
Squash/Handball	Average	350–600/hour
Swimming	Average	400–1000/hour
Tennis	Singles	275/hour
Tennis	Doubles	225/hour
Walking	2/12 mph	250/hour
Walking	Up Stairs	1,050/hour

Based on average energy expenditure for a 150-pound person.

COMMON QUESTIONS ABOUT DIET AND WEIGHT

Is there such a thing as an addiction to food?

Some people have a psychological addiction to food in the sense that they use food to relieve discomfort, depression, boredom, or anxiety. This behavior is similar to the way people use drugs, alcohol, and smoking. However, we must be careful when we talk about food addictions because the method of recovery is so different. For example, if you are addicted to cocaine, the treatment is to stop taking the drug—to withdraw from the source of your addiction. But you can't stop eating food. And if you try to eat very little food, you'll find that it backfires (as we described earlier in this chapter). Some researchers have detected abnormal brain chemistries associated with eating disorders. They have tried using opioid blockers to inhibit binge eating.

If you use food as a way to alter your mood, and feel intense cravings at certain times of stress or when you are unhappy, your treatment probably needs to focus on other issues besides food. Food is not the problem since it is not really an addictive substance. You need to explore, preferably with the help of a professional, the psychological and social factors leading to your eating behavior.

Will drinking more water help me to avoid too much water loss when I'm dieting?

Drinking water will not replace the water that is lost from your cells when you're on a very low-calorie diet. It will only be excreted by your kidneys.

Are formula diets safe?

Liquid diets should never be used for quick weight loss. In my opinion, using a liquid food substitute only reinforces the inability to relate to food in a healthy way. Statistically, most people who have lost weight on formula diets regain it, plus more.

How effective is behavior modification in controlling eating behavior?

Behavior modification can help jump-start a healthy eating lifestyle. If over a long period of time, you have developed poor eating habits, you might find that certain careful routines help change your attitudes about food—especially while you are getting used to new practices. Many women find food journals helpful. Others find that following specific patterns works. For example, only eating at a certain time of day, always setting the table and sitting down when you eat, or only buying foods at the supermarket that are on your list. Ask yourself, "Am I really hungry? Am I really hungry for this particular food? Will my hunger be gone when this food is gone?" If you are hungry, eat. If you really want a cookie, have just one. If you are not really hungry, change your environment and wait ten minutes. You'll find that the urge to eat leaves. After a while, you'll learn to identify true hunger and accept that you'll have the impulse to nervously eat without having to act upon it.

Weight loss best occurs when calories are not consumed in excess and when the source of those calories is a low-fat, high-carbohydrate diet. Weight loss accomplished through exercise has been shown to be more reliable in keeping weight off, and it improves cardiovascular health. But the body is very efficient—it only uses 100 calories to run one mile. You can burn more calories by eating after you exercise.

Do drugs help weight loss?

Recent studies show that fenfluramine, a drug related to amphetamines, is effective in helping to lose weight. However, it can cause depression in some people, even after they discontinue its use. To date, no long-term studies have been done on its safety or efficacy.

RESOURCES

ORGANIZATIONS
Food and Drug Administration
Consumer Inquiries
5600 Fishers Lane
Rockville, MD 20857
301-443-3170

Center for Science in the Public Interest
1501 16th Street, NW
Washington, DC 20036
202-332-9110

Bureau of Health Care Delivery and Assistance
Health Resources and Services Administration
Public Health Service
5600 Fishers Lane
Rockville, MD 20857
301-443-2320

Community Nutrition Institute
2001 S Street, NW
Washington, DC 20009
202-462-4700

PUBLICATIONS

*Consuming Passions: Feminist Approaches to Weight Preoccupations and
    Eating Disorders*
edited by Catrina Brown and Karin Jasper
Second Story Press, 1993

Beauty Secrets: Women and the Politics of Appearance
by Wendy Chapkis
South End Press, 1986

The Obsession
by Kim Chernin
Perennial Library, 1982

Fat Chance! The Myth of Dieting Explained
by Jane Ogden
Routledge, 1992

The Beauty Myth: How Images of Beauty Are Used Against Women
by Naomi Wolf
Anchor Books, 1991

Radiance Magazine
P.O. Box 31703
Oakland, CA 94604
415-482-0680
(A quarterly magazine for large women)

Tufts University Diet & Nutrition Letter
80 Boylston Street, Suite 353
Boston, MA 02116
617-482-3530

17

DEPENDENT NO MORE
Staying Strong and Addiction Free

~~~~~~~~

A physician colleague of mine recently complained about a woman patient who was continuing to smoke during pregnancy. "I must admit, I feel very annoyed and impatient with her," she said. "She's an educated woman. She knows the hazards. She wants a healthy baby. We've been through it a dozen times. But she still smokes. I have to tell you, I find myself being angry and resentful." Another colleague, normally a caring, compassionate doctor, admitted, "I have a problem feeling sympathy for people who deliberately take substances that they know will hurt them, then come to me expecting that I'll magically make them well."

Most doctors I know, myself included, have felt frustration and deep concern when we see our patients ingesting dangerous substances—smoking, drinking too much alcohol, or abusing drugs. It's hard not to be judgmental—to equate "bad" behavior with being bad. Doctors complain that it's a real struggle to be an advocate for a patient who seems on the face of it to be intent upon self-destruction. How can a woman care about her health when she makes the conscious choice to abuse it?

This judgment comes from trying to make a simple black-and-white, cause-and-effect correlation between attitude and behavior. But the issues are more complex. When I see a woman who smokes, drinks excessively, or abuses drugs, I always start with the premise that she is not a masochist. She doesn't want to hurt herself. In every case, there is a perceived benefit that is so strong it outweighs the negatives. My task as an advocate and partner is to discover what my patient thinks she is gaining, to explore her fears of quitting, and to help her achieve replacement behavior that will address her needs in a healthy way.

Substance abuse among women—whether tobacco, alcohol, or drugs—is an urgent problem that has typically been underplayed in research and treatment. One reason is that the progression of substance abuse is a quieter and more tangled matter for women. It is intricately linked with socialization, life stresses, and the daily reinforcement of stereotypes. It's not surprising that substance abuse is a pressing health issue for women when you consider that we are socialized to be dependent. Throughout our lives the message is reinforced: You can't do it alone. You don't have the resources you need. You're incomplete on your own. Your strength is not inside you. Many women respond to feeling unfulfilled and empty by reaching beyond themselves for a crutch or a magic solution that will lift them above their sadness or sense of inadequacy. For some women, this takes the form of involvement in dependent relationships. Others become obsessed with their work. But for growing numbers of women, the crutch of choice is a substance.

IS THERE A DEPENDENT PERSONALITY?

I have had women say to me, "I'm a dependent personality." Again, they're convinced that they smoke, overeat, drink too much, or abuse drugs because they cannot do otherwise. They lurch through life without control or direction, helplessly falling in and out of relationships with abusive, addicted, or chronically uncommitted men, and they believe the fault lies in a core addiction that transcends all others: The addiction to being a dependent self. Adopting the definition of the day, many of them define themselves as "codependent" personalities.

Codependency entered our language during the 1980s. It was used initially to describe people—almost always women—who were in relationships with alcoholics or drug abusers. The codependent was the enabling partner—the one who made the addictive behavior possible by supporting the person who was addicted. If the alcoholic or drug abuser was dependent on the use of a substance, his partner was likewise dependent on being a caretaker, on smoothing the disruptions and making things all right. In its genesis the codependency movement was empowering for women. It supplied courage and support to those whose self-esteem had hit bottom and who could find no options but to stay with their alcoholic or drug-addicted partners. It countered their sense of personal failure and blame by reassuring them that their partner's behavior was not their fault. It helped them to be strong.

However, the codependency movement was not without problems, especially as it evolved beyond substance abuse issues. Suddenly, women were being told that every life dilemma was rooted in an inner pathology. Women who had never been addicted to substances were suddenly being told they were "addicted" to bad relationships, "addicted" to food, "addicted" to love. The language of pathology was not empowering for many women because it made them feel as though their very natures were twisted—that they were a bundle of forces beyond their control. Women began to accept the label of being codependent whenever they experienced a crisis.

Codependency cannot be viewed as a catchall explanation for dysfunctional behaviors in women. It does, however, remind us that the socialization of some women has led to a "learned helplessness" that has been nurtured by generations of tradition and ritual. This learned helplessness is clearly an entry point to unhealthy behaviors.

In the study and treatment of specific substance addictions, some experts have found that identifying a woman as having an addictive personality actually adds to her sense of hopelessness. It can also mask real problems. For example, it has been learned that up to 74 percent of all women substance abusers have been sexually abused at some time in their lives. This knowledge dramatically changes the way women addicts must be viewed—and takes away the stigmatizing label of "addictive personality."

Rather than saying that some women have "addictive personalities," it is more useful to remind ourselves of the social experiences that can rob women of self-esteem or lead to posttraumatic stress disorder (PTSD). We cannot treat the symptoms until we treat the cause.

It is urgent that we bring some light to this subject because every day in America, women are killing themselves with substance abuse. And the Big Three dependencies that we must address are smoking, alcohol, and drugs.

WOMEN WHO SMOKE

If you ask a woman why she smokes, she will rarely reply, "I'm addicted to nicotine." Rather, she will offer a positive explanation, describing a perceived benefit such as:

"I smoke to keep my weight down."

"I smoke to calm my nerves."

"I smoke to boost my energy."

"I smoke because it relaxes me."

Young girls who take up the habit are strongly influenced by all of these perceptions—especially the relationship of smoking to weight control. Every day in America, some three thousand young women join the 21.6 million women who smoke. Adolescent girls are picking up the habit at a rate exceeding adolescent boys, and 90 percent of smokers begin smoking before age twenty-one. It is estimated that one out of every five high school senior girls smokes. If this trend continues, women smokers will outnumber men smokers by the year 2000. Students who smoke cigarettes have also been found to use alcohol and illicit drugs. Caucasian adolescent girls are more likely to start smoking than African-Americans or Latinas, and overall lifetime use continues this pattern: 73 percent Caucasians, 63 percent African Americans, and 52 percent Latinas. The reasons young girls start smoking, in spite of increased public awareness of the health hazards, are rooted in complex social factors. These include:

1. FAMILY ROLE MODELS. Women seem to be more strongly influenced than men by growing up in households with parents who smoke.

2. STYLE PERCEPTIONS. Women who smoke are still perceived, at least in the abstract, to be more attractive than nonsmokers. In one revealing survey of sixth graders, both boys and girls rated male smoker models as less good-looking and desirable, while rating female smoker models as slightly more good-looking and desirable.

3. MEDIA SEDUCTION. The tobacco industry's seduction of women began full swing during the 1970s when the Marlboro man was joined by the Virginia Slims woman. But the association of smoking with independence, excitement, and sexuality among women has been around for a lot longer. For example, movies produced during and after World War II almost always showed strong male heroes smoking. Traditional "good" women

such as housewives never smoked. But the more exciting, independent career women did.

4. PERCEIVED BENEFITS. These include weight control, stress reduction, and the energy-lifting qualities that women believe cigarettes to have.

The benefits are clearly quite compelling because research has shown that most young women feel sick after smoking their first cigarette and continue to suffer adverse effects throughout their smoking lives. Surely they would not accept the vicious side effects if they did not think it was worth it. Remember, women are not masochistic. The tobacco industry has been able to help people over the initial unpleasantness of smoking. Since the industry knows that the more distasteful the first smoking experience, the less likely it is that a person will try again, it has developed "lite" cigarettes and marketed them most aggressively among women. (Where else have we allowed drug dealers to "cut" their products legally in order to enhance addiction?)

When it comes to women's health, smoking is a wolf in sheep's clothing. Any perception that smoking makes you look better, feel better, or appear more stylish or attractive to others is a lie. Although women's entry point to cigarette smoking is social, the hook is chemical. Nicotine is an addictive substance. In fact, among chemical dependencies, cigarette smoking is one of the most difficult to overcome.

What happens when you smoke a cigarette? Each cigarette contains about ten milligrams of nicotine; between one and two milligrams is delivered directly to the lungs. Once it is absorbed, it travels quickly to the brain, then is metabolized rapidly by the liver. Studies have shown that this metabolic process occurs more rapidly in men than in women, resulting in higher levels of nicotine in women smokers' systems. Over time, women experience more damaging effects than men, even though overall they smoke less.

As you have learned in previous chapters of this book, smoking is a primary risk factor in virtually every major health crisis to afflict women.

Smoking is one of the leading factors in the development of coronary artery disease, particularly potent in younger women; smoking carries three times the risk for stroke and six times the risk for burst blood vessels in the brain—again, most notable in young smokers.

Smoking causes lung damage and pulmonary problems more rapidly in women than in men.

Smoking has an antiestrogenic effect, negating the protective effects of estrogen and causing earlier menopause. Furthermore, the benefits of ERT at menopause are almost totally negated in women who smoke, and smokers over thirty-five who take oral contraceptives risk heart attacks and strokes. Lung cancer has now surpassed breast cancer to become the leading cause of cancer death in women. The lung is not the only organ to be placed at risk for cancer. Women who smoke risk cancer of the bladder, cervix, head, neck, and esophagus, as well as leukemia.

New studies suggest that smoking is a key factor in the development of cataracts as well as Graves' disease (hyperthyroidism). It is possible that the increasing rate of smoking among women will actually take away the extra years of life that women have led, compared with men.

THE MEDICAL COMPLICATIONS OF SMOKING

Coronary artery disease
Lung cancer
Esophageal cancer
Cervical cancer
Head and neck cancer
Bladder cancer
Cancer of the larynx
Emphysema, chronic bronchitis, asthma
Osteoporosis
Cataracts
Hyperthyroidism
Early ovarian failure (menopause)
Fetal damage/miscarriage
Low birth weight babies
Babies with Sudden Infant Death Syndrome (SIDS)
Respiratory problems in children
Death from all causes

Women need not smoke themselves to be put at risk for these illnesses. The dangers of "passive smoke," that produced by family members, are being increasingly documented. Precancerous lesions have been found in the lungs of women married to smokers, and up to 17 percent of lung cancer in nonsmokers can be attributed to environmental smoke during childhood.

Women smokers do more than place their own health at risk. There is an increasing body of evidence that children are harmed when their mothers smoke. The damage begins with low birth weight in infants born to smokers. It continues in a number of effects of "passive" smoking—that is, living in a household with a smoker. Environmental smoke causes 300,000 cases of bronchitis and pneumonia in children every year. Children under eighteen months have more colds and middle-ear fluid when their parents smoke. Children of smokers suffer more frequent respiratory infections and asthma. There is also a link to behavioral problems. In one report, children whose mothers smoked at least one pack of cigarettes a day during and after pregnancy had three times as many behavioral problems, such as hyperactivity, as other children.

Tobacco use is the single most preventable cause of disease and death!

How to Quit

It is very hard for women to quit smoking. Research shows that they are more sensitive to the chemical effects of nicotine than men, and their withdrawal symptoms are more severe. In addition, the perceived benefits of smoking are much stronger for women. A socialization toward dependency coupled with fear of weight gain strengthens women's resistance to quitting. Nevertheless, as the evidence piles up about the health hazards of smoking, many women are reaching the conclusion that they cannot continue to damage themselves with this habit, no matter how beloved it has become.

Respiratory disease experts have defined a path to quitting that includes four stages:

1. **Not yet ready to quit.**

2. **Thinking about quitting.**

3. **Ready to quit.**

4. **Staying smoke free.**

Most of the smokers I see are at stage two. They're thinking about quitting. They say they want to quit. But they're afraid. Often they've tried before and failed, and wonder if they have it in them ever to be successful.

The most common fear is weight gain. People who quit smoking do tend to gain weight owing to the combination of a temporary slowdown in metabolic rate and a frequent change in eating habits. But the average weight gain is not really that great, and it usually isn't permanent. What lurks beneath the fear of weight gain is really the fear of losing control.

Women view smoking as a mood stabilizer and a crutch that keeps them from falling apart. They tend not to trust their own inner resources, but rely on external means of support to keep them even. When I talk to smokers about their fear of gaining weight, they strongly believe that they won't be able to stop themselves from binging on food if they can't grab a cigarette when the urge strikes. "What will I do about my oral fixation?" one woman asked me—as though it were a certainty that she would have to put something in her mouth several times an hour to replace the cigarettes she normally smoked in that period.

Although smoking is legal, it is becoming less socially acceptable in most circles. Women who continue to smoke often feel a great deal of shame, especially if they have children who are being affected. Nobody really enjoys being addicted to a substance. Smoking is an embarrassing public admission that they can't control their health behavior.

But when I work with women who want to quit smoking, I focus on the positive benefits, not a reinforcement of their shame. It's my goal to help them find replacement rewards rather than focus on the deprivation. It's important to find out what the smoker feels she is gaining from her habit, educating her about the ways in which the benefit is a false one, and then emphasizing the greater benefits to be gained by not smoking. Each person's experience is unique. However, in addition to the obvious health benefits, the woman who quits smoking may find:

▶ Greater energy (contrary to myth, smoking actually depletes energy)
▶ Clearer sense of taste and smell
▶ Fuller breathing capacity
▶ No more coughing
▶ Cleaner breath
▶ Clearer skin
▶ More freedom to go anywhere without being concerned about smoking
▶ Elimination of mess and tobacco smell
▶ Greater social acceptance
▶ A sense of accomplishment, control, and pride

Once a woman is ready to quit, there are two issues to resolve in helping her remain smoke free. The first is the nicotine addiction itself. In many respects, this is the easiest part of the task. Although nicotine is highly addictive, the addiction disappears within two weeks of not smoking. More difficult is the habit of smoking. All smokers create regular rituals around smoking.

"I start every morning with a cigarette and a cup of coffee."

"When the phone rings, I grab a cigarette."

"If something upsets me, I need a cigarette to calm me down."

"I always relax with a cigarette after dinner."

Over time, these events become associated with smoking. The link is so strong that when a women stops smoking, she may continue to crave cigarettes long after she has completed the nicotine withdrawal. That is why it is the consensus of treatment professionals that the best way to stop smoking—and remain smoke free over the long term—is to join a support group and be instructed in behavior modification. Even though the patch, acupuncture, hypnosis, and other quitting methods can be effective in the beginning, long-term success is more certain when behavior modification is learned and support groups are joined.

WOMEN WHO ABUSE ALCOHOL

Beverly was a fifty-three-year-old widowed woman who came to me with multiple complaints. I immediately recognized her as someone I had seen in the newspapers because of her involvement with various charities. I found her to be charming and intelligent, a lovely, fashionable woman who obviously took great pride in her appearance. But I also saw the strain behind her eyes and the nervous twisting of her hands as she talked.

Beverly told me that for months she had been depressed and unable to perform her normal activities. At night, she had trouble sleeping, even though she felt exhausted. Lately, she had been avoiding friends and social occasions and spending most of her time alone at home.

I began to ask Beverly some questions about her life, which she answered easily and honestly. Only when I asked about alcohol did she hesitate. She said she didn't usually drink that much, but always had at least two or three glasses of wine in the evenings. Sometimes she drank more to help her sleep or because she was depressed.

From her description, I believed that Beverly might have an alcohol problem—even though she rarely got "drunk." Alcohol has increasingly become an addictive substance for older women, especially when they live alone and are depressed. As a doctor with many patients who are older women, I have grown very sensitive to the signs. But although Beverly had been to several other doctors before coming to see me, I was the first one to ask her about alcohol.

Alcohol is the hidden scourge of women in America. Like Beverly, women tend to abuse alcohol in private, then take great pains to hide their problem. Even though women alcoholics make extensive use of the health care system for a wide variety of ailments, they often fail to mention alcohol consumption—and doctors fail to ask.

There are significant gender differences in the way women and men use and abuse alcohol. Beverly was an example of a typical woman drinker. For most of her life, alcohol had never been especially prominent. She started drinking in earnest following her husband's death because she felt she needed something to ease the stress. At first, her drinking did just that. But within a few months, alcohol became the source of her stress and depression, not a relief from it.

Alcohol abuse, especially among older women, is kept secret because the stigma is so great. Women in our society are expected to meet high standards of behavior. When they fail to do this—for example, by drinking excessively—they are not treated as being ill but as being immoral. In the public mind, alcohol use by women is associated with unrestrained sexual activity, even though the evidence is just the reverse. For one thing, it is more typical for women alcoholics to drink alone and to be older; the mean age of women at treatment centers is forty-four years old. Women alcoholics are not out cruising bars, although younger women often drink to enhance their social skills, and lesbians frequent bars to meet other women.

A study conducted by researchers at the University of North Dakota found that not only does alcohol not make women promiscuous, it makes them more likely victims of the alcohol-induced aggression of others. The woman who drinks becomes a target, not an initiator. Yet when robbery, rape, battery, or other violence occurs against her, she is blamed for making herself vulnerable. She is scolded: "This wouldn't have happened if you had been sober."

Like most biases against women, this one has a long history. In ancient Rome, alcohol consumption by women was punishable by death because it was believed that it made them lascivious. This attitude has continued over the centuries; in some countries, women are still put to death if they are caught drinking. In our own country, women who seek help for addiction problems in some states are defined by law as child neglectors. By coming forward to receive treatment, they are at risk of losing their children. No wonder alcoholic women are driven into the closet! Shame and fear compel them to hide a behavior that is linked to immorality and is dangerous to their physical welfare and their family security.

The Poisonous Process

Like most addictive substances, alcohol is a great deceiver whose actual effects are exactly the opposite from the drinker's expectations. Women who drink in order to calm themselves or feel better, grow more depressed instead. Women who drink in order to heighten sexual arousal and enjoy sex more find instead that they are less easily aroused, have less satisfying orgasms, and over time lose all interest in sex.

Research shows that women drink alcohol as a form of self-medication against stress, to dull dissatisfaction with life, and to bury painful memories—often involving violence or sexual abuse. (It is estimated that 45 percent of women in alcoholic treatment programs begin as battered wives.) But any relief is only temporary. For women, more so than men, alcohol dependency is a rapid downward spiral that begins with pleasure and ends with pain.

In recent years, a number of studies have been published that indicate a strong genetic factor in male alcohol abuse. The genetic link in women is less clear. The risk factors for alcohol abuse in women are largely environmental. For women, alcohol abuse is usually secondary to depression, and this profile makes the disease more difficult to recognize. While alcohol abuse in men usually manifests itself with antisocial behavior (including violence), women's depressive profile keeps their problem hidden.

Alcohol is more intoxicating in lower amounts for women than it is for men. On average, women drink 45 percent less alcohol than men, but experience the same degree of impairment. Blood alcohol levels rise rapidly and this effect varies across the menstrual cycle, being strongest premenstrually and the least severe during menstruation. One reason for the increased toxicity in women is that they have a lower volume of body water than men; since alcohol is water soluble, it is less diluted in women than in men. Also, women have less of a stomach enzyme that deactivates alcohol. These factors might be the reason why women suffer more serious health effects than men with a much lower alcohol intake. For example, although a high percentage of heavy drinkers are male, 40 percent of all patients suffering cirrhosis of the liver are women. In general, women get organ damage drinking less heavily than men, in a shorter period of time, and at lower blood alcohol levels. Alcohol also raises estrogen levels, which may be the reason for its connection to breast cancer. Certain alcoholic beverages, like bourbon, also contain plant estrogens, which may contribute to higher estrogen levels.

An alcoholic woman's life span is reduced by fifteen years because of liver disease, alcohol-related accidents, and suicides. Drinking women have four times the mortality rate of nondrinking women.

Although Caucasian women drink more heavily than African-American women, African-American women alcoholics have a higher mortality and report more alcohol-related health problems. In addition, the rate of fetal alcohol syndrome is seven times higher with African-American women. More than 70 percent of Latina women are abstainers, yet almost the same number of Latino men are alcohol drinkers—an example of cultural/gender influences. Only 6 percent of Latina women have alcohol-related problems. Alcohol consumption among Asian-Americans is the lowest of all ethnic groups in the United States. Native Americans experience considerable variability in drink-

---

THE COMPLICATIONS OF ALCOHOLISM

Cirrhosis of the liver
Accidents
Suicide
Hypertension
Obesity
Anemia
Malnutrition
Amenorrhea
Miscarriage
Early menopause
Infertility
Breast cancer
Fetal alcohol syndrome

ing patterns. Some tribes totally abstain while others have disproportionately heavy alcohol consumption patterns. Alcohol-related problems are among the ten leading causes of death for Native Americans and Alaskan Natives; these include unintentional injuries, chronic liver disease and cirrhosis, homicide, and suicide.

What is the dividing line between a woman who drinks alcohol "socially" and a woman whose alcoholic consumption is a health hazard? The answer is, there is no clear dividing line. Since women can be intoxicated with even small amounts of alcohol, there's no way to say that one, two, or three drinks is under or over the line.

GENDER DIFFERENCES IN ALCOHOL ABUSE

Women who abuse alcohol have a different social and biological profile from that of men. While these factors may not have a direct causative effect, they are often present in women who abuse alcohol.

1. Women are more likely to have alcoholic role models in their nuclear families and to have alcoholic spouses.
2. Women's drinking problems usually occur later in life.
3. Women consume less alcohol than men (although with the same effects), and are less likely to engage in aggressive social behavior or public drunkenness.
4. Women progress rapidly from the onset of drinking through later stages of alcoholism.
5. Women tend to begin drinking heavily in response to a traumatic event or stress.
6. Women alcoholics experience more stigmatization than men.
7. Women alcoholics tend to be separated or divorced. Alcohol disrupts their relationships to a greater degree than it does men's.
8. Women suffer more liver cirrhosis in response to heavy drinking.
9. Alcoholic women are generally characterized as feeling more guilty, anxious, or depressed than men.

Getting Help

Alcoholism is more easily picked up in men, whose manifestations are more public. They might lose a job or be sent into treatment by an employer; the diagnosis and treatment program might come via the criminal justice system in reference to drunk driving or violent behavior. But alcoholic women present more subtly, utilizing the health care system to deal with medical or family problems that might not be linked with alcohol abuse. Women alcoholics are hiding in doctors' offices, hospitals, and clinics. Many doctors fail to elicit the history and ignore laboratory abnormalities that are tip-offs. Women don't present themselves to detox programs as men do. They go to doctors talking about depression, anxiety, and many physical complaints. This places them at dual risk since a prescription of sedatives might be added to their daily cocktails by doctors who are unable or unwilling to address the real problem.

If a woman is lucky enough to have a health care provider identify her alcoholism as a problem, she may still lack adequate treatment since women-centered programs are not available. Women are, by and large, poorer than men, and financial barriers to treatment are great. (Legal barriers also get in the way; in some states, women alcohol abusers are defined by law as child neglectors.) Treatment centers make no allowance for women's need for child care.

Once a woman is in a program, her road to recovery is often different from a man's. A woman may appear sicker or less motivated if male patterns are used as the norm. And unrecognized prior histories of abuse may hinder a woman's ability to recover. Alcoholics Anonymous, a powerful treatment model, was developed by men and is more successful with men.

You may recall Penny, the overweight, hypertensive woman who was panic stricken about losing her hair. I promised her we would get to the bottom of her hair loss and her depression, and I was committed to being her advocate. I told her we would experiment with different blood pressure medications until we found one that worked for her. A few weeks after that visit, Penny suddenly showed up in my office determined to tell the truth. I ushered her in and sat down to listen.

"I just couldn't do it," she said miserably.

"Do what?" I wondered.

"Go through all the medication changes, or have you make a decision that was based on a lie," she said, barely able to look at me. She then told me that she had been drinking heavily for quite some time, and she was terrified that her drinking was making her very sick. "I have to stop," she said. "Look at me. My hair is falling out. I'm bloated . . ." She started to cry. "I'm so sorry I lied to you."

I had asked Penny about her drinking habits several times, and she had always assured me that she didn't drink. I hadn't caught the signs, although I had been on the lookout, and that shows how difficult detection can be.

"I know it feels shameful to have this kind of problem," I told her. "I assume that's why you lied. But I'm glad you came in today because it means you understand that we are partners in making you better, and that process begins with the truth."

Women ask me, "How do I know if I have a problem?" That's not an easy question to answer. From a medical standpoint, statistics suggest that above two drinks a day raises a risk. There is consensus on the fact that pregnant women should not drink alcohol at all. But beyond that, the best guide is your own sense of whether or not alcohol has become a problem—as well as the input from those who are close to you.

WOMEN WHO ABUSE DRUGS

Roxanne had a familiar story to tell. As she sat across my desk, her fifty-five-year-old face burning with shame, she hesitantly admitted the secret she had been desperately trying to keep for more than thirty years. When she was a young mother, her doctor prescribed amphetamines to help her lose weight and to lift her energy. Roxanne continued to use the drugs, not so much for weight control, but because she found that without them she was depressed and fatigued. When her own doctor stopped prescribing, she went elsewhere. Over the years, Roxanne never had a problem finding doctors who would give her the amphetamines. She laughingly told of one "diet doctor" who had willingly given her pills during a period when her weight was very low. "Unless he was blind, he couldn't have thought I really needed to lose weight," she said. "I went to him for years, and he never mentioned diet or exercise or my weight. He just gave me the pills."

In time, Roxanne found that she had to take more pills to gain the same effects, and often she felt nauseated, dizzy, and sleep-deprived. Recently, she had tried to stop taking the pills because her heartbeat was rapid and she was afraid she might have a heart attack. For the first time, she came face to face with the level of her addiction.

"I feel like the worst kind of drug addict," she told me miserably. She was deeply ashamed, but she also blamed the doctors. "Why didn't they stop me?" she asked. "Why didn't they know how bad this could get?"

I didn't have a ready answer for Roxanne. But I knew her experience was not unusual. It was clear to me that our profession has silently supported the use of prescription drugs by women for a long time. Today, we see the legacy of rampant prescription drug use during the 1950s in the addiction problems that still plague women from that era. Then, pills were the "magic bullets" for every discomfort—from insomnia to anxiety to boredom to depression. Women didn't stop to wonder why their lives were not working. Doctors didn't encourage them to find their source of self-esteem and pleasure from within; nor did they search beyond the symptoms to seek deeper causes, such as sexual abuse or domestic violence. Doctors easily prescribe pain medicine for back pain and headaches instead of fully exploring the psychosocial contributions to a chronic pain syndrome.

One might think the days of *Valley of the Dolls* are long passed. But even now, doctors are more inclined to prescribe drugs than to take the time to work through more complex solutions when women present with depression or related symptoms. Women still receive the bulk of prescription mood-altering drugs. Women use the health care system more than men, and according to studies, physicians are more inclined to diagnose female complaints as being treatable by drugs. Bias coupled with poor training in treating psychosocial problems encourage doctors to prescribe drugs.

The heavy prescription of mood-altering drugs also makes sense when you consider that the average office visit with a physician is about fifteen minutes—hardly enough time to dig for deeper issues. That fifteen minutes typically ends with the writing of a prescription, which satisfies both the doctor and the patient that something has been done. Seventy-one percent of female adolescents who ever used tranquilizers had them prescribed by a doctor, and older women receive prescriptions for tranquilizers two and a half times more often than older men. Serious health consequences are related to tranquilizer use in older women: suicide, insomnia, impaired thought processes, and instability of gait leading to falls and fractures.

I believe that one reason drug treatment programs are so heavily oriented toward men is that our profession expects and even encourages women to be drug dependent. The tradition of medicalizing women's normal life problems has created an attitude that a woman with a problem should be helped with drugs. I sometimes wonder if this is because it's so much easier to medicate than to open up a Pandora's box of women's issues.

Like alcoholism, women often find the path to drug addiction by way of depression and the need to alter mood. That's true with prescription drugs as well as illegal drugs.

According to the National Institute on Drug Abuse's 1990 National Household Survey on Drug Abuse, 32 percent of women have used illegal drugs at some time in their lives. Substance abuse is directly linked with other poor health behavior, such as high-risk sex and smoking. Substance abuse in pregnancy can lead to poor fetal outcomes like fetal alcohol syndrome and sudden infant death. Obstetrical complications are higher in drug-addicted women. And cocaine use has been linked to sudden death in pregnant women.

Whether they are prescription or illegal drugs, the abuse of substances to self-medicate or anesthetize one's emotional pain is an epidemic among women. The medical and social establishments are complicit in the abuse. Poor women and women of color, victimized by the culture of poverty, often become sex workers to support themselves and their children. They are at high risk of substance abuse in the exchange of sex for drugs. The hypersexuality associated with crack and cocaine use also puts women at risk for unprotected sex.

In 1991, 9 percent of women reported ever using cocaine. Cocaine is highly addictive, and after a brief period of euphoria, is associated with agitation and depression. Complications of cocaine use include impulsivity, high blood pressure, seizure, cardiac arrhythmia, heart attack, and sudden death. Cocaine use in pregnancy is associated with miscarriage, fetal death, premature labor, congenital malformations, sudden infant death syndrome (SIDS), and addicted babies.

Our national fiction about drugs says that they are something "losers" use. Many times, it is just the opposite.

Sally was twenty-six years old, a thin, eager apprentice newspaper journalist who worked long days and nights, including most weekends, in order to break into a highly competitive field. She first came to my office for a normal checkup, and when I took her history, everything appeared normal. She had never had any health problems before. But later, as she was sitting on my examination table, Sally suddenly burst into racking sobs. "I think I have a drug problem," she cried, shaking with disbelief. "I'm so scared!"

This was an emergency. I calmed Sally down and gently suggested that she get dressed so we could talk in my office. I assured her that I was going to listen to her and do what I could to help.

By the time Sally joined me in my office, she had stopped crying. In fact, she seemed relieved to have made the revelation which, she assured me, she hadn't expected to do. The admission had just poured out of her.

Sally told me that she had always been a high achiever in school, and from an early age she had known she wanted to be a journalist. She had landed a great job with a news magazine, but felt it was now in jeopardy. A new boyfriend had introduced her to cocaine so they could have "hot sex." Not only did it make sex better, Sally found that she really got into her writing when she was high. But after some initial rushes of creativity, she began to get frazzled and more focused on getting high than on writing. She didn't feel well when she was not using cocaine. She felt exhausted, depleted, and edgy. And she required more and more of the drug. Not only was she becoming physically dependent, she was now going through large sums of money to support her habit. Sally was alarmed at how the drug seemed to be controlling her life. Her performance at work was suffering, and her bank account was rapidly emptying. She was at a loss to know how to break the cycle and gain control of her life again.

Sally was a young woman with a clear sense of herself, and she was determined that her emerging dependence on cocaine would get nipped in the bud before it destroyed her life. But her experience caused me to reflect on how vulnerable women are, at home, in the bedroom, and in the workplace, by virtue of the expectation of perfection and compliance. It seems to me that women are faced with a double whammy when it comes to addiction. On one hand, they are made to feel as if they need something outside their own self and power to help them function; on the other hand, they are told that they must perform better—yes, become "superwomen"—in order to stay even in the tough, competitive world. No wonder a magic pill seems like such a good idea.

COMMON QUESTIONS ABOUT ADDICTIONS

I only smoke one or two cigarettes a day, usually in the evening. Will this small amount harm me?

It may surprise you that smoking up to five cigarettes a day still increases your risks for CAD and cancer—although it certainly doesn't approach the level of a pack-a-day smoker. But I suggest you ask yourself what the one or two cigarettes are giving you that you need, and see if you might find that benefit elsewhere. As long as you are smoking at all, you are participating in the habit of smoking; you may socialize with smokers and therefore pick up secondhand smoke. Finally, smoking is an addiction, even at your level. By stopping altogether, you can break the addiction's hold on you.

Are nicotine patches a good way to stop smoking?

Research shows that combined with a support group, transdermal nicotine replacement therapy can be quite effective; alone, the long-term success rate is only about 15 percent. Nicotine patches help relieve the initial withdrawal cravings by releasing steady amounts of nicotine into the system over a twenty-four-hour period. The recommended duration of use is about three months, with declining levels of nicotine. The patch does not, however, reduce other symptoms of withdrawal such as hunger and weight gain.

Since nicotine patches must be prescribed by a doctor, I suggest you talk to yours about the pros and cons. Be alert to conditions like CAD or hypertension that might make you a poor candidate for this therapy.

Nicotine gum is also available. Women may require higher doses than men to avoid withdrawal symptoms.

My mother was an alcoholic. Do I have a higher risk of becoming one?

Studies have shown that women who grew up in alcoholic homes are more likely to become alcoholics themselves. The primary reason is that during your formative years your primary adult role model—your mother—dealt with stress or sadness or anger by drinking alcohol. You never learned another way to deal with anxiety because she couldn't teach you. It's therefore easier for you to repeat her behavior. However, this is by no means inevitable. On the contrary, if you are educated about the dangers of alcoholism and have taken independent steps to strengthen your self-esteem, your mother's alcoholism may never be a risk factor for you.

If a doctor prescribes a drug, isn't it safe?

Most psychotropic medications are generally safe. The issue is not whether they will cause harm; rather, it's whether they are being used too randomly to treat anxiety and depression without the adjunct support of psychotherapy or without dealing with underlying environmental triggers. Dependency can lead to higher amounts of antianxiety drugs, and unpleasant and potentially harmful withdrawal symptoms. Sedatives can act together with alcohol to cause extreme drowsiness, leading to falls and car accidents. Remember, most drugs have been studied only in men, without regard to women's menstrual cycles or hormonal status. Many psychoactive drugs need to be used in smaller doses for women, since they have twice the side effects in women as in men. Some drugs need to be prescribed with a special sensitivity to women's cycles. For example, drug levels of lithium, tricyclic antidepressants (TCAs), and Prozac may drop by as much as 53 percent premenstrually, and may need to be adjusted to maintain a therapeutic level. Some antidepressants show better effects in men than in women. Imipramine, a TCA, is one. However, TCAs may be more effective in treating pain in women than in men. Women generally need lower doses of antipsychotic medicines. Be aware that benzodiazapines (such as Valium) may have different levels for women who use oral contraceptives, and may contribute to psychomotor problems in the week before menses.

Not all psychoactive drugs are addictive. Major tranquilizers are not, and neither are antidepressants used to treat depression or panic disorders. The real concern for addiction is in the benzodiazapine class of drugs—Valium, Xanax, and pain medications like codeine and percoset, etc.

RESOURCES

SMOKING
American Cancer Society
800-ACS-2345

National Cancer Institute
800-4-CANCER

Smokers Anonymous
2118 Greenwich Street
San Francisco, CA 94123

ALCOHOL
Adult Children of Alcoholics
P.O. Box 3216
Torrance, CA 90505
310-534-1815

Al-Anon
P.O. Box 862
Midtown Station
New York, NY 10018-0862
212-302-7240

Alcoholics Anonymous
P.O. Box 454
Grand Central Station
New York, NY 10017
212-870-3400

DRUGS
Cocaine Anonymous
3740 Overland Avenue, Suite G
Los Angeles, CA 90032
800-347-8998

Narcotics Anonymous
P.O. Box 9999
Van Nuys, CA 91409
818-780-3951

GENERAL
Co-Dependents Anonymous
P.O. Box 14537
Minneapolis, MN 55414
612-537-6904

Hazeldon Foundation (Support for chemical dependencies)
P.O. Box 176
Center City, MN 55012
800-328-9000

American Lung Association
1740 Broadway
New York, NY 10019
800-586-4872

18

TAKING CARE

From Mother to Daughter to Mother

~~~

Every morning, I rise early and am in full motion almost before my feet hit the floor. The first couple of hours of my day are a frenzied blur. By the time I get two rambunctious boys off to school and take my daily run, there's barely time for a shower and a quick breakfast before I'm off to the office. I imagine that I am like most working mothers. I cherish those few minutes when I can relax and think about myself, or work on projects like this book that mean so much to me. Each free moment is like a breath of pure oxygen to my system. And I struggle not to feel irritated or resentful when the phone rings with yet another demand, or a small voice calls me from the other room.

There was a time, when I was younger, that I felt I could conquer any and all challenges. When I heard women talk about the stresses of marriage and motherhood, I didn't think they were talking about people like me. I thought they were talking about people who had big problems and few resources. Little did I know that stress can be a collection of mundane events that stretch out forever—the apples and cookies hurriedly purchased late Sunday when I remember it's my turn to send a school snack; the lost mittens and hats that have to be replaced this minute; the inevitable grocery stop on the way home from work; the dozens of details that steal time away from the chance to simply enjoy my children.

Every day, I perform many roles, and I try to give myself completely to each one. Sometimes I long for a simpler life, but when I really think about it, I realize how much I relish my caretaker roles—how much I love being a mother to these two funny, smart, lively little boys; how good it feels to be married to a man who is my partner; how rewarding it is to be a doctor and make a daily difference in people's lives.

Women are, as we have always been, the caretakers for the people in our lives—the cogs in the wheels that keep families and communities running. In the past, that position was much simpler. Today, we are not just the caretaker wives and mothers. Many of us will sacrifice careers and leisure pleasures to become the caretakers of elderly parents. Most women can expect to be taking care of someone for most of their lives.

Since we're at the center of the action, much is expected of us. When things go wrong in a family or community, women bear the brunt of the blame. Today, we are experiencing a backlash against working women, single mothers, and feminist activists that is eerily reminiscent of the period before women's emancipation. Then, women who failed to comply with traditional roles were ridiculed, ostracized, or hospitalized for insanity. People thought a woman was crazy to prefer education and a career to a lifetime of backbreaking work, soul-deadening isolation, and the rigors of bearing many children. Now, there is a growing outcry against women who assert themselves in society. A highly popular radio personality was applauded when he coined the term "feminazis" to describe women who openly seek equality in our institutions. Until recently deleted from psychiatry's list of official diagnoses, the diagnosis of "self-defeating personality disorder" was given to women who are frustrated by sexual harassment, discrimination, and failure to succeed in a male-patterned world.

Single mothers who raise their children alone, at great personal and financial cost, are not praised for having the courage and commitment to perform a difficult task on their own. Rather, they are chastised for not trying harder to make their marriages work, even if that means remaining with men who abuse them. Mothers who work outside the home—and most do, at least part-time—are blamed for everything from crime on the streets to teen sex and drug addiction.

It is clear to me that society points a finger at women in order to justify its own neglect. Mothers are easy targets when it comes to passing out blame, but rarely does anyone think to ask what role the men play, or "Where are the fathers?"

The real issue is not whether women should work, or whether single mothers are good or bad. These are realities that cannot be denied. The very complexity of our times makes it impossible to turn back the clock—even if we wanted to. We should be asking what it means for a society to embrace its responsibility to women and children; to shed its institutional biases; and to support the life and well-being of all its citizens.

The social context in which we live is very relevant to the question of health, and that is precisely why women and teenage girls are suffering. If staying well were simply a matter of following the prescriptions for healthy living outlined in this book, the women of America would be glowing with good health. But health care itself must change to better reflect our needs, and that is a long way from happening.

Even so, we must not be paralyzed by the inadequacies of the system. The process of change begins with the personal commitment we bring to bettering our personal health while we rattle the cages of the health care system. Our role as the appointed caretakers need not sap our energy. Instead, it can empower us to begin the process of change in our own homes.

CARING FOR THE EMERGING GENERATION

As women strive to get better care for ourselves, we are also aware of the next generation newly emerging into womanhood. What kind of world will our daughters inherit? What can we do to insure that their experience of the health care system will be better than our own? What can we do to help our own daughters make the choices that will further their well-being? If you are the mother of a daughter, these questions are of urgent interest to you.

Because I am a woman doctor and a mother myself, my patients often talk to me about their children. In particular, women talk about their daughters. Often, with the wisdom of hindsight, they see how they might have avoided health problems if only someone had taught them that lifetime health begins in youth. "When I was twenty, I was invincible," one woman laughed. "Smoking, drinking, experimenting with drugs, casual sex. It never occurred to me that something bad might happen to me. I was lucky. I managed to get through it unscathed. But now I look at my fifteen-year-old and I remember how I felt then. How do I communicate to my daughter that she's not invincible?"

Women are frightened by the times we live in. They're worried about being able to hold it together for their adolescent children. Under any circumstances, adolescence is a time of great upheaval. The dramatic biological changes that accompany this transition have been the same for millenia. But the social context in which they occur is very different now, and it continues to change rapidly—not necessarily for the better. Changes in the economic structure, the family, the media, and local communities have affected the way adolescents live and interact with their peers, families, and the rest of society.

People in my profession once thought it was sufficient to treat the health or illness of the individual—as though good health was an isolated entity, unrelated to larger societal forces. Today, the picture has grown more complex. The leading causes of death among adolescents and young adults are accidents, suicide, and homicide—all violent events. We know that many teenagers engage in unprotected sex, smoke cigarettes, and abuse alcohol and drugs. Providing guidance to your daughter means taking into consideration all the social forces that place her at risk, especially the pressure to be sexual.

I find it interesting that a nation that claims to care so deeply about its children so easily ignores their needs. Like women, children and adolescents find the health care system sadly lacking. Much of the sickness and death that occurs among young people is entirely preventable and attributable to unhealthy behavior. Yet, physicians have been found to engage in far fewer prevention activities than established guidelines recommend. Not only have they not been trained to give advice to teens about nutrition, risky sexual behaviors, substance abuse, and the like, but given the current fee reimbursement structure, it is not cost effective for them to spend time on these issues.

In 1990, adolescents made an estimated sixty million visits to private physicians—mostly as a result of school-required physicals, although the most frequent reason for older teenage girls was prenatal visits. Yet relatively few of these visits included preventive services such as diagnostic screening or counseling. Vision exams, Pap tests and breast palpations, and cholesterol measurements were performed in fewer than 5 percent of adolescent visits; blood pressure readings were taken in fewer than one-third of the visits. Health promotion counseling on HIV transmission, breast self-exams, and nutritional guidelines were performed in fewer than two percent of adolescent visits. Two-thirds of the time, no counseling was provided at all, a real problem, given the prevalence of violence, abuse, eating disorders, and substance abuse in adolescents.

The startling inadequacy of current preventive services becomes more apparent when we study recently published national data of teenagers' health status: One-third of students in grades nine to twelve reported having smoked cigarettes in the previous month; one-fifth of high school students said they smoked every day. Yet smoking cessation advice was provided in only 1 percent of adolescent physician visits.

In 1991, 54 percent of ninth through twelfth graders reported having had sexual intercourse at least once; 19 percent said they'd had four or more partners; 55 percent reported not using condoms. Even in light of these disturbing figures, fewer than 1 percent of doctors counsel teens about risks associated with HIV transmission. And although half of girls ages fifteen to twenty are sexually active, only 6.1 percent of them receive Pap tests.

Only 25 percent of accredited American medical schools include a required course in preventive medicine, and those that do spend less than forty hours on instruction. Without training, many physicians don't know how to approach sensitive topics with their patients. Although 80 percent of doctors treating pre-teens and teenagers reported that they routinely inquired about and provided anticipatory guidance regarding puberty and menstruation, only half of them initiated discussions about sexuality, and substantially fewer inquired about depression, incest, or child abuse. Remember, doctors are people with their own beliefs, inhibitions, and prejudices. They must be given the information and skills necessary to truly care for today's patients.

Adolescents don't have much access to health care on their own, and many of them would prefer to avoid using health services rather than risk their parents knowing the confidential details about behavior and diagnoses. Consider this: If parental knowledge were mandatory, many adolescents would not seek medical care for depression, birth control, sexually transmitted diseases, or drug use. Nearly half of the unmarried females attending Planned Parenthood clinics in ten states reported they had not informed their parents. Of these, 80 percent said they would not seek counseling or care if parental knowledge were required, although almost all of them said they would continue having sexual relations.

Parental knowledge and consent has become a hot topic in recent years—particularly in the context of sexual behavior, birth control use, and abortion. Many people staunchly believe that parents have a right to know about their teenagers' behavior, and certainly should know when their children seek medical care. But this belief assumes that all family environments are loving and nurturing, that parents are well educated about health behavior, and that teens can always assume that their parents will support their best interests. With child abuse and neglect endemic conditions in American families, we can safely say this perfect vision is unrealistic.

It's also important to understand that the need for privacy and confidentiality is part of the normal process of adolescent development. Girls, in particular, keep health concerns private from their families, while boys keep them private from their peers. Girls find it easier to disclose confidential information to health providers than boys do. Yet our doctors aren't asking. Although mandatory consent laws may be well meaning and are designed to enhance family unity and improve parent-child communication, these laws tend to increase health risks to adolescents by delaying medical care. Confidentiality is also an issue when family practitioners treat adolescents who may be reluctant to divulge information to a physician who is also caring for their parents.

BE AN ADVOCATE FOR YOUR DAUGHTER

How can you help your daughter maneuver the tricky territory of adolescence and emerge as a strong, healthy adult?

The most important thing you can do is be a good role model. Although adolescents are notoriously defiant when it comes to accepting advice from their parents, you remain the most important role model your daughter has. You are the one she looks to for a sense of what it means to be an adult woman. They way you approach life, develop your own sense of self, and relate to others can show her what is possible.

Another aspect of role modeling is your health behavior. Many studies have shown that unhealthy behavior, such as smoking, excessive drinking, and drug use, start early in life—and that this behavior is more likely to be adopted by adolescents if their parents engage in it. When it comes to smoking, this is particularly true for girls; a higher percentage of girls than boys become smokers if their parents smoke. Studies have also shown that the earlier a child begins to smoke, the higher her risk of nicotine addiction. And lung cancer mortality is highest among adults who began smoking before age fifteen.

Be a model of nutritional good sense. A mother recently complained to me that her twelve-year-old daughter was already dieting to lose weight. "She's a beautiful girl," she groaned. "Why does she think she has to starve herself to get skinnier? I've tried to talk to her about it, and I get nowhere. She's determined to lose ten pounds."

I asked this mother, who was slender herself, "Have you ever dieted to lose weight?" She shrugged. "Well, of course, who hasn't? You know, I stop eating for a couple of weeks every year to get rid of those extra pounds after the holidays. That's normal."

I could see that she wasn't making the connection between her own behavior and her daughter's. She didn't realize that her annual diet sent a strong and clear message: Dieting is normal. Women eat too much and have to starve themselves to stay slim. Being slim is more important than eating nutritious meals. And it is often a girl's first diet that puts her at risk for eating disorders.

Another woman, whose fourteen-year-old daughter was hospitalized with anorexia nervosa, recalled how her husband used to tease the girl about her weight, even nicknaming her "Pudge." She defended her husband—"He didn't mean anything by it. It was just his affectionate name for her"—but admitted that the teasing had an impact.

If good nutrition and exercise are priorities in your home, your daughter will be more inclined to adjust her life to healthy behavior—especially if you are clear about the direct link to lifelong health. Help your daughter understand how a good nutrition and exercise program instituted early on will eliminate risk factors, like osteoporosis, later in life. Help her develop a positive relationship to food as a source of energy and strength, and not as an enemy or a replacement for love and support. If your daughter does not get stuck in a yo-yo dieting syndrome early in life, chances are she won't have to worry about becoming overweight. Teach her that starvation diets only lead to rebound weight gain, and that the more she diets, the harder it will become to lose weight. Set an example by being comfortable with your own body, accepting the changes it goes through in the course of life.

The natural process of a girl's growth includes the drive to establish one's own sense of self while remaining connected to others—differentiating without separating. This drive begins at the "terrible twos" when your child's favorite word is No! By the time of adolescence, your daughter is a full-fledged individual. During this period, adolescents establish their individuality in ways that can try your patience and terrify you. You might wonder how you can impart important lessons when your teenager challenges everything you say. But if you remember your own adolescence, you might recall how false your bravado was—how much you needed to be seen, heard, and understood. Help your daughter feel as though she has someone in her corner—you. Balance the freedom she needs to make independent choices with a sense of security that you're there to back her up. Allow her to differentiate without needing to separate. Reinforce her self-esteem every chance you get. This is a time when she's very vulnerable to social and sexual signals that bombard her from all sides. She may feel anguish if her looks don't conform to the "pretty" teen ideal; she might try to be more compliant and appear less bright than she is because smart girls aren't as popular; she might be pressured into unhealthy behavior because she doesn't want to be different. Developmental psychology, from a woman-centered perspective, describes adolescent girls as "going underground"—a loss of self that takes years to reverse; sometimes that self doesn't re-emerge until a woman is in her forties, sometimes never. A teenage girl's life is a minefield of pressures and choices—and the glue that will hold her together is a sense of self-esteem.

Girls with low self-esteem have higher rates of teenage pregnancy. Be realistic about sexuality. There isn't a mother alive who doesn't hope her daughter will avoid having sex until she's mature, but the admonition, "Just say no," falls woefully flat as a strategy. Be open with your daughter about sexual responsibility, and be frank about what constitutes an emotionally and physically fulfilling sexual relationship. Speak about sexuality as a state of mind, not a condition of the body. Support the efforts of schools and communities to provide information about safe sex, and to make condoms available. Studies have shown that providing condoms does not in itself promote sexual activity among adolescents. In fact, when condoms are distributed as part of an HIV prevention strategy, it tends to delay sexual activity.

Discuss the risk of unwanted pregnancy as a separate issue from sexually transmitted disease. Avoid moralizing; rather, protect your daughter's interests by describing the medical and emotional dangers of teenage pregnancy. Teen pregnancies have more complications and often result in premature and low birth weight infants. Studies have shown that pregnant teenage girls who choose to maintain their pregnancies often do more poorly in life than those who have abortions. A study by the Johns Hopkins School of Hygiene and Public Health, released in 1990, tracked 334 pregnant girls age seventeen and younger and found compelling evidence that those who had abortions did better educationally, economically, and emotionally, and had fewer subsequent pregnancies. Teen motherhood fosters a cycle of poverty.

Teach your daughter the responsibilities that come along with her reproductive powers. Teach your sons sexual responsibility and to be respectful of girls' bodies and minds. In a woman-centered system, women would take an active role in deciding when to reproduce. Pregnancy would be a planned event in a woman's life. Contrast this ideal with the current situation, where pregnancy happens to girls because of poor access to birth control, poor education about using it, and pressure from boys and men who bear no responsibility.

Be on the lookout for depression. With all the biological and social forces overwhelming them, adolescents can and do become severely depressed. In fact, suicide among adolescents has increased 156 percent since 1960, and now ranks as the third leading cause of death among fifteen- to twenty-four-year-olds. Depression can be an outcome of abuse or addiction. It is exacerbated by unhealthy behavior. It is more likely when an adolescent has low self-esteem. Adolescents don't have the emotional maturity or memory to realize that the pain they feel on a momentary basis is not necessarily permanent. A failed exam, a lost boyfriend, or any "normal" disappointment can seem huge and irreversible. You can help your daughter by letting her know that she's strong and terrific, that failure and disappointment are natural aspects of life, and that the pain and disappointment won't last forever. A parent who responds to a failed exam by saying, "You'll never make anything of yourself," or to a lost boyfriend with, "You should try harder to get along," is just reinforcing esteem-crushing stereotypes. Even parents who consider themselves supportive and encouraging may not realize the unstated pressures and expectations that can make a girl feel inadequate. A patient of mine who is a very loving and involved parent, recently broke down crying in the middle of a physical exam. This was the year her daughter was applying to private high schools. A shy and studious girl, she had never given her parents any cause for concern. My patient told me that she was coming home from work one day and saw a crowd standing outside her apartment building. She looked in the direction of their stares and saw her daughter standing on a ledge outside their twelfth-story apartment. Later, she learned this was not the first incident. It was a rude awakening! She simply hadn't known, hadn't seen the signs of desperation beneath the mask of her daughter's quiet demeanor.

Provide your daughter with a safe environment. Safety is the fundamental need of all children, yet every day childhood sexual abuse confines thousands of young girls to lifetimes of emotional pain and physical health problems. Twenty-six out of every thousand teenage girls are victims of abuse.

Exposure to violence is another problem for young people today—the result of the decline in our communities and the regular exposure to violent acts on television. Increasing numbers of American families keep guns in their homes, and there has been a rise in accidental deaths among children and teenagers as a result. People say they purchase guns to keep their families safe, but the evidence is growing that households with guns are less safe for women and children. Furthermore, those who argue that television violence does not have consequences forget that our children's generation is the first ever to be raised with such an unrelenting exposure to violence. Television is a relatively recent invention, and what little is known about its long-term effects is slow to enter medical practice. However, we cannot pretend that the images our children see every day leave no impression. Limit the amount of time your children watch TV, and make an effort to discuss the images they see, especially regarding violence among people and toward women. Make television watching an opportunity to reinforce positive ideas, and openly examine what TV tells us about social attitudes. For example, when you see a rape victim on television being blamed because she was dressed provocatively, you can use the opportunity to educate your daughter about the consequences of dress and behavior, while discussing how society blames women victims rather than the perpetrators of violence.

Finally, show your daughter that you value yourself and find value in the work you do—whether that work is as a home caretaker or in a job away from home. If you go to a job every day, don't feel guilty. Daughters of working mothers do better academically, are more independent, and are more likely to pursue careers themselves. Sons show better cognitive development. Children of both sexes have less rigid views of sex roles, especially daughters. Know that the choices you have made for your own life will directly influence your daughter. Take advantage of the opportunity to make that influence positive.

CARING FOR THE PREVIOUS GENERATION

Edith was a perimenopausal woman who had been experiencing intermittent vaginal bleeding for some time. She was very skittish about having tests done, but her gynecologist finally convinced her to have a sonogram, which showed a possible endometrial cancer. The gynecologist then did an endometrial biopsy in her office, after which Edith started to bleed profusely.

When the gynecologist called me, she was at her wit's end. "Will you talk to her?" she asked. "Edith refuses to go into the hospital."

"Don't be intimidated by your patient," I told the gynecologist. "This woman needs to get to an emergency room now. Does she understand the consequences of her not going?"

The gynecologist said she would try again, but she called me back five minutes later. "She won't go to the hospital," she said. "Can you see her?"

So, Edith came into my office, and she was very upset, but I saw right away that she was not an ignorant woman. She was a fourth grade teacher, an educated person who seemed to understand a great deal about her health risks. We talked about her frustration with the medical system and her nervousness about her condition. And it finally came down to the fact that she was the sole caretaker for her demented mother. "You wonder why I'm reluctant to go to the hospital," she said. "This isn't a trivial thing." I was beginning to understand where Edith was coming from, and I began to examine her, thinking about how I could convince her to go to the hospital. Suddenly, she looked up at me from the examining table, and she said in a tortured voice, "Doctor, you don't know me. This is the first time that you're meeting me, so you don't know how I normally behave. But do you know how terrible it is to be all alone?" She sighed and gave me a long, pleading look. "You do understand that, don't you?"

And suddenly I did see. Edith was an unmarried woman with no family of her own. She was the sole caretaker of her demented mother. And there was no one to care for her when she had a problem. She was lying weeping on my examining table, not because she was bleeding or even because she had cancer. She was weeping from the existential pain of being alone. The weight of her responsibility for her illness and for her mother was heavier because she had no one with whom she could share it. And like so many women, she was asking, "Who will care for me?"

Caring for elderly parents has become a permanent part of women's role. By the year 2050, nearly 30 percent of the population will be over sixty-five, and the number of people over age eighty-five will triple between 1980 and 2020.

Today, the older married woman typically outlives her husband and survives well into her seventies and even eighties. Although her life expectancy is longer, she is often plagued by numerous health problems that require care—such as Alzheimer's disease, frailty, osteoporosis, osteoarthritis, cancer, cardiovascular disease and stroke, diabetes, urinary incontinence, and any number of disabilities. Unfortunately, many physicians are not sufficiently aware of important issues in older women's health, or of how women differ from men in the diagnosis and treatment of disease. There is frequent age bias against women—seen, for example, in the unaggressive treatment of diseases such as CAD, or in the avoidance of screening tests for older women.

A major problem for elderly women is functional decline—the general inability to be fully mobile and care for oneself. When we look at the risk factors for functional decline we see a list of predominantly preventable and intervenable causes: low income, number and severity of chronic diseases, alcohol, smoking, obesity, inactivity, visual impairment, and use of tranquilizers. Frailty itself has no precise scientific meaning, but most gerontologists (physicians who specialize in the care of the elderly) agree that the crucial biological characteristic is the progressive reduction in the capacity of the organism to withstand stress. It is a state of vulnerabilty and lack of resilience—a result of the combined effects of biologic aging, disease, and disuse. New studies show that what was once thought of as a natural part of aging is really the result of sedentary living. Inactivity saps our reserves in all parts of our bodies. Exercise throughout our entire life span is a must to protect against frailty. Data are also emerging about estrogen's role in maintaining good cognitive function and memory in aging women.

Often women misjudge their true exercise levels and don't realize what it takes to get the moderate intensity exercise for aerobic conditioning along with the resistance training to improve muscle mass. They may not know how to sustain exercise when they can no longer exercise in their accustomed way. And realistically, there are many other barriers to an actaive life—arthritic pain, angina, demands from an ailing spouse, incontinence, and lack of facilities, transportation, or money.

What is even less appreciated is the rapid functional decline that comes with bed rest. This is important for elderly women who are hospitalized. As we discussed earlier, one day of bed rest can cause the same loss of aerobic capacity as one year of sedentary living.

Rachel was a sixty-two-year-old woman with a degenerative gene disease that weakened her arms and legs. She was single, worked avidly, and followed a physical therapy regimen to keep her going. Every year, she saw a gynecologist who was in the habit of performing routine screening ultrasounds on all of her menopausal patients. One of these routine screenings revealed an ovarian cyst, and Rachel was hospitalized for a complete hysterectomy. Her postoperative course was complicated by fever and antibiotic-induced diarrhea. She spent ten days in the hospital, mostly in bed.

When Rachel left the hospital, she felt grateful that the cyst had proven to be benign not cancerous. But she was physically devastated by the functional loss of activity. Rachel needed subsequent surgery for another problem, but this time I had her do physical therapy beforehand to enhance her strength, and I made sure the physical therapist was involved from the day of Rachel's admission to the hospital. It made a big difference in her recovery.

Seven percent of people under age seventy are severely impaired, and the percentage rises to 22 percent over age eighty-five—a group expected to triple in size between 1980 and 2020. Most of these are women, although the usual caregiver for an elderly man is his elderly wife. When you think about it, the cultural standard of women marrying older men is completely inappropriate based on the reality. It's a custom derived from the male preference for younger and more fertile wives. But in the majority of cases, the younger wife becomes a widow, left alone in a world that doesn't encourage intimate social networks, isolates her from her extended family, and is incapable of caring for her needs.

Elderly women caregivers are often in poor health themselves. They visit doctors more frequently, have more depression, and take more mood-altering drugs. In all, the cause is the perceived lack of support, not just the burden of caretaking.

THOSE IN THE MIDDLE

Wives, daughters, and daughters-in-law are the primary caregivers to our elderly, not hospitals or nursing homes. The bulk of responsibility falls on the shoulders of middle-aged women—what has become known as the "sandwich generation." Not only are many of them part of the paid labor force out of necessity, but their roles as unpaid caregivers to dependent older people have been added to existing responsibilities as wives, mothers, homemakers, and grandmothers.

When sons and other male relatives do provide help, it is often through assistance with transportation and handiwork—the equivalent of "taking out the garbage" in the scheme of larger demands.

Who is this woman in the middle? She is a woman in midlife, caught between two needy generations and torn between the competing demands of her multiple roles. Her roles as a paid worker outside the home and an unpaid caregiver to dependent parents have been added to her traditional roles of wife, homemaker, mother, and grandmother. And the two universes of home and work put her in the middle of a reality that has not yet been realistically addressed by our community and its social institutions.

She is on average forty-nine years old, and her context and needs are unique. When she asks for help, she is usually seeking emotional support. When her male counterpart asks for help, he means with the chores. Women caregivers feel more burdened by the role than male caregivers. They experience significantly greater declines in their own health than men in similar roles. And in general, the greatest sufferers are daughters, not wives—again reflecting the larger burden of being in the middle. A quarter of these women actually give up their paid work to become full-time caregivers. This contributes to the cycle of dependency and poverty among older women because of lost future benefits for health and retirement. Most, however, continue working and sacrifice free time and opportunities to socialize.

Social policies reinforce this role. Medicare reimbursements force hospitals to discharge elderly patients more quickly, thereby sending them home sicker. Most of these costs are then borne by the patient and the patient's family. Caretaking by a relative is not reimbursable by most insurers, and where it is, the caretaker is not allowed to have any outside job.

Health professionals, in their interactions with women, often reinforce the idea that women are caretakers; in fact, they depend on it to get the job done. They promote the idea of home-care management and the transfer of responsibility and costs from the system to the family. Yet the economic contribution of women goes unrecognized since caretaking is seen to be part of domestic work. The ideology of women as caretakers serves the interests of the family and society at large—both socially and economically. The question is, does it serve the interests of women?

Women are a majority of the population and a majority of the workforce. Employment practices need to be changed to reflect women's ways. Flexible time, job sharing and parent-care sabbaticals without loss of benefits need to be introduced. And in addition to financial support, caregivers need better in-home support and the freedom to take needed breaks from caregiving. Extended family structure and cultural influences make it feel less burdensome to Latinas, Asian-Americans, and African-Americans. But too often, social supports fail.

"Who cares for me?" It is a question I hear every day, in one way or another, from my female patients. Women today are more eager than ever to practice good health, to function with strength and vitality, and to avoid the decline that afflicted previous generations. But too often, instead of healthy, vital women, I see women who have exhausted their emotional and physical reserves—women who once wanted it all, but now feel as though they have very little; women who once stood on the front lines of a movement for equality, but now find that they have grown invisible.

Women are tired. They're resentful. Often, they feel trapped.

Beth, a forty-year-old divorced woman, kept returning to see me because she just couldn't shake a persistent cold. With each visit, she looked increasingly pale and weary. We spent some time talking about her life, and she related a familiar story.

"When I was thirty-six, I decided to divorce my husband," she told me. "He was not a bad man, just neglectful. He made me feel like I was the least important person in his life. I felt I deserved more, and when I got up the courage to take my twelve-year-old daughter and leave him, I was so proud of myself. I discovered that I was never as lonely by myself as I had been sitting in a room with this silent man. But now I wonder how liberated I really am."

Beth told me about her struggle to make ends meet with a grueling full-time job; how her ex-husband rarely paid child support and only occasionally visited their daughter; how long work hours made it impossible to monitor her daughter's behavior or take an active part in her life; how last year her father died, leaving her disabled seventy-two-year-old mother in her care; how the pressures just kept piling up.

"My daughter is graduating from high school next year," she said wistfully, "and then she'll go away to college. I feel as if I've let her down in some way. I wonder if the decision I made to divorce my husband was selfish—if I was looking out for my own happiness at my daughter's expense. I love my mother, but I resent having this new responsibility. Lately, I've had this bad cold and I'm worried about it. What if I really get sick? Who will take care of me?"

As soon as she said those words, Beth blushed. "That sounds so self-centered," she said guiltily. I applauded her. "Yes, you're being self-centered—finally. Good for you!"

I didn't have a ready answer for Beth's dilemma. But I do know one thing: Unless women start taking care of themselves, all the effort they pour into their families, jobs, and communities will deplete rather than energize them. If women don't begin to see that their own health comes first, and become outspoken advocates of their care, they will once again be victims instead of innovators.

Caring for Yourself

The decision to take care of yourself and not put yourself last is the most important one you can make. Consider the following actions as the stepping stones to future vitality

▶ Take care of your future by staying healthy—leading a healthy lifestyle and making good health care choices. Engage in good preventive health practices and use this book as a guide to appropriate health screening.

▶ Take care of your future by remaining financially independent. Many elderly women are poor because they worked at home for no pay or in poorly paid jobs. They earned little and acquired few pension rights. Elderly widows are often left with no pension when their partners die. Financial autonomy is essential, even for married women. Learn how to manage money, save, and invest to be financially secure in your older years.

▶ Take care of yourself by maintaining large social networks. Given the growing numbers of divorced, never married, and widowed women, we must redefine our ideas about extended family. Social networks are a crucial part of the quality of life for older people. Women need to broaden their ideas about intimacy, both emotional and physical, so that intimate relationships remain with them or can be started anew in their older years. Living alone needs to be replaced with communal living, which can take many forms—living with a friend, living in a communal house, or living in a complex of single apartments. After a lifetime of working toward connections—in families, in jobs, in social groups, in political organizations—we must not become isolated because our partners die and our children move away. We must value each other and value ourselves.

Let's make a commitment to take care of ourselves so that we can have the lives we deserve. And let's make a further commitment that we will not leave our daughters a legacy of invisibility within the system. In order to stop being invisible, we must be seen and heard, and we must see and hear ourselves. We must become "self"-centered. Let us redefine our role as caretakers. We have always taken this role to mean that we put ourselves last on the list, meeting everyone else's needs before we look to our own. I am now proposing that we cannot meet the needs of others, much less our own needs, unless we start by taking care of ourselves.

We must not be afraid to move beyond equality and into a world of respected difference—where difference is not the same as unequal. This difference must be reflected in our social institutions, for without being accountable to reflect women's way, these institutions cannot serve us.

The first women's health movement at the turn of this century allowed difference to be defined as separate, affirming women's reproductive and nurturing roles in society. The second women's health movement of the 1960s reclaimed reproductive health in the context of women's empowerment. In the current women's health movement, we are now poised at the threshold of a major social transformation. Women are showing their political power with their votes, their dollars, and their presence in corporate boardrooms. Furthermore, as more women join the ranks of medical professionals, we can expect forces inside and outside of medicine to collaborate in making our health care system truly reflect who we are and be responsive to our needs.

This book is designed to foster that collaboration, to empower you to be your own health advocate as we encourage medicine to do the same.

Appendix

Your Health Journal

Use this journal to keep track of your medical profile.

FAMILY HISTORY AND ENVIRONMENT

Keep a record of illnesses experienced by family members:

Current or Past Illness	Mother	Father	Siblings
Hypertension			
Coronary artery disease			
Stroke			
Diabetes			
Hyperlipidemia			
Osteoporosis			
Alzheimer's disease			
Cancer:			
Lung			
Breast			
Colon			
Ovarian			
Uterine			
Cervical			
Melanoma			
Other			

Current or Past Illness	Mother	Father	Siblings
Communicable diseases:			
TB			
HIV			
Hepatitis			
Physically disabled			
Mentally disabled:			
Inadequate nurturer			
Low self-esteem			
Poor/distorted body image			
Depression			
Major psychiatric disorder			
Violence:			
Abused			
Abuser			
Incarceration			
Nutrition:			
Obesity			
Chronic dieter			
Eating disorder			
Substance abuse:			
Alcohol			
Tobacco			
Illicit drugs			
Prescription drugs			

PERSONAL HISTORY
Social and Environmental History

Factor	Type	Date
Intrauterine exposures:		
Hormones		
Toxins		
Infections		
Trauma		
Violence:		
Childhood sexual abuse		
Childhood physical abuse		
Rape		
Sexual exploitation		
Sexual harassment		
Victim of trauma		
Witness to trauma		
Battering		
Dysfunctional family:		
Non-nurturant home		
Unsafe environment		
Unstable household		
Toxic exposures:		
Home:		
Tobacco		
Radon		
Lead		
Occupational		

Factor	Type	Date
Medical:		
Fluoroscopy		
Childhood radiation		
Chemotherapy		

PERSONAL BEHAVIORS/RISKS

Behavior	Description	Dates
Substance use:		
Tobacco		
Illicit drugs		
Prescription drugs		
Alcohol		
Caffeine		
Eating:		
Chronic dieting		
Anorexia		
Bulimia		
Dietary restrictions		
Dietary adequacy:		
Calories		
Fiber		
Fat		
Calcium		
Protein		
Sexual behavior:		
Age of first sex		
Number of partners		
Safe sex practices		
Unsafe sex practices		
Sexual identity comfort		
Sex work		
STDs		

Behavior	Description	Dates
Presence of intimacy		
Sexual dysfunction		
Exercise:		
Sedentary		
Moderately active		
Athletic		
Excessive exercising		
Caretaking:		
Children		
Parent/extended family		
Partner		
Medication:		
Past		
Present		
Over the counter		
Supplements		
Allergic reactions		

HEALTH/UTILIZATION OF MEDICAL SERVICES

Immunizations:	Completed	Booster
Childhood		
Measles		
Mumps		
Rubella		
Tetanus		
Diphtheria		
Polio		
HIB		
Pneumococcal		
Hepatitis B		
Influenza		
Travel vaccination		

Reproductive health:	Description
Onset of menses	
Menstrual problems	
Age at menopause	
Menopausal problems	
Fertility	
Age at first pregnancy	
Number of pregnancies	
Miscarriages	
Abortions	
Stillbirths	
Complications of pregnancy	
Complications of delivery	
Infertility	
Diagnostic procedures	
Therapeutic procedures	
Infertility drugs	
Diagnosed cause	
Contraception type	
Number of years	
Complications	

Medical conditions:	Diagnosis	Treatments
Medical		
Surgeries		
Hospitalizations		
Transfusions		

PERIODIC SCREENING FOR EARLY DETECTION

Screening	Date	Abnormal results
Blood pressure (most medical encounters; yearly after forty)		
Cholesterol/triglycerides		
Childhood		
Teens		
Young adult		
Adulthood		
Diabetes (for high-risk groups such as markedly obese, family history, gestational diabetes)		
Fasting plasma glucose		
Glycohemoglobin		
Osteoporosis (bone density testing for high risk)		
Tuberculosis (every one to three years)		
Childhood		
Adulthood to age thirty-five		
After age thirty-five		
Lung cancer (may want yearly chest X ray for smokers and at intervals for those exposed to bystander smoke)		
Breast cancer (mammogram every other year during forties; yearly after fifty; high risk yearly after forty)		
Colon cancer (fecal occult blood yearly after forty; sigmoidoscopy every three years after fifty; colonoscopy for high risk every five years after forty)		
Cervical cancer (yearly Pap smear after sexual initiation; every six months for HIV positive)		

Screening	Date	Abnormal results
Uterine cancer (no screening tests, but abnormal bleeding should be evaluated with transvaginal ultrasound and/or endometrial sampling)		
Ovarian cancer (no screening tests available, but high risk with transvaginal ultrasound and CA125)		
Vulvar cancer (yearly inspection)		
Melanoma/skin cancer (regular complete skin check)		
Thyroid (palpation for nodules yearly, especially for women with prior upper body irradiation)		
Oral cavity (regular inspection)		
Sexually transmitted diseases (all sexually active women should be screened; high-risk women should be screened for HIV)		
Dental disease (regular checkup)		
Eye exam, glaucoma screening		

Notes for the Doctor:

Notes

The development of this book involved hundreds of journal articles, reports from government agencies and research institutions, books, and other resources. In addition, at the back of each chapter there is a list of resources—including organizations, books, and newsletters—that can be contacted for further information. The following selected references relate to studies and statistics that are mentioned in the text.

Gender issues in research and treatment:

Bennett, J. C., "Inclusion of Women in Clinical Trials—Policies for Population Subgroups," *The New England Journal of Medicine* vol. 329, July 22, 1993.

Bickel, Janet, M.A., and Phyllis Kopriva. "A Statistical Perspective on Gender in Medicine." *Journal of the American Medical Women's Association*, vol. 48, No. 5, September/October, 1993.

Clancy, Carolyn M., M.D., and Charles T. Massion, M.D. "American Women's Health Care—A Patchwork Quilt With Gaps." *Journal of the American Medical Association,* vol. 268, No. 14, October 14, 1992.

Hamilton, Jean A., "Biases in Women's Health Research." *Women and Therapy,* vol. 12, 1992.

Rodin, Judith, and Jeannette R. Ickovics. "Women's Health-Review and Research Agenda as We Approach the 21st Century," *American Psychologist,* September 1990.

The role of estrogen in preventing heart disease:

Sacks, Frank M., M.D., at al. "Effect of Postmenopausal Estrogen Replacement on Plasma Lp(a) Lipoprotein Concentrations." *Archives of Internal Medicine* vol. 154, May 23, 1994.

Wenger, N. K., L. Speroff, and B. Packard. "Cardiovascular Health and Disease in Women," *The New England Journal of Medicine* vol. 329, July 22, 1993.

The negative effects of secondhand smoke:

Editors. *Primary Care and Cancer,* special reports, vol. 330, Nos. 112 and 113, February and March, 1994.

Environmental Protection Agency/Surgeon General. "The Health Consequences of Involuntary Smoking," 1992.

Special effects of lung cancer in women:

Ernster, Virginia L., Ph.D. "The Epidemiology of Lung Cancer in Women," Department of Epidemiology and Biostatistics, September 10, 1993.

Recommendations for mammography:

Editors. *Women's Health Watch.* "Mammography: What to Do?" Harvard Medical School, May, 1994.

Miller, Anthony B., M.B., F.R.C.P. "Mammographic Screening Guide for Women 40 to 49 and Over 65 Years Old." Studies conducted by the Breast Cancer Detection Demonstration Project, Department of Preventive Medicine and Biostatistics, AEP, vol. 4, No. 2, March 1994.

Solin, Lawrence J., et al. "The Importance of Mammographic Screening Relative to the Treatment of Women with Carcinoma of the Breast." *Archives of Internal Medicine,* vol. 154, April 11, 1994.

Treatment of women with colorectal cancer:

Myers, Ronald E., Ph.D., and Paul Engstrom, M.D. "Primary and Secondary Prevention of Colorectal Cancer," *Primary Care and Cancer,* vol. 14, No. 2, February 1994.

The role of nutrition in cancer prevention:

Hunter, D. J., et al. "A Prospective Study of the Intake of Vitamins C, E, and A and the Risk of Breast Cancer." *The New England Journal of Medicine,* vol. 329, No. 4, July 22, 1993.

Wynder, Ernst L., M.D., and Leonard A. Cohen, Ph.D. "Nutritional Opportunities and Limitations in Cancer Research." *Oncology,* November, 1994.

Unnecessary Caesarians:

Study published by the Public Citizen Health Research Group, May, 1993.

Physician ignorance of domestic violence issues:

Family Violence Prevention Fund. "California Hospital Emergency Departments Respond to Domestic Violence." Survey published August 1993.

The impact of domestic violence on women's health:

Reports by the National Health Initiatives on Domestic Violence; and Southern California Injury Prevention Research Center, University of California Los Angeles, School of Public Health, 1994.

Sorenson, Susan B., Ph.D., and Audrey F. Saftlas, Ph.D. "Violence and Women's Health—The Role of Epidemiology," AEP, vol. 4, No. 2, March 1994.

Understanding the female libido:

Tieffer, Leonore. "Historical, Scientific, Clinical, and Feminist Criticism of The Human Sexual Response Cycle or Model," *Annual Review of Sex Research,* vol. 2, 1994.

Index

B

R

S